Topics in Anti-Cancer Research

(Volume 5)

Edited by

Atta-ur-Rahman, ***FRS***
University of Cambridge
UK

&

Khurshid Zaman
Bentham Science Publishers
USA

Bentham Science Publishers Ltd.
Executive Suite Y - 2
PO Box 7917, Saif Zone
Sharjah, U.A.E.
Email: subscriptions@benthamscience.org

BENTHAM
SCIENCE

CONTENTS

INTRODUCTION

The fifth volume of this series entitled "Topics in Anti-Cancer Research" presents an overview of recent developments in the field of cancer. The topics covered include regulatory policies, cell based anticancer drug delivery systems, anticancer agents targeting heat shock proteins, and tumor homing peptides (THPs) for treatment of cancer.

PREFACE

The fifth volume of the Book series entitled "Topics in Anti-Cancer Research" is based on new contributions from eminent scientists working in the field of cancer research and therapy. The topics presented cover recent advances in cancer drug development targeting carbonic anhydrase IX and XII.

Frost *et al.* discuss the roles of carbonic anhydrase IX and XII in stabilizing pHe in physiological conditions and their use in anti-cancer targets. Studies on the recent patents of CA IX and XII targeted inhibitors are also discussed, especially with reference to sulfonamide-based small molecule inhibitors, derivatives of boron cluster compounds, metal complexes of poly(carboxyl)amine-containing ligands, nitroimidazole-, ureidosulfonamide and coumarin-based compounds and G250 and A610 monoclonal antibodies for cancer therapy.

Zhu *et al.* present an analysis of patents and patent applications associated with cancer drug development in China including existing regulatory policies, data and trend of Chinese domestic anti-cancer drug patents, exploration of Chinese applicants in other countries and recent case study of liver cancer. Bosnakovski has reviewed the promising field of cell based anti-cancer drug delivery systems and studied recent patents and current developments.

Tutar discuss the potential role of heat shock proteins in the metabolic processes of cancer cells and the interaction of heat shock proteins with other proteins and kinases to inhibit cancer cells leading to apoptosis, for better therapy. Patents using this mechanism are also reviewed.

Dhama *et al.* reviewed the data of recent searches and patents on tumor homing peptides (THPs) functioning for targeted drug delivery in cancer cell and the significance of THPs in cancer therapy.

We expect that these topics on new drug targets, drug delivery approaches and techniques in cancer research & therapy will prove to be of great interest to researchers and scientists in the field of cancer and its treatment.

The editors are obliged to the authors for their excellent and timely contributions and to the reviewers for their thorough reviewing, which has enabled us to improve the quality of these chapters. We also extend our thanks to Mr. Mahmood Alam and Mrs. Rafia Rehan, as well as other colleagues of Bentham Science Publishers, for their rigorous participation and support in the accomplishment of the present eBook.

Atta-ur-Rahman, FRS
Kings College
University of Cambridge
Cambridge
UK

&

Khurshid Zaman
Bentham Science Publishers
USA

List of Contributors

Ackova, Darinka G.	Department of Pharmacy, Faculty of Medical Sciences, University Goce Delcev - Stip, Krste Misirkov bb, 2000 Stip, R. Macedonia Email: darinka.gorgieva@ugd.edu.mk
Bayram, Banu	Health Sciences Department, Nutrition and Dietetics Department, Health Sciences University, Istanbul, Turkey Email: banu.bayram@sbu.edu.tr
Bosnakovski, Darko	Faculty of Medical Sciences, University "Goce Delcev" Stip, Krste Misirkov bb, 2000 Stip, R. Macedonia Email: darko.bosnakovski@ugd.edu.mk; darko@umn.edu
Dhama, Kuldeep	Division of Pathology, ICAR-Indian Veterinary Research Institute, Izatnagar, Bareilly, Uttar Pradesh - 243122, India Email: kdhama@rediffmail.com
Fan, Xinhong	Tongji Law School, Shanghai 200092, P.R. China Email: fanxh33@126.com
Frost, Susan C.	College of Medicine, Department of Biochemistry and Molecular Biology, University of Florida, Box 100245, Gainesville, FL 32610, USA Email: sfrost@ufl.edu
Gao, Ruru	Department of Chemistry, Tongji University, Shanghai 200092, P.R. China Email: gaoruru1991@163.com
Khandia, Rekha	Department of Biochemistry & Genetics, Barkatullah University, Bhopal-462 026, Madhya Pradesh, India Email: rekha.morchhale@gmail.com
Mboge, Mam Y.	College of Medicine, Department of Biochemistry and Molecular Biology, University of Florida, Box 100245, Gainesville, FL 32610, USA Email: mammboge@ufl.edu
McKenna, Robert	College of Medicine, Department of Biochemistry and Molecular Biology, University of Florida, Box 100245, Gainesville, FL 32610, USA Email: rmckenna@ufl.edu
Munjal, Ashok K.	Department of Biochemistry & Genetics, Barkatullah University, Bhopal-462 026, Madhya Pradesh, India Email: ashokmunjal70@yahoo.co.in
Özgür, Aykut	Faculty of Natural Sciences and Engineering, Department of Bioengineering, Gaziosmanpaşa University, Tokat, Turkey Email: aykutozgur@gmail.com
Qin, Leyang	Tongji University Library, Shanghai 200092, P.R. China Email: qinleyang@126.com

Sachan, Swati	Immunology Section, ICAR-Indian Veterinary Research Institute, Izatnagar, Bareilly- 243 122, Uttar Pradesh, India Email: swatisachan@gmail.com
Shen, Jinhua	Tongji University Library, Shanghai 200092, P.R. China Email: jhshen@lib.tongji.edu.cn; shenjinhua111@126.com
Smilkov, Katarina	Department of Pharmacy, Faculty of Medical Sciences, University Goce Delcev - Stip, Krste Misirkov bb, 2000 Stip, R. Macedonia Email: katarina.smilkov@ugd.edu.mk
Sun, Lichun	Department of Medicine, Tulane University Health Sciences Center, New Orleans, LA 70002, USA Email: peptide612@gmail.com, lsun@tulane.edu
Tiwari, Ruchi	Department of Veterinary Microbiology and Immunology, College of Veterinary Sciences, UP Pandit Deen Dayal Upadhayay Pashu Chikitsa Vigyan Vishwavidyalay Evum Go-Anusandhan Sansthan (DUVASU), Mathura-281001, Uttar Pradesh, India Email: ruchi.vet@gmail.com
Tutar, Lütfi	Faculty of Arts and Sciences, Department of Molecular Biology and Genetics, Ahi Evran University, Kırşehir, Turkey Email: lutfitutar@gmail.com
Tutar, Yusuf	Cumhuriyet University, Faculty of Pharmacy, Department of Basic Sciences, Division of Biochemistry, Sivas, Turkey Email: ytutar@cumhuriyet.edu.tr; ytutar@yahoo.com
Yang, Feng	Tongji University Library, Shanghai 200092, P.R. China Email: fyang@lib.tongji.edu.cn
Zhang, Gengping	Tongji University Library, Shanghai 200092, P.R. China Email: gpzhang@lib.tongji.edu.cn
Zhu, Guohua	Tongji Law School, Shanghai 200092, P.R. China Email: Chonghu666@163.com

Topics in Anti-Cancer Research

(Volume 5)

CHAPTER 1

Advances in Anti-Cancer Drug Development Targeting Carbonic Anhydrase IX and XII

Mam Y. Mboge*, **Robert McKenna** and **Susan C. Frost***

University of Florida, College of Medicine, Department of Biochemistry and Molecular Biology, Box 100245, Gainesville, FL 32610, USA

Abstract: The microenvironment within a solid tumor is heterogeneous with regions being both acidic and hypoxic. As a result of this, cancer cells upregulate genes that allow survival in such environments. Some of these genes are pH regulatory factors, including carbonic anhydrase IX (CA IX) and in some cases XII (CA XII). CA IX helps to maintain normal cytoplasmic pH (pHi) while simultaneously contributing to the extracellular pH (pHe). CA XII is also thought to be responsible for stabilizing pHe at physiological conditions. Extracellular acidification of the tumor microenvironment promotes local invasion and metastasis while decreasing the effectiveness of adjuvant therapies, thus contributing to poor cancer clinical outcomes. In this review, we describe the properties of CA IX and CA XII that substantiate their potential use as anticancer targets. We also discuss the current status of CA isoform-selective inhibitor development and patents of CA IX/XII targeted inhibitors that show potential for treating aggressive tumors. Some of the recently published patents discussed include sulfonamide-based small molecule inhibitors including derivatives of boron cluster compounds; metal complexes of poly(carboxyl)amine-containing ligands; nitroimidazole-, ureidosulfonamide-, and coumarin-based compounds; as well as G250 and A610 monoclonal antibodies for cancer treatment.

Keywords: Bicarbonate transport, cancer therapeutics, carbonic anhydrase, carbonic anhydrase IX, carbonic anhydrase XII, CO_2 transport, coumarins, drug development, ERα, estrogen response element, HIF-1α, hypoxia response element, immunotherapy, pH regulation, prognostic marker, RNAi technology,

* **Corresponding authors Mam Y. Mboge and Susan C. Frost:** University of Florida, College of Medicine, Department of Biochemistry and Molecular Biology, Box 100245, Gainesville, FL 32610, USA; Tel +1 352 294-8386, Fax +1 352 392-2953, E-mails: mammboge@ufl.edu, sfrost@ufl.edu

Atta-ur-Rahman and Khurshid Zaman (Eds.)

sulfonamides, therapeutic target, tumor microenvironment, zinc metalloenzymes.

1. INTRODUCTION

Carbonic anhydrase (CA, EC 4.2.1.1) is a family of metalloenzymes (mainly zinc) that catalyze the reversible hydration/dehydration of CO_2 to bicarbonate: $CO_2 + H_2O \rightleftharpoons HCO_3^- + H^+$ via a two-step ping-pong mechanism. Present in both prokaryotes and eukaryotes, these enzymes have evolved into six distinct classes: α, β, γ, δ, ζ, and η [1 - 21]. Of these classes, only α-CAs are present in humans, of which fifteen isoforms are encoded [1, 9, 22]. Among these isoforms, only twelve coordinate a zinc in the active site and are catalytically active (CAs I–IV, CAs VA–VB, CAs VI–VII, CA IX, and CAs XII–XIV). Isoforms VIII, X, XI are termed CA-related proteins (CARPS) as they lack at least one amino acid in the active site to coordinate the zinc and therefore are catalytically inactive. The active human CA isoforms differ in kinetic properties along with cell and tissue distribution. CAs play crucial roles in many physiological processes including CO_2 and bicarbonate transport between metabolizing tissues and lungs, pH and CO_2 homeostasis, bone resorption, and electrolyte secretion [1, 9, 11 - 13, 22]. Of the human isoforms, only the membrane-associated isoforms IX and XII have been implicated in tumorigenicity, cancer metastasis, and as clinical prognosticators [19 - 25]. In this chapter, the characteristics, expression patterns, and functions both in normal and neoplastic tissue of the cancer associated CA IX and CA XII will be discussed. We will also discuss the anti-cancer targeting strategies for both isoforms.

1.1. Active Site Structure and Catalysis of CA IX and CA XII

The amino acids that form the active site of α-CAs are highly conserved, and at the core of the active site is a zinc (Zn^{2+}) ion that is essential for catalysis (Fig. (**1**)) [25 - 27]. The zinc is located at the base of a 15Å deep active site cleft and is tetrahedrally coordinated by three histidines (His94, His96, His119; CA II numbering used throughout this manuscript unless otherwise specified) and a water/hydroxyl [28 - 30]. The first step of catalysis in the hydration direction is the nucleophilic attack by the Zn-bound hydroxyl group on CO_2 to produce

HCO^-_3. The HCO^-_3 is then displaced by an active site water and released. In the second step of catalysis, the Zn-bound water is regenerated to a hydroxyl through the transfer of a proton mediated by a highly ordered solvent network and conserved histidine residue (His64) found in most isoforms, termed the proton shuttle residue [1, 25, 31].

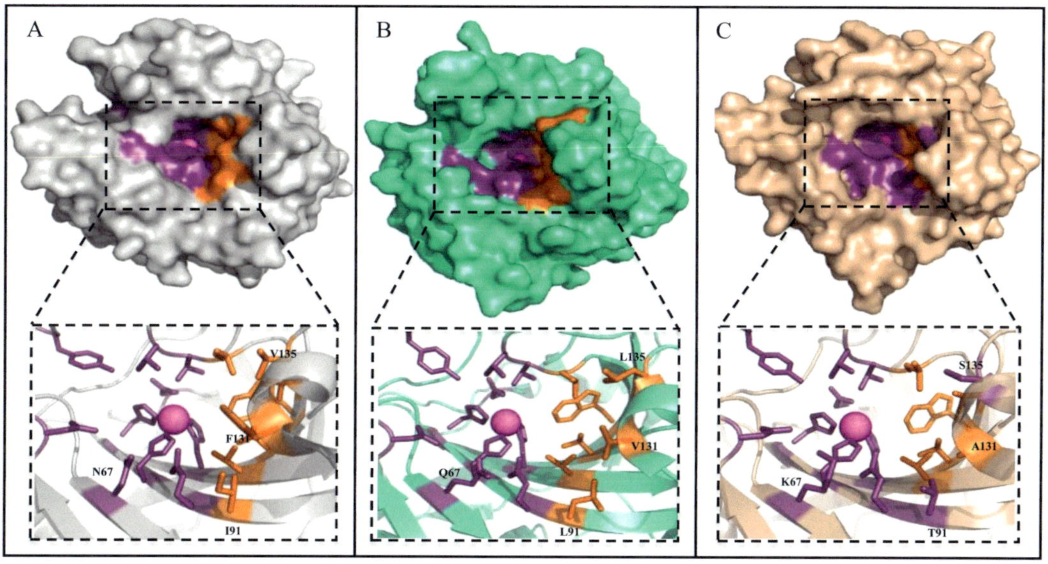

Fig. (1). Structure of human α-CAs. Surface depiction of (A) CA II, PDB ID 3KS3 (grey), (B) CA IX, PDB ID 3IAI (green), C) CA XII, PDB ID IJCZ (wheat). Active site zinc (magenta sphere), hydrophilic (purple) and hydrophobic (orange) residues are shown. Residues within the active site that are different between these CAs are labeled (CA II numbering). CA II (N67, I91, F131, V135), CA IX (Q67, L91, V131, L135) and CA XII (K67, T91, A131, S135).

The proton transfer step is the rate-limiting step in this catalysis reaction. Isoforms CA II, CA IX and CA XII exhibit extremely fast catalytic activity (Table **1**) [1, 22]. It is thought that this catalytic efficiency is in part due to the ability of His64 to shuttle protons with a low energy barrier between an inward (pointing towards the active site) and outward (pointing away from the active site) conformations [1, 25, 31]. The active sites of CAs also exhibit a divided active site cleft with a hydrophobic and a hydrophilic side (Fig. (**1**)). The hydrophobic side supports the pathway for substrate and product entry and exit, while the hydrophilic side provides the amino acids that define an ordered solvent network for proton transfer [32].

Table 1. Catalytic Efficiency, Distribution and Associated Diseases of CA II, IX and XII [1].

Isozyme	K_{cat} (s^{-1})	K_M (mM)	K_{cat}/K_M (M^{-1} s^{-1})	Oligomeric State	Tissue/Organ Localization	Subcellular Localization/Associated disease
CA II	1.4×10^6	9.3	1.5×10^8	Monomer	RBC, kidney, brain, lung, testis, osteoclasts, eye, GI tract	Cytosol/ Glaucoma, epilepsy, edema, altitude sickness
CA IX	3.8×10^5	6.9	5.5×10^7	Dimer	GI mucosa, tumors	Transmembrane/ Cancer
CA XII	4.2×10^5	12.0	3.5×10^7	Dimer	Eye, tumors, reproductive epithelia, intestines, and kidney	Transmembrane/ Cancer, glaucoma

Although there is high conservation of amino acid type and position lining the active sites of the CAs, X-ray crystallography studies have identified at least four amino acids within the active site (positions 67, 91, 131 and 135) that differ between CA II, CA IX and CA XII (Fig. (**1**)) [32]. These differences could be used to design CA isoform specific inhibitors to CA IX and XII and reduce other off target inhibition of CAs, particularly the ubiquitous CA II.

1.2. Biochemical and Biophysical Properties of CA IX and CA XII

CA IX and CA XII are transmembrane glycoproteins with their N-termini facing the extracellular milieu (Table **1**) (Fig. (**2**)) [33 - 36]. The *CA9* and *CA12* genes are mapped to chromosome 9p12-13 and 15q22, respectively [33 - 36]. CA IX is 414 amino acids (aa) in length, consisting of a signal peptide (37aa), a proteoglycan-like (PG) domain (59aa), a catalytic domain (257aa), a transmembrane domain (20aa), and a C-terminal intracellular domain (25aa) [35 - 38]. CA XII is shorter in length (354aa) and divided into only four distinct domains, as the PG domain is absent [39]. These include a 269aa catalytic domain, a 26aa transmembrane domain, and a 28aa C-terminal intracellular domain. For both isoforms, the signal peptide domain is cleaved in the mature protein [39]. Mass spectroscopic analysis indicates that CA IX has distinct *N*-linked and *O*-linked glycosylation sites at Asn309 and Thr78, respectively [40]. Similarly, CA XII is also a glycoprotein but containing two *N*-linked glycosylation sites at Asn52 and Asn136. Intermolecular disulfide bonds stabilize

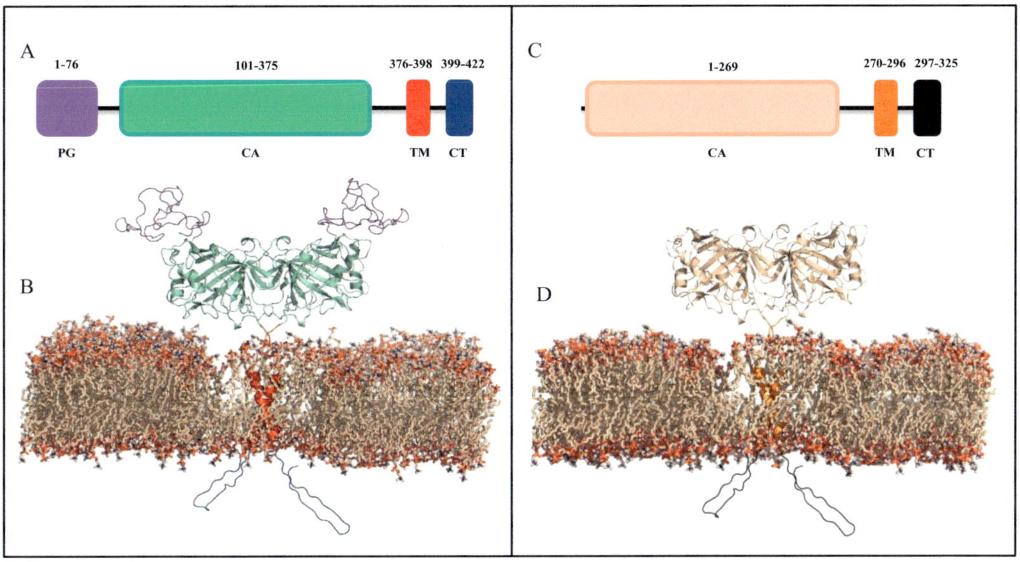

Fig. (2). Schematic and structural models of CA IX* and XII. (A) CA IX domains include the proteoglycan-like domain (PG, purple), catalytic domain (CA, cyan), a transmembrane anchor (TM, red), and intracellular C-terminal domain (CT, blue). (C) CA XII domains include the catalytic domain (CA, wheat), the transmembrane domain (TM, gold), and intracellular C-terminal domain (CT, black). (B) Homodimeric membrane bound form of CA IX includes the extracellular PG and CA domains (purple and green), the TM anchor (red), and the CT domain (blue). (D) Homodimeric membrane bound form of CA XII includes the CA domain (wheat), the TM anchor (gold), and the CT domain (black). The TM domains are predicted to form helix-helix interactions within the lipid bilayer. The CT domains are predicted to exist as unstructured loops. * Structural model of CA IX provided by Brian Mahon [21].

both isoforms: between Cys 119-Cys299 in CA IX and between Cys23-Cys203 in CA XII [39, 40]. If the sequences of the catalytic domains of CA IX and CA XII were aligned, these two Cys residue pairs would be at the same position. Three phosphorylation sites have also been confirmed on the intracellular domain of CA IX corresponding to Thr443, Ser448, and Tyr449 [2, 40, 41]. Although present in CA XII, studies have yet to show phosphorylation of the analogous Tyr residue. These post-translational modifications in CA IX are thought to play important roles in modulating catalytic activity and signaling [2, 40, 41]. The molecular weight of CA IX is predicted to be 49.5kDa, but it migrates as a doublet with molecular weights of 54 and 58kDa, both of which are glycosylated [34, 42]. The observed differences in molecular weight may result from differences or deletions in primary sequence. This is supported by data showing that two molecular weight species exist after removal of the *N*-linked glycans [42]. Under non-reducing conditions, both CA IX and CA XII are obs-erved in their homodimeric forms [33, 42]. Interestingly, soluble forms of both CA IX (consisting of only the PG and CA domains) and CA XII have been observed in culture medium of highly invasive tumor cell lines and the sera of cancer patients [43 - 45]. Although the purpose of the secreted form is not fully understood, recent studies suggest an involvement in cell signaling. Moreover, circulating forms of CA IX have shown great potential as biomarkers for therapeutic outcomes in cancer patients [46 - 49].

1.3. Regulation of CA IX and CA XII Expression in Cancer

Expression of CA IX is modulated by hypoxia-inducible factors (HIFs) in response to decreased oxygen levels and increased cell density [50, 51]. HIF-1, typically associated with aggressive tumors, consists of a heterodimeric complex of α- and β-subunits (HIF-1α and HIF-1β) [1, 50 - 52]. Formation of the HIF-1 complex mediates a transcriptional response to hypoxic stress by interacting with target genes such as the *CA9* gene that contain hypoxia response elements (HRE) in the promoter region [50]. HIF-1α expression is tightly regulated and activated by both hypoxia-dependent and hypoxia-independent oncogenic signaling. It can be down-regulated by hydroxylation-induced proteosomal degradation via von Hippel Lindau tumor suppressor protein (VHL), which mediates protein ubiquitination. HIF-1α may also be inactivated by the Akt-mammalian target of rapamycin (mTOR) signaling pathway [53 - 55].

Under normoxic conditions, although constitutively expressed, HIF-1α is rapidly degraded or inactivated by preventing interaction with its transcriptional co-activators [56]. Under hypoxic conditions however, hydroxylation and degradation is prevented, which in turn inhibits VHL binding to HIF-1α. Non-hydroxylated HIF-1α binds with transcriptional co-activators and is translocated to the nucleus for heterodimerization with HIF-1β, producing HIF-1. HIF-1 then binds to target genes that contain a HRE site, inducing transcription of glucose transporter 1 (GLUT1) and glucose transporter 3 (GLUT3), vascular epidermal growth factor (VEGF), insulin-like growth factor-2 (IGF2), ATP-binding cassette transporter B1 (ABCB1), sodium-hydrogen exchanger (NHE-1) and CA IX, among others [55 - 60]. Expression of these hypoxia-induced genes are involved in regulating iron, glucose and cell matrix metabolism, cell proliferation and viability, vascular remodeling and plasticity, cell adhesion, angiogenesis, pH regulation and other cellular processes [55, 57 - 60].

In contrast to CA IX, CA XII expression, though observed under hypoxic conditions, is not controlled by HIF-1α. Studies have shown that CA XII is robustly regulated in breast cancer cells by estrogen via estrogen receptor alpha (ERα) [61]. This regulation involves a distal estrogen-responsive enhancer region that communicates with the transcriptional start site of the *CA12* gene via intrachromosomal looping [61]. The interaction between estrogen and ERα occurs through the estrogen response element (ERE) and results in the recruitment of RNA polymerase II and receptor co-activators. These cause changes in histone acetylation and enhanced transcription of the *CA12* gene [61].

Estrogens stimulate normal cell growth and proliferation thus increasing the frequency of mutations and chromosomal aberrations. The effects of estrogenic steroid hormones are largely mediated through interaction and activation of ERα and estrogen receptor beta (ERβ). Estrogens are potent modulators of the pathophysiology, homeostasis, and development of many tissues such as skeletal, cardiovascular, adipose breast, male and female reproductive tracts. Cumulative exposure of estrogens (specifically ERα) causes an increased risk of cancer [61 - 64].

1.4. Functions and Expression of CA IX and CA XII in Normal Tissue

CA IX expression in normal tissues is restricted to stomach and epithelial tissues of the gut particularly the basolateral surfaces of the crypt enterocytes of the duodenum, jejunum and ileum of the small intestine [65, 66]. In the large intestine, CA IX expression is restricted to the base of the glands in the cecum and colon [65, 66]. However, abundant levels of CA IX are observed in developing embryonic tissues of the gut epithelium, skeleton muscle and lung, most of which are decreased in adult tissue [67]. The biological and molecular functions of CA IX include carbon dioxide and bicarbonate transport, acid base balance, and signal transduction.

In contrast, expression of CA XII has been observed in many organs and at different developmental stages with high expression reported for the pancreas, appendix, colon, rectum, kidney, prostate, intestine, and activated lymphocytes, moderate expression in oral mucosa, esophagus, urinary bladder, breast, vagina, cervix, uterine, endometrium and skin [68, 69]. Its biological functions range from facilitating the directed movement of bicarbonate in cells to maintenance of an internal steady state concentration of chloride ions within an organism or cell. Similar to CA IX, CA XII is also involved in chemical reactions and pathways involving small molecule metabolism.

1.5. Functions and Expression of CA IX and CA XII in Neoplastic Tissue

Although CA IX expression in normal tissues is limited, it has been observed in a many aggressive tumors including the brain, breast, bladder, cervix, colon, colorectal, head and neck, pancreas, kidney, lung, ovaries, stomach oral cavity, B and T-cell lymphomas [67, 69 - 72]. In advanced renal cell carcinomas (RCC) high CA IX expression seems to correlate to better response to IL-2 therapy [73]. However, no consensus has been reached thus far about its potential to predict clinical outcome in RCC [73 - 76]. Nevertheless, CA IX overexpression in most cancers is linked to poor prognosis, chemotherapeutic resistance, and poor clinical outcome [23]. This expression is attributable to the existence of hypoxic regions within solid tumors linked to defective tumor vasculature, which results in insufficient blood supply to certain areas. In response to this, tumor cells make oncogenic alternations in metabolism and express genes that are essential for survival [23, 24, 55 - 60]. These clonogenic transformations result in expansion of cells with more aggressive phenotypes and increased metastatic potential.

CA IX is upregulated in these tumors in response to hypoxia and, because its enzymatic activity is to facilitate the conversation of CO_2 to HCO^-_3 and H^+ in the presence of H_2O, it functions to maintain physiological pH inside the cell (pHi) while simultaneously regulating the extracellular pH (pHe). Moreover, membrane ghost studies show that the hydration activity (conversion of CO_2 to bicarbonate and a proton) increases as pH increases. However, at pH values lower than ~6.8, the dehydration (conversion of bicarbonate to CO_2 and water) reaction is favored

[52]. This supports the hypothesis that CA IX balances the pHe of the bicarbonate system within the range (6.5 to 6.8) that favors cancer cell survival and aggression while causing apoptosis of surrounding normal cells. While it is well known that extracellular acidification promotes tumor invasion and metastasis [23, 24], the reasons for this are not completely understood.

CA XII is optimally active at higher pH values (pKa of ~7.1) than CA IX (pKa of ~6.3), so it is therefore considered to be responsible for stabilizing pHe under more physiological conditions, which in turn contributes to more favorable outcomes at least in breast cancer [77]. At pH values lower than ~6.8, CA XII is shown to be inactive (unpublished data). Because its expression is tightly regulated by estrogen, CA XII is strongly associated with luminal cancers of the breast (Estrogen receptor (ER)/Progesterone receptor (PR)-positive) and better clinical outcomes than patients with Human epidermal growth factor receptor II (Her2) and the triple negative phenotype (ER/PR)-negative [61, 78, 79]. The latter represents a more aggressive form of breast cancer that is strongly associated with CA IX expression. Cancers other than breast cancer show variability in CA XII as a prognostic marker: good prognosis in lung cancer, equivocal prognosis in brain, and poor prognosis in colorectal cancer [80 - 82]. High expression of CA XII has been observed in glioblastomas, astrocytomas, lung carcinomas, urinary bladder transitional cell carcinomas ductal breast carcinoma cells and T-cell lymphomas, with moderate to low expression observed in cells obtained from ovarian cyst adenocarcinoma and metastatic breast adenocarcinoma [69, 72, 80, 82]. Recent studies have shown an upregulation of CA XII on the surface of chemoresistant cells, suggesting its potential as a therapeutic target to overcome chemoresistance in cancer cells [83].

2. CA IX AND CA XII AS ANTI-CANCER TARGETS FOR THERAPY

CA IX and CA XII both play important roles in tumor progression, acidification and metastasis, suggesting that both make important therapeutic cancer targets [23, 24, 50]. There are several factors that make them attractive therapeutic targets. Their catalytic domains face the extracellular milieu (Fig. (**2**)) thus eliminating many drug delivery complications often exhibited by cytosolic targets.

In addition, constitutive expression of CA IX is limited which reduces the potential for off target effects on normal tissue [65, 66]. Hence, targeting CA IX/CA XII alone, or in combination and with other therapies, may prove beneficial in fighting specific cancers with high CA IX/CA XII expression. Importantly, knockdown of CA IX in xenograft models resulted in decreased primary tumor growth and metastatic potential as well as an increase in tumor susceptibility to treatment [84]. As a result, interest in developing inhibitors against CA IX and CA XII are being explored by many research and pharmaceutical groups.

2.1. CA IX and CA XII Targeted Inhibitor Drug Design

The α-CAs are similar in both amino acid sequence and structure. These similarities lead to difficulties in the design of CA inhibitors (CAIs) that are isoform selective, as the majority of the active site residues are both identical in amino acid type and spatial location [32]. Hence, the lack of differences leads to inhibitors targeting multiple isoforms. In designing selective inhibitors against CA IX or CA XII, binding to CAII may also occur leading to decreased inhibitor effectiveness and unwanted side effects. Therefore, the design of highly selective CAIs for CA IX and CA XII requires the exploitation of active site differences, interaction with residues near the active site, and/or reduced cell permeability [32].

Since both isoforms expose their catalytic sides to the extracellular environment, designing targeted membrane impermeable inhibitors may also prove useful. Both the catalytic and inhibitory mechanisms of the α-CAs have been studied extensively and have aided in designing potent CA inhibitors that have a wide range of clinical applications. A typical CAI has three components; a zinc-binding group (ZBG), a linker region (heterocyclic or benzene ring), and a variable "tail" region [27, 32]. The zinc-binding CAIs can be divided into two groups based on their coordination to the metal: those that form tetrahedral adducts and interact directly with the zinc (e.g., sulfonamides and bisulfites), and those that form trigonal-bipyramidal adducts through binding to the zinc-bound hydroxyl/water (e.g., cyanates and formates) [19, 20, 27, 31, 85 - 88]. Both types of zinc binding

CAIs effectively prevent catalysis [19, 20, 27, 89].

2.1.1. Classical CAIs

There are two types of "classical" CA inhibitors. These differ in their coordination of the catalytic zinc. The sulfonamides and their isosters (sulfamides/sulfamates), which are the most studied of the CAIs, interact directly with the zinc by forming tetrahedral adducts [19, 27, 85, 88]. The second type of classical CAIs include the metal chelating anions that bind to the zinc in three different geometries: a trigonal-bipyramidal, a distorted tetrahedral, or a tetrahedral geometry [19, 27, 88].

2.1.1.1. Sulfonamide Based Inhibitors

The "classical" inhibitors include drugs such as: acetazolamide, brinzolamide, dorzolamide, metazolamide, and zonisamide [1, 85, 87]. Sulfonamides and their isosters bind in deprotonated forms to the zinc, displacing the zinc-bound hydroxyl/water while maintaining a tetrahedral coordination about the active site [85, 86]. These inhibitors have been used to treat a range of diseases from glaucoma to epilepsy. More recently, the focus has been on applying these inhibitors in cancer treatment [20, 90 - 95]. However, few show selective inhibition for a single isoform including CA IX/CA XII (Fig. (**3**)) [1, 9, 27].

These inhibitors are now considered as first/second generation CAIs, which form compact structures to interact deep within the CA active site cavity (Fig. (**4**)). But even within these compounds some, such as celecoxib, saccharin, and valdecoxib, show slightly higher affinity for CA IX/ CA XII over off target CA II (Fig. (**3**)) [1, 9, 27]. Hence, to design more CA isoform specific inhibitors that target CA IX and CA XII, the minor differences in the active site residues have to be taken into consideration. For example, compound 18, which belongs to a class of positively charged membrane impermeant compounds, is a potent inhibitor of both CA IX and CA XII and is under investigation as a target for CA IX (Fig. (**3**)) [94, 96].

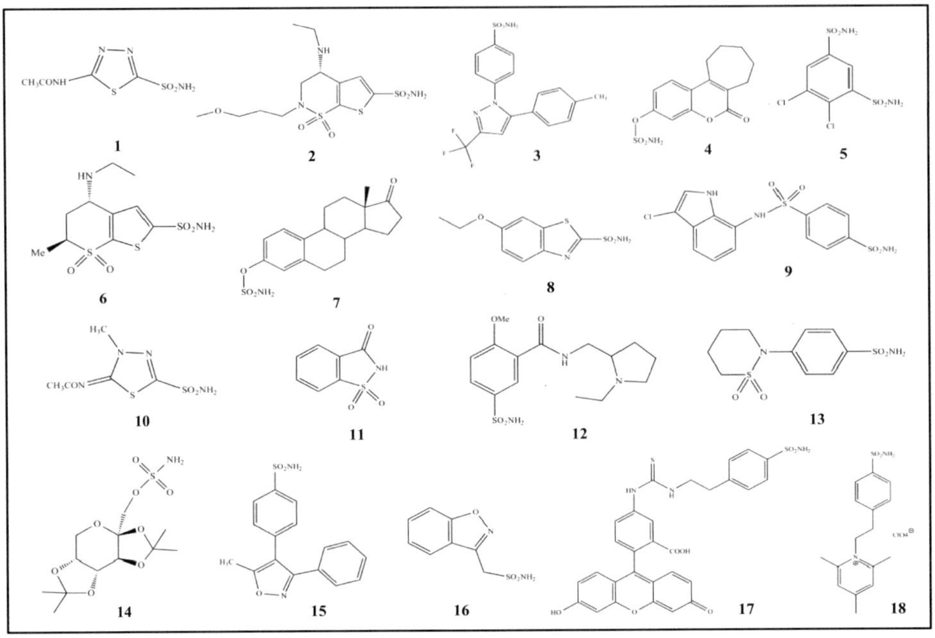

	Name	Ki(nM) CA II	Ki(nM) CA IX	Ki(nM) CA XII
1	Acetazolamide	12	25	5.7
2	Brinzolamide	3.0	37	3.0
3	Celecoxib	21	16	18
4	COUMATE	21	34	12
5	Dichlorophenamide	38	50	50
6	Dorzolamide	9.0	52	3.5
7	EMATE	10	30	7.5
8	Ethoxzolamide	8.0	34	22
9	Indisulam	15	24	3.4
10	Methazolamide	14	27	3.4
11	Saccharin	5,900	100	630
12	Sulpiride	40	46	3.9
13	Sulthiame	9.0	43	56
14	Topiramate	10	58	3.8
15	Valdecoxib	43	27	13
16	Zonisamide	35	5.1	11,000
17	Sulfonamide derivative	45	24	5.0
18	Sulfonamide derivative	21	14	7.0

Fig. (3). Structures of carbonic anhydrase inhibitors 1-18 and inhibition data. Structure of inhibitors 1-18 (top). Inhibition data with selected sulfonamide and sulfamate-based inhibitors against isozymes IX and XII (bottom). Values given to 2 significant digits [1].

A B C

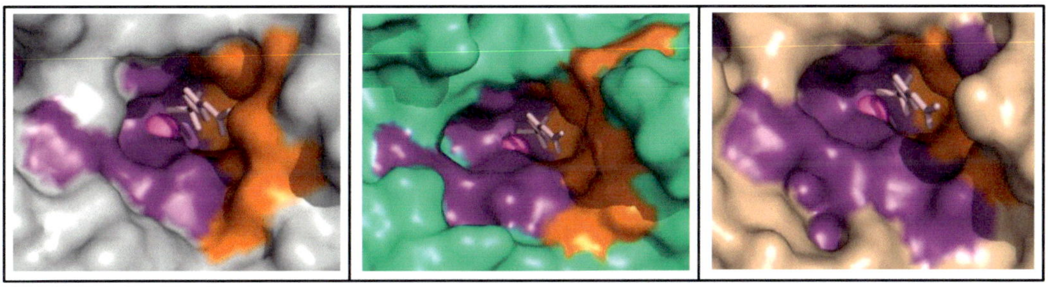

Fig. (4). Structure of human α-CAs bound to acetazolamide, a "classical" sulfonamide inhibitor. Surface depiction of acetazolamide bound to (A) CA II, PDB ID 3HS4 (grey), (B) CA IX, PDB ID 3IAI (green), and (C) CA XII, PDB ID IJCZ (wheat). Active site zinc (magenta sphere), hydrophilic (purple) and hydrophobic (orange) residues are shown.

2.1.1.2. Metal-chelating Anions

The metal-chelating anions, unlike the sulfonamides and their isosters, may bind to the zinc in one of three possible geometries: a trigonal-bipyramidal geometry, a tetrahedral geometry, or in a distorted tetrahedral geometry [87]. The ability to bind in multi-faceted geometries is due primarily to the structural features of the ligand. These inorganic anions are weaker CA inhibitors than sulfonamides [30, 86, 87, 97].

2.1.2. Non-Classical CAIs

The "non-classical" CAIs include both small molecule inhibitors and several biologics such as monoclonal antibodies and RNAi based molecules [21, 72, 98 - 107]. Some "non-classical" small molecule CA inhibitors do not bind directly to the zinc and they include thiocarbonates, phenols, coumarins, and polyamines (Fig. (**5**)) [1, 27]. The carbohydrate based sulfonamide derivates and steroid sulfatases [98 - 104] bind the zinc but have additional moieties (longer variable tail regions) that allow for greater isoform specificity [105, 106].

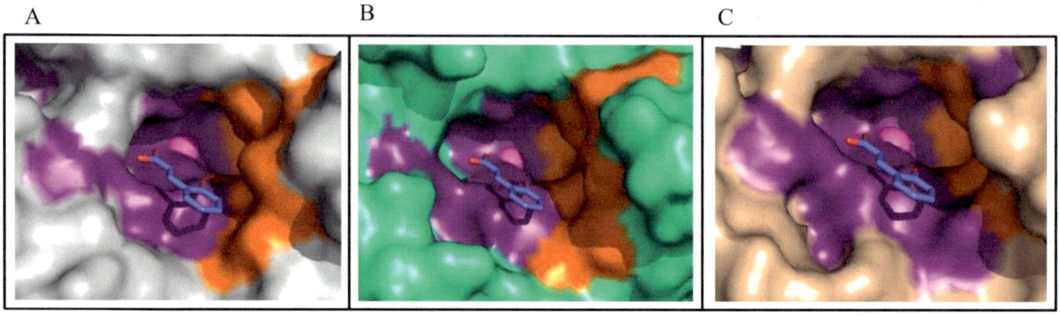

Fig. (5). Structure of human a-CAs bound to a "non-classical" sulfonamide inhibitor. Surface depiction of a substituted coumarin bound to the active site of (A) CA II, PDB ID 5BNL (grey), (B) CA IX, PDB ID 3IAI (green), (C) CA XII, PDB ID IJCZ (wheat). Active site zinc (magenta sphere), hydrophilic (purple) and hydrophobic (orange) residues are shown.

2.1.2.1. Carbohydrate-Based Sulfonamides

The carbohydrate-based sulfonamide derivatives and steroid sulfatases are derived from classic sulfonamide CAIs and may exhibit antitumor & antimitotic activities [105 - 107]. These compounds have primary sulfonamides attached to mono- or disaccharide moieties instead of an aromatic ring [102, 108, 109]. The inhibitors exhibit high affinity for CA IX/CA XII and their sugar moieties cause reduced membrane permeability and thus greater selectivity for targeting the extracellular facing of both tumor associated isoforms [100, 102, 103, 106, 107]. The observed lack of membrane permeability exerted by these CAIs may be attributed to their high molecular weights, and bulky sugar tails that are not easily transported. Furthermore, the presence of sugar moieties maintains water solubility and good bioavailability [102, 108, 109].

2.1.2.2. Immunotherapy

In addition to small molecule inhibitor development, there are several biologics used for CA inhibition. Mouse monoclonal antibodies such as VII/20, M75, G250 (that recognize the PG domain of CA IX) and more recently 6A10 (that recognizes CA XII) show great potential for anti-cancer therapy [110 - 113]. These antibodies are highly selective for binding to, and internalization by, CA IX/CA XII-expressing cancer cells. The use of antibody-based targeting systems to deliver cytotoxic payloads or radiolabeled antibodies to tumor cells provides an alternative approach to targeted therapy [21, 114 - 116]. Ligand conjugates consisting of either bivalent small molecules or a CA IX-specific, ligand-dye conjugate linked to a cytotoxic drug (maytansinoid DM1) were shown to specifically target tumor tissue and deliver the cytotoxic agent [114].

Recently, a Phase II clinical trial was initiated for use of Lutetium 177- labeled anti CA IX monoclonal antibody girentuximab (cG250) in patients with advanced clear cell renal cell carcinoma (ccRCC) [115, 116]. For the aforementioned tumor type, the radiolabeled chimeric monoclonal antibody cG250 was extensively investigated both for radioimmunodetection and radioimmuno therapy (RIT). Results from these studies show significant antitumor effects and less toxicity to normal cells [115, 116]. These effects were observed because of the specific targeting of cG250 to CA IX expressing lesions, which is a potent antibody-based carrier for tumor-targeted delivery of β-emitting radionuclides [115, 116].

Phage display technology has also been utilized for the development of novel peptide based CA IX-specific antibodies with the ability to potently inhibit CA activity and induce endocytosis [117]. These antibodies have the advantage of specifically disrupting the catalytic activity of the enzyme and induce surface CA IX internalization into endosomes. These novel peptide based antibodies thus target CA IXs tumorigenic functions, including pH regulation [112, 118]. New monoclonal antibodies against human recombinant CA XII for immunodetection and immunotherapy are also currently being developed and characterized [119, 120].

Recently, clinical trial data have been reported for use of chimeric antibody (CAR) engineered T cells against CA IX for treatment of metastatic ccRCC [121]. Results from these studies show that CA IX targeting CAR T cells exert antigen-specific effects *in vivo* and induce liver toxicities at low doses of T-cells [121]. This illustrates the potency of receptor modified T cells. The observed antigen-directed "on target" toxicity was successfully prevented by pretreatment with G250, consequently blocking antigen sites in off target organs and allowing higher T cell doses [121]. However, the effects of this therapeutic strategy on long-term patient survival are yet to be reported.

2.1.2.3. RNAi Technology

Several studies have utilized RNAi technology to modulate CA IX expression in several cancers [84, 122, 123]. The mechanism of RNAi uses the endogenous miRNA pathway that regulates protein expression by gene silencing through post-transcriptional mechanisms [123 - 125]. Ultimately, this activates translational repression and induces mRNA cleavage or degradation [123 - 125]. Typically, efficient siRNAs are designed with exact base complementation to the target mRNA and induce complete degradation. In contrast, shRNAs are typically exported to the cytosol and processed to form viable siRNA [124]. Successful knockdown of CA IX by siRNA or shRNA mediation has been shown to reduce growth, proliferation, and enhance the effects of commonly used inhibitors in several types of cancers [21, 40, 70, 84, 126 - 128].

Specifically, knockdown of CA IX using shRNA strategies in human breast cancer cells, when implanted into mouse mammary tissue, significantly inhibited primary tumor growth and metastasis formation [84]. A similar effect was noted in the 4T1 breast tumor model. The 4T1 mammary carcinoma is a "transplantable" mouse tumor cell line that is both tumorigenic and metastatic. When compared to the 4T1 shRNA control (non-silencing RNAi) group, the 4T1 shCA IX (CA IX-silencing RNAi) group showed 100% survival post tumor inoculation [84]. Furthermore, RNAi delivery systems designed to successfully deliver siRNA or shRNA to target cells, such as viral vectors or liposomes, promote siRNA longevity and evade inciting an immune response [21, 124]. As such, RNAi technology shows promise as a novel cancer therapeutic option or can possibly be used as an alternative to developing isoform specific CAIs in certain selected cancers. However, more research is needed to validate the use of RNAi technology as a viable option for therapy.

3. RECENT PATENTS FOR USE IN CANCER THERAPY

This section discusses recent patents granted during 2012-2016 on CA IX and CA XII for the use of small molecule inhibitors and immunotherapy for cancer treatment. It also includes some of the CA IX/CA XII inhibitors that are currently in clinical trials for treatment of the several cancers.

3.1. Small Molecule Inhibitors

3.1.1. Derivatives of Boron Cluster Compounds (Patent: WO2013060307)

The invention described in this patent, published by Prague *et al.*, describes derivatives of boron cluster compounds and their pharmacologically acceptable salts and solvents and their specific inhibitory effects on CA IX [129]. The patent includes methods of synthesis, use, diagnosis and/ or therapy for CA IX expressing cancers [129 - 132]. The selective inhibition achieved by these novel compounds is because of a parallel presence of two substituted structural factors [131, 132]; the boron containing clusters (as a hydrophobic pharmacophore) and a group capable of binding to the active site of the enzyme. In the case of CA IX, the substituted group is a sulfonamide [129].

X-ray crystallography studies of one of the boron cluster derivatives, in complex with CA II (resolution: 1.60 Å), showed that the compounds bind tightly to the active site of CA II [129]. However, the inhibition efficacy of the compounds *in vitro,* assayed using conventional colorimetric methods, showed greater specificity for CA IX than CA II. The cytotoxicity of the derivatives was also tested on cancer cells versus normal cells. The results showed consistently less cytotoxicity to normal cells in comparison to tumor cells [129]. In order to demonstrate pharmaceutical exploitation of the compounds in this invention, the maximum tolerated dose and limiting toxicities of two promising CA IX inhibitors were tested in mice. The dose limiting toxicities observed included drowsiness, apathy, and local irritation [129]. However, the maximal tolerated dose observed and achieved supports further pharmacological use of the CA IX inhibitors for cancer therapy.

3.1.2. Metal Complexes of Poly(Carboxyl) Amine Containing Ligands (Patent: WO2013103813)

As described in this patent filed by Molecular Insight Pharmaceuticals, the invention is directed to the synthesis and use of metal complexes of poly(carboxyl)-amine containing compounds [133, 134]. The metal complexes include radionuclide and non-radionuclide metal complexes such as Pt, Zn, ^{64}Cu, ^{186}Re, ^{188}Re and ^{99m}Tc [135]. These compounds are specific inhibitors of CA IX and may find use as candidate agents for imaging tumors and chemotherapy [133]. Biological studies for the compounds described in this invention were performed in cell culture to determine binding affinity and in human xenograft bearing mice for analysis of tissue biodistribution [133].

The *in vitro* binding affinity studies showed that radionuclide complexes of these compounds are potent inhibitors of CA IX with IC_{50} values in the nanomolar range. In contrast, the free (uncomplexed) compounds exhibit 2-250-fold higher IC_{50} values than the corresponding complex [133]. Tissue distribution studies of the CA IX inhibitors *in vivo* showed that the compounds were detected in blood, heart, liver, lungs, spleen, small and large intestine, stomach, kidneys and skeletal muscles [133]. Especially high concentrations of the inhibitor were detected in the kidney and liver of mice. Results from these studies also showed rapid clearance of the CA IX inhibitors from non-tumor tissue [133]. According to the inventors and results discussed, these compounds are suitable candidate agents for imaging and targeting tumor tissues with high expression of CA IX.

3.1.3. Nitroimidazole Based Compounds (Patent: WO2014030142)

Lambin *et al.* recently patented nitroimidazole-containing compounds for use in radiotherapy (Fig. (**6**)) [96, 136, 137]. The basic principle of irradiation is to damage the cancer cells to such an extent that they will die. The irradiated cells form free radicals and immediately damage the DNA or react with oxygen, creating reactive oxygen species that damage the cell. Under hypoxic conditions when there is little to no oxygen present, less reactive oxygen species are formed and the irradiation is not as effective. Studies have shown that extracellular acidosis also makes tumors less sensitive to irradiation treatment [138]. Nitroimidazole scaffolds are well known radiosensitizers and this patent describes the development of dual drugs that can selectively inhibit CA IX and enhance hypoxic tumor sensitization toward cancer therapy [137, 139]. These compounds include a panel of sulfonamide/sulfamide/sulfamate derivates containing 2- or 5-

nitroimidazoles moieties [140]. Note that compound 6-1 (Fig. (**6**)) has no inhibitory effect on CA activity because it is not a sulfonamide derivative (NH_2 is substituted for CH_3). Crystallographic studies show binding of these novel nitroimidazole compounds in the active site cavity of CAs. These structural studies were validated *in vitro* in HT29 and HeLa cell lines, where selective CA IX inhibition reduced hypoxia induced tumor acidosis [140].

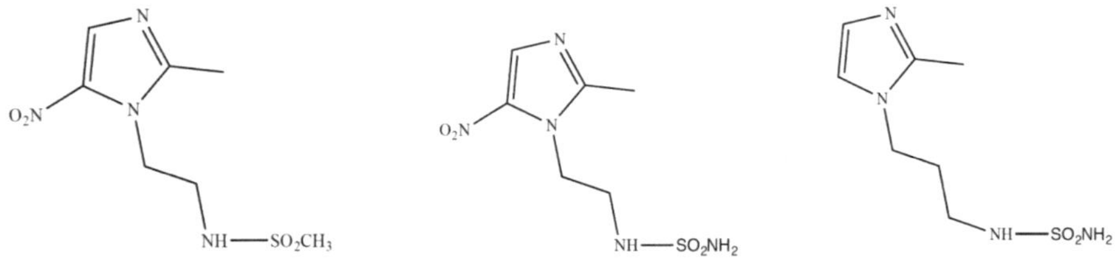

Compounds	CA II (nM)	CA IX (nM)	CA XII (nM)
6-1	> 2000	> 2000	> 2000
6-2	10.1	20.4	8.1
6-3	52	21	37

Fig. (6). General structural formulae of patented nitroimidazole compounds.

In vivo studies using nitroimidazole and sulfonamide duel targeting drugs show reduced extracellular acidification, reduced tumor growth at non-toxic doses, and increased tumor sensitization to irradiation in a CA IX dependent manner [139]. These compounds, as described in the patent, are potent inhibitors targeted against CA IX that increase the sensitivity of tumor cells to radiation suggesting a novel approach to drug design [137]. Thus, specifically targeting CA IX in hypoxic tumors using nitroimidazole derivatives can be developed as a new strategy for therapeutic intervention in cancer.

3.1.4. Ureido-Sulfonamide Based Compounds (Patent: WO2012021963)

Metasignal Therapeutics Inc. patented therapeutic ureido-sulfonamide compounds with the formula R-Q-Ar--SO_2NH_2 (Fig. (**3**): Compound 18) wherein R is an aryl, hetaryl, alkyl or cycloalkyl group, Q is the group -L(CH2)n-, wherein n = 0, 1 or 2 and L is the group - NHCXNH-, -NHC(S)SNH-, -NHCONHCSNH- or -SO2NH-,

X is O or S and Ar is a C6-C10 aromatic or a heteroaromatic group that contains at least one heteroatom of oxygen, nitrogen or sulfur [141, 142]. Two compounds of this series: 4-{[(3nitrophenyl) carbamoyl] amino} benzene sulfonamide (Fig. (**7-1**)) and 4-{[(4-fluorophenyl) carbamoyl] amino} benzene sulfonamide (Fig. (**7-2**)) selectively inhibit CA IX and CA XII, and have been shown to effectively inhibit hypoxic tumor growth, suppress metastases, and impair and deplete cancer stem cells in mammals [84, 126]. *In vitro* studies showed a significant decrease in invasion and/or induced cell death when treated with an ureido-sulfonamide derivative. Furthermore, inhibition of CA IX activity impaired maintenance and depleted the cancer stem cell population in human breast cancer [126]. A reduction in tumor growth and size was also observed with studies performed *in vivo* [84, 143]. One of the ureidosulfonamide derivatives (Fig. (**7-3**)) under the name SLC-0111 is currently in Phase I clinical trials initiated by SignalChem

Lifesciences Corp. (SLC) in Vancouver, British Columbia (2014- NCT02 215850). The first arm of this study evaluates the safety of SLC-0111 in dose escalation studies in patients with advanced solid tumors [139]. The second arm of this clinical trial will focus on treating only patients whose tumors express CA IX. SLC is also developing a backup small molecule inhibitor of CA IX (SLC-021) and in collaboration with the National Research Council of Canada, a monoclonal antibody (SLC-0131) targeting CA IX. Both programs are in the preclinical development stage.

3.1.5. Coumarin Based Compounds (Patent: WO2012070024)

Metasignal Therapeutics Inc. also recently patented novel coumarins, thiocoumarins, and glycosylated coumarins, and their use as inhibitors of carbonic anhydrase IX and XII for treatment of hypoxic and metastatic cancer (Fig. (**8**)) [144]. Unsubstituted coumarins/thiocoumarins are nonselective to most CA isoforms and bind in hydrolyzed form at the entrance of CA active site with no interaction with the zinc ion (Fig. (**8-1**)) [98]. However, substituted coumarins are selective for membrane-bound CA isoforms due to the addition of bulky tail moieties. Coumarins are considered mechanism-based inhibitors, which undergo enzymatic hydrolysis of the lactone moiety to give the corresponding 2-

hydroxycinnamic acid. The latter is responsible for CA IX inhibition in the high nanomolar range by means of the occlusion of the entrance to the enzyme site [27, 108, 145].

7-1

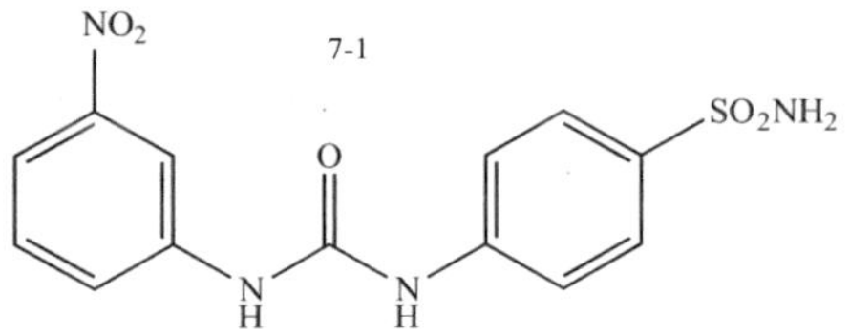

7-2

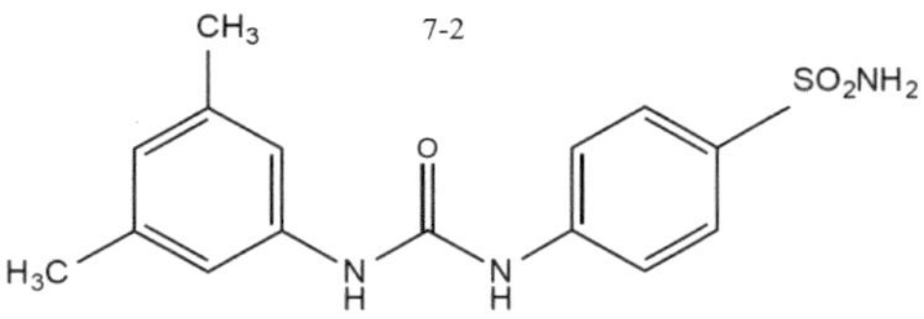

7-3

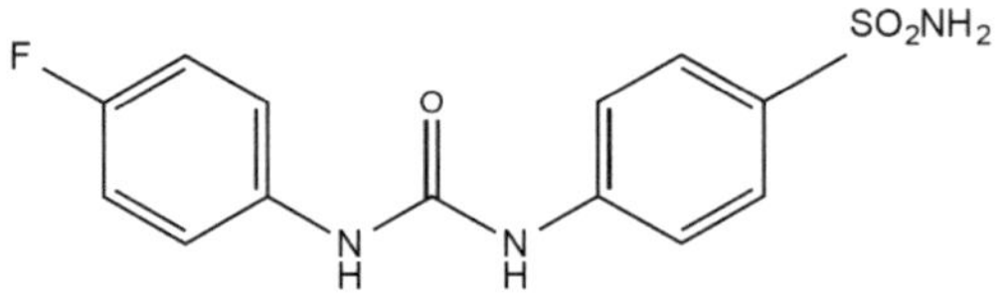

Compounds	CA II (nM)	CA IX (nM)	CA XII (nM)
7-1	15	0.9	5.7
7-2	1765	6.9	6.2
7-3	960	45.1	4.5

Fig. (7). Structure of ureido-sulfonamide compounds.

8-1

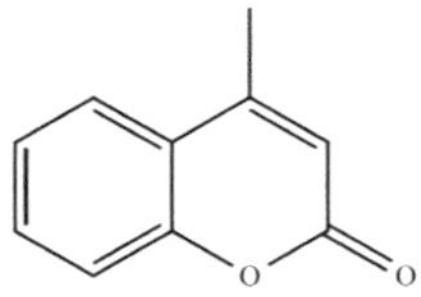

8-2

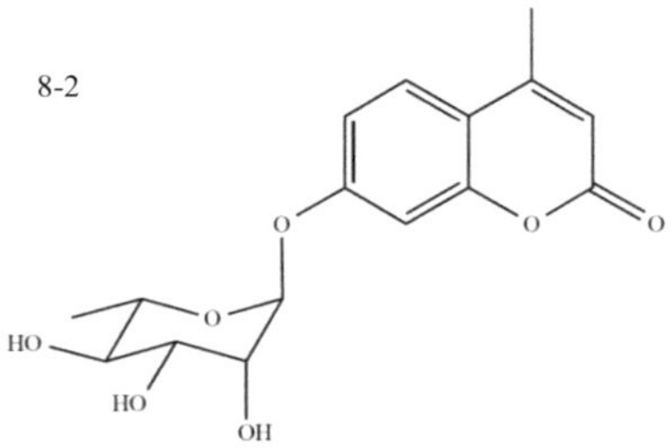

8-3

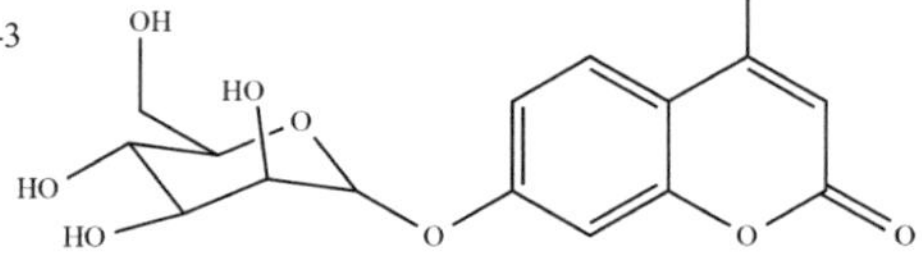

Compounds	CA II (nM)	CA IX (nM)	CA XII (nM)
8-1	> 100	-	-
8-2	> 100	201	108
8-3	> 100	9.2	43

Fig. (8). Structure of coumarin based compounds. (A) General structural formula of coumarin/thiocoumarins. (B) and (C) Glycosyl-substituted derivatives.

In this patent, the inventors claimed 40 novel (thio) coumarin derivatives substituted at positions C4 (hydrogen, cyano, methyl, *O*-allyl), C6 (hydrogen, hydroxy, *O*-allyl, *O*- glycosyl, etc.) and C7 (hydrogen, hydroxy, O-allyl, O-glycosyl, linker + heterocycles, such as 1,2,3 trizole, coumarin, pyridinium, aryl, imidazole or branched chains) of the main ring [144]. Among the different strategies developed in order to design selective hCA IX inhibitors, the 'sugar approach' represents one of the most promising tools and was used in this patent to decorate some of the coumarin-based inhibitors. These substituted derivatives contain bulky glycoside moieties, which decrease membrane permeability and exert multiple inhibitory effects. Addition of a sugar moiety also improves the biophysical & biochemical properties such as water solubility and bioavailability of these compounds [107, 144, 146].

The glycosylated coumarins strongly attenuate primary tumor growth and the formation of metastasis in 4T1 mouse model expressing high levels of CA IX [147]. Conversely, no such effects were observed in a breast cancer cell with limited CA IX expression. These selective inhibitors were also effective in limiting colonization to the lungs. One of the glycosyl coumarin derivatives was also shown to inhibit the action of cancer stem cells within breast tumors [84, 126]. The use of carbohydrate scaffolds in the design of CA inhibitors has desirable physicochemical properties for the treatment of metastatic cancer [145].

3.2. Antibody

3.2.1. Monoclonal Anti CA IX G250 Antibody (Patent: WO2007065027A2)

Patents were filed and clinical trials conducted for the use of antibodies that recognize and target CA IX [148]. These antibodies (mAbG250 & derivatives) alone or in combination with IL-2 or IFN-alpha, have been studied extensively in clinical settings for use in cancer therapy [149 - 151]. The G-250 antibody was patented for treatment of G250/CA IX antigen-expressing tumors, in particular renal cell carcinoma, using G250-antigen-specific antibodies as an adjuvant treatment modality to high-risk patients diagnosed with non-metastatic disease [148].

Since then, G250 antibodies and a chimeric version of G250 (cG250) have been used in combination with cytokines, cytotoxins and radionuclides to elicit antibody dependent cytotoxicity, as well as receptor-mediated internalization allowing for targeted delivery of various therapeutic payloads [115, 116]. This approach thus increases therapeutic efficacy by mediating tumor cell destruction and decreased cytotoxicity of surrounding normal tissue [115, 116]. Phase I and II clinical trials demonstrate that the cG250 antibody (RENCAREX) is safe, well tolerated, and able to positively impact disease burden alone and together with cytokines [152]. These studies recently completed Phase III clinical trials as adjuvant therapy aimed at reducing recurrence in surgically treated renal cell carcinoma (RCC) patients who have a high risk of relapse [139].

However, results from the Phase III trials showed that the antibody did not meet its primary end point. The analysis showed no improvement in median disease free-survival following RENCAREX treatment compared with placebo. However, a biomarker analysis showed that response to treatment was directly correlated to CA IX expression. The patient population with high CA IX levels treated with cG250 showed a clinically and statistically significant improvement when compared to placebo and patients with low CA IX score. Therefore, an immunotherapy for anti-CA IX ccRCC in the adjuvant setting may still be an option.

A Phase I trial was recently completed and a Phase II trial initiated for the treatment of metastatic ccRCC with Leutetium-177 (^{177}Lu)-cG250/Girentuximab [115, 116]. The Phase I trials were designed to access the maximum tolerated dose, dosimetry, pharmacokinetic and incidence of human anti-chimeric antibody formation [116]. Results from these dose escalation studies were very promising as (^{177}Lu)-cG250 radioimmuno- therapy was generally well tolerated and resulted in disease stabilization in the majority of patients [116]. Because of these encouraging results, a Phase II trial was initiated in patients with advanced ccRCC [115]. Interim results of this ongoing radioimmunotherapy trial are also promising in terms of clinical response in patients with progressive metastatic ccRCC. The toxicity profile of (^{177}Lu)-cG250 seems to be generally mild, apart from transient myelotoxicity [115]. Final analysis of the Phase II trials will shed more light on the therapeutic efficacy and safety of this treatment modality in patients with metastatic ccRCC.

3.2.2. GM-CSF (Patent: US20130230483)

More recently, a chimeric molecule comprised of a granulation macrophage colony-stimulating factor (GM-CSF) was patented for the treatment of renal cell carcinomas, cervical and bladder cancers [153]. The GM-CSF is a monomeric glycoprotein that functions as a cytokine and is secreted by fibroblasts, endothelial cells, T cells, mast cells, natural killer cells, and macrophages. It facilitates development of the immune system and promotes defense against infections [153]. The GM-CSF molecule attached to a CA IX variant (CA IXv) serves as a kidney cancer specific antigen and, as indicted in the patent application, provides a highly effective "vaccine" that raises an immune response directed against renal cell cancers [153 - 155]. Results from preclinical studies showed that this fusion protein induced specific cytotoxic T lymphocytes *in vitro* and inhibited tumor growth in severe compromised immunodeficiency disease (SCID) mice injected with human carcinoma cell line stably transfected with the fusion protein [155]. The GM-CSF and CA IX chimeric molecule can be used as a traditional vaccine or in adoptive immunotherapeutic applications.

3.2.3. Monoclonal Anti CA XII 6A10 Antibody (Patent: WO2011138279)

Although there are currently no CA XII-specific monoclonal antibodies in clinical trials, a recent patent was filed for use of 6A10 monoclonal antibody to specifically target CA XII [156]. This antibody was generated from stable monoclonal hybridoma producing IgG antibodies that bound to the surface of lung cancer cells [157]. The 6A10 monoclonal antibody showed > 20 times higher specificity for human CA XII than CA IX [157]. Results from these studies also showed that 6A10 inhibited exofacial CA activity in CA XII expressing cancer cells in nanomolar concentrations, without interacting with normal peripheral blood mononuclear cells [113, 157].

The mechanism of action for this antibody appears to be through inhibition of the catalytic activity of CA XII rather than on antigen binding per se. *In vitro*, 6A10 exerts growth limiting effects on tumor spheroids under hypoxic culture conditions where CA XII was active and where its catalytic activity was likely rate limiting [113, 157]. Results from studies *in vivo* corroborate the *in vitro* findings suggesting that membrane bound CAs are critical for cancer cell physiology. Specifically, the tumor xenograft model of breast cancer used in these studies displayed a significant delay in tumor outgrowth when 6A10 was administered [113, 157]. This clearly establishes the importance of targeting CA XII as a therapeutic approach in cancer treatment.

4. CURRENT & FUTURE DEVELOPMENTS

CA IX and CA XII are promising targets for systemic anticancer therapy [23, 24, 27]. Due to the limited presence of CA IX in normal tissue and its upregulation in many tumor types, it has gained significant attention since its discovery [67, 70, 82]. However, the physiological properties of CA XII and its overexpression in tumors have also incited research interest [69, 80, 82, 83]. CA IX expression and in some cases CA XII have been associated with poor prognosis and tumor progression to metastasis as a consequence of their roles in pH regulation [23, 24, 50, 82]. CA IX functions to balance pH_i while simultaneously contributing to acidification of the tumor microenvironment. In contrast, CA XII is believed to operate more efficiently at physiologic pHe [23, 24, 77]. The actions of both enzymes are important for metabolic regulation, cell motility, chemoresistance and metastatic behavior in solid tumors [23 - 25].

Furthermore, inhibition of CA IX/CA XII activity by either small molecules or specific antibodies in several cancers has proven to slow overall tumor growth and metastatic properties [84]. Many classes of CA IX/CA XII inhibitors have been extensively studied in the preclinical setting and demonstrated promising results [1, 9, 27, 108]. Most specifically, patents have recently been published for use of sulfonamide based small molecule inhibitors to target CA IX/ CA XII for the treatment of cancer. Some of these include derivatives of boron cluster compounds, metal complexes of poly(carboxyl)amine containing ligands, nitroimidazole, ureidosulfonamide and coumarin based compounds [129, 133, 137, 141, 144]. These inhibitors have increased specificity and selectivity for tumor associated CA IX and CA XII over other possible off target CAs [129, 133, 137, 141, 144]. One possible reason for the increased isoform selectivity observed, as in the case of coumarin derivatives, is the addition of bulky tail moieties such as sugars that decrease membrane permeability and increase bioavailability [89, 144]. These patented compounds have shown great promise as anticancer agents by inhibiting tumor growth, metastasis, and enhancing tumor sensitization towards chemotherapy both *in vitro* and *in vivo* [129, 133, 137, 141, 144]. To this extent, one the ureidosulfonamide derivatives (SLC-0111) is currently in Phase I clinical trials for the treatment of solid tumors expressing CA IX [91, 139, 141].

Antibody-based targeting of CA IX and CA XII is another strategy that is currently being used for isoform specific and selective inhibition. These monoclonal antibodies include G250 (the first CA IX targeted inhibitor to reach clinical trials for the treatment of cancer), the anti CA XII 6A10 antibody, and GM-CSF a chimeric glycoprotein attached to a CA IX variant [148, 153, 155, 156]. This chimeric molecule serves as a kidney cancer-specific antigen and provides a highly effective "vaccine" that raises an immune response directed against renal cell cancers [153]. Although, the G250 antibody did not meet its primary end point goals in a Phase III clinical trial, it however showed a direct correlation between CA IX expression and response to treatment. Since then, the G250 antibody and a chimeric version cG250 have been used in combination with cytokines, cytotoxins and radionuclides to elicit antibody dependent cytotoxicity and receptor induced internalization allowing for targeted delivery of various therapeutic payloads [115, 116]. This approach increases therapeutic efficacy by mediating tumor cell destruction and decreased cytotoxicity of surrounding normal tissue as observed with (^{177}Lu)cG250/Girentuximab which, is currently in Phase II clinical trials [115].

Although concerns still remain about off-target toxicities of CA inhibitors, mainly because of possible interactions with intracellular CAs and lack of isoform specificity [32], much progress has been made towards designing and developing CA IX/CA XII selective inhibitors. Most of these show great promise as anti-cancer therapeutics [32]. Despite such progress and promise, no CA IX or CA XII inhibitors have yet been approved for use in a clinical setting for the treatment of cancer. Moving forward, more attention should be focused on knocking down CA IX and CA XII expression using RNAi technology as a possible therapeutic approach for treating cancer [21]. The development of RNAi technology and RNAi delivery systems to completely eradicate CA IX/CA XII expressing in tumor cells may be more therapeutically beneficial than targeting activity alone. This will also prevent off target toxicities from inhibition of other CA isoforms. Alternatively, CAIs (alone or conjugated to cytotoxic agents) or siRNA can be used in combination with chemotherapy or radiation to combat chemoresistance, decrease tumor metastasis and improve patient outcome and survival. While preclinical evidence suggests that these concepts have great potential for success, more attention to clinical research is required to bring benefit to cancer patients.

CONFLICT OF INTEREST

The authors confirm that they have no conflict of interest to declare for this publication.

ACKNOWLEDGEMENTS

The authors acknowledge support from the National Institutes of Health, Project CA165284 (SCF) and Minority Supplement CA165284-03S1 (MYM).

REFERENCES

[1] Supuran CT. Carbonic anhydrases: Novel therapeutic applications for inhibitors and activators. Nat Rev Drug Discov 2008; 7(2): 168-81. [http://dx.doi.org/10.1038/nrd2467] [PMID: 18167490]

[2] Ditte P, Dequiedt F, Svastova E, *et al.* Phosphorylation of carbonic anhydrase IX controls its ability to mediate extracellular acidification in hypoxic tumors. Cancer Res 2011; 71(24): 7558-67. [http://dx.doi.org/10.1158/0008-5472.CAN-11-2520] [PMID: 22037869]

[3] Brown BF, Quon A, Dyck JR, Casey JR. Carbonic anhydrase II promotes cardiomyocyte hypertrophy. Can J Physiol Pharmacol 2012; 90(12): 1599-610. [http://dx.doi.org/10.1139/y2012-142] [PMID: 23210439]

[4] Sly WS. The membrane carbonic anhydrases: From CO_2 transport to tumor markers. EXS 2000; 90(90): 95-104. [PMID: 11268540]

[5] Aspatwar A, Tolvanen ME, Parkkila S. Phylogeny and expression of carbonic anhydrase-related proteins. BMC Mol Biol 2010; 11: 25. [http://dx.doi.org/10.1186/1471-2199-11-25] [PMID: 20356370]

[6] Chegwidden W R, Dodgson SJ, Spencer IM. The roles of carbonic anhydrase in metabolism, cell growth and cancer in animals. EXS 2000; 90(90): 343-63.
[PMID: 11268523]

[7] Hilvo M, Innocenti A, Monti SM, De Simone G, Supuran CT, Parkkila S. Recent advances in research on the most novel carbonic anhydrases, CA XIII and XV. Curr Pharm Des 2008; 14(7): 672-8.
[http://dx.doi.org/10.2174/138161208783877811] [PMID: 18336313]

[8] Henry RP, Swenson ER. The distribution and physiological significance of carbonic anhydrase in vertebrate gas exchange organs. Respir Physiol 2000; 121(1): 1-12.
[http://dx.doi.org/10.1016/S0034-5687(00)00110-9] [PMID: 10854618]

[9] Supuran CT. Carbonic anhydrases-an overview. Curr Pharm Des 2008; 14(7): 603-14.
[http://dx.doi.org/10.2174/138161208783877884] [PMID: 18336305]

[10] Biswas UK, Kumar A. Study on the changes of carbonic anhydrase activity in insulin resistance and the effect of methylglyoxal. J Pak Med Assoc 2012; 62(5): 417-21.
[PMID: 22755300]

[11] Sterling D, Reithmeier RA, Casey JR. Carbonic anhydrase: In the driver's seat for bicarbonate transport. JOP 2001; 2(4) (Suppl.): 165-70.
[PMID: 11875254]

[12] Purkerson JM, Schwartz GJ. The role of carbonic anhydrases in renal physiology. Kidney Int 2007; 71(2): 103-15.
[http://dx.doi.org/10.1038/sj.ki.5002020] [PMID: 17164835]

[13] Henry RP. Multiple roles of carbonic anhydrase in cellular transport and metabolism. Annu Rev Physiol 1996; 58: 523-38.
[http://dx.doi.org/10.1146/annurev.ph.58.030196.002515] [PMID: 8815807]

[14] Chaput CD, Dangott LJ, Rahm MD, Hitt KD, Stewart DS, Wayne Sampson H. A proteomic study of protein variation between osteopenic and age-matched control bone tissue. Exp Biol Med (Maywood) 2012; 237(5): 491-8.
[http://dx.doi.org/10.1258/ebm.2012.011374] [PMID: 22619369]

[15] Frasseto F, Parisotto TM, Peres RC, Marques MR, Line SR, Nobre Dos Santos M. Relationship among salivary carbonic anhydrase VI activity and flow rate, biofilm pH and caries in primary dentition. Caries Res 2012; 46(3): 194-200.
[http://dx.doi.org/10.1159/000337275] [PMID: 22508543]

[16] Gilmour KM. Perspectives on carbonic anhydrase. Comp Biochem Physiol A Mol Integr Physiol 2010; 157(3): 193-7.
[http://dx.doi.org/10.1016/j.cbpa.2010.06.161] [PMID: 20541618]

[17] Kuo WH, Yang SF, Hsieh YS, Tsai CS, Hwang WL, Chu SC. Differential expression of carbonic anhydrase isoenzymes in various types of anemia. Clin Chim Acta 2005; 351(1-2): 79-86.
[http://dx.doi.org/10.1016/j.cccn.2004.07.009] [PMID: 15563874]

[18] Del Prete S, Vullo D, Fisher GM, *et al.* Discovery of a new family of carbonic anhydrases in the malaria pathogen Plasmodium falciparum--the η-carbonic anhydrases. Bioorg Med Chem Lett 2014; 24(18): 4389-96.

[http://dx.doi.org/10.1016/j.bmcl.2014.08.015] [PMID: 25168745]

[19] Supuran CT, Winum JY. Designing carbonic anhydrase inhibitors for the treatment of breast cancer. Expert Opin Drug Discov 2015; 10(6): 591-7.
[http://dx.doi.org/10.1517/17460441.2015.1038235] [PMID: 25891195]

[20] Supuran CT, Winum JY. Carbonic anhydrase IX inhibitors in cancer therapy: an update. Future Med Chem 2015; 7(11): 1407-14.
[http://dx.doi.org/10.4155/fmc.15.71] [PMID: 26230880]

[21] Mahon BP, Pinard MA, McKenna R. Targeting carbonic anhydrase IX activity and expression. Molecules 2015; 20(2): 2323-48.
[http://dx.doi.org/10.3390/molecules20022323] [PMID: 25647573]

[22] Silverman DN, Lindskog S. The catalytic mechanism of carbonic anhydrase - implication of a rate limiting protolysis of water. Acc Chem Res 1988; 21: 30-6.
[http://dx.doi.org/10.1021/ar00145a005]

[23] McDonald PC, Winum JY, Supuran CT, Dedhar S. Recent developments in targeting carbonic anhydrase IX for cancer therapeutics. Oncotarget 2012; 3(1): 84-97.
[PMID: 22289741]

[24] Neri D, Supuran CT. Interfering with pH regulation in tumours as a therapeutic strategy. Nat Rev Drug Discov 2011; 10(10): 767-77.
[http://dx.doi.org/10.1038/nrd3554] [PMID: 21921921]

[25] Supuran CT. Structure and function of carbonic anhydrases. Biochem J 2016; 473(14): 2023-32.
[http://dx.doi.org/10.1042/BCJ20160115] [PMID: 27407171]

[26] Fisher SZ, Maupin CM, Budayova-Spano M, *et al.* Atomic crystal and molecular dynamics simulation structures of human carbonic anhydrase II: Insights into the proton transfer mechanism. Biochemistry 2007; 46(11): 2930-7.
[http://dx.doi.org/10.1021/bi062066y] [PMID: 17319692]

[27] Supuran CT. How many carbonic anhydrase inhibition mechanisms exist? J Enzyme Inhib Med Chem 2016; 31(3): 345-60.
[http://dx.doi.org/10.3109/14756366.2015.1122001] [PMID: 26619898]

[28] Pocker Y, Sarkanen S. Carbonic anhydrase: structure catalytic versatility, and inhibition. Adv Enzymol Relat Areas Mol Biol 1978; 47: 149-274.
[PMID: 31766]

[29] Krishnamurthy VM, Kaufman GK, Urbach AR, *et al.* Carbonic anhydrase as a model for biophysical and physical-organic studies of proteins and protein-ligand binding. Chem Rev 2008; 108(3): 946-1051.
[http://dx.doi.org/10.1021/cr050262p] [PMID: 18335973]

[30] Eriksson AE, Jones TA, Liljas A. Refined structure of human carbonic anhydrase II at 2.0 A resolution. Proteins 1988; 4(4): 274-82.
[http://dx.doi.org/10.1002/prot.340040406] [PMID: 3151019]

[31] Supuran CT, Scozzafava A, Casini A. Carbonic anhydrase inhibitors. Med Res Rev 2003; 23(2): 146-89.

[http://dx.doi.org/10.1002/med.10025] [PMID: 12500287]

[32] Pinard MA, Mahon B, McKenna R. Probing the surface of human carbonic anhydrase for clues towards the design of isoform specific inhibitors. Biomed Res Int 2015; 2015: 453543. [http://dx.doi.org/10.1155/2015/453543]

[33] Whittington DA, Waheed A, Ulmasov B, *et al.* Crystal structure of the dimeric extracellular domain of human carbonic anhydrase XII, a bitopic membrane protein overexpressed in certain cancer tumor cells. Proc Natl Acad Sci USA 2001; 98(17): 9545-50. [http://dx.doi.org/10.1073/pnas.161301298] [PMID: 11493685]

[34] Pastorek J, Pastoreková S, Callebaut I, *et al.* Cloning and characterization of MN, a human tumor-associated protein with a domain homologous to carbonic anhydrase and a putative helix-loop-helix DNA binding segment. Oncogene 1994; 9(10): 2877-88. [PMID: 8084592]

[35] Opavský R, Pastoreková S, Zelník V, *et al.* Human MN/CA9 gene, a novel member of the carbonic anhydrase family: Structure and exon to protein domain relationships. Genomics 1996; 33(3): 480-7. [http://dx.doi.org/10.1006/geno.1996.0223] [PMID: 8661007]

[36] Grabmaier K, Vissers JL, De Weijert MC, *et al.* Molecular cloning and immunogenicity of renal cell carcinoma-associated antigen G250. Int J Cancer 2000; 85(6): 865-70. [http://dx.doi.org/10.1002/(SICI)1097-0215(20000315)85:6<865::AID-IJC21>3.0.CO;2-Q] [PMID: 10709109]

[37] De Simone G, Supuran CT. Carbonic anhydrase IX: Biochemical and crystallographic characterization of a novel antitumor target. Biochim Biophys Acta 2010; 1804: 494-09.

[38] Alterio V, Hilvo M, Di Fiore A, *et al.* Crystal structure of the catalytic domain of the tumor-associated human carbonic anhydrase IX. Proc Natl Acad Sci USA 2009; 106(38): 16233-8. [http://dx.doi.org/10.1073/pnas.0908301106] [PMID: 19805286]

[39] Türeci O, Sahin U, Vollmar E, *et al.* Human carbonic anhydrase XII: cDNA cloning, expression, and chromosomal localization of a carbonic anhydrase gene that is overexpressed in some renal cell cancers. Proc Natl Acad Sci USA 1998; 95(13): 7608-13. [http://dx.doi.org/10.1073/pnas.95.13.7608] [PMID: 9636197]

[40] Hilvo M, Baranauskiene L, Salzano AM, *et al.* Biochemical characterization of CA IX, one of the most active carbonic anhydrase isozymes. J Biol Chem 2008; 283(41): 27799-809. [http://dx.doi.org/10.1074/jbc.M800938200] [PMID: 18703501]

[41] Dorai T, Sawczuk IS, Pastorek J, Wiernik PH, Dutcher JP. The role of carbonic anhydrase IX overexpression in kidney cancer. Eur J Cancer 2005; 41(18): 2935-47. [http://dx.doi.org/10.1016/j.ejca.2005.09.011] [PMID: 16310354]

[42] Li Y, Wang H, Tu C, Shiverick KT, Silverman DN, Frost SC. Role of hypoxia and EGF on expression, activity, localization and phosphorylation of carbonic anhydrase IX in MDA-MB-231 breast cancer cells. Biochim Biophys Acta 2011; 1813(1): 159-67. [http://dx.doi.org/10.1016/j.bbamcr.2010.09.018] [PMID: 20920536]

[43] Kobayashi M, Matsumoto T, Ryuge S, *et al.* CAXII is a sero-diagnostic marker for lung cancer. PLoS One 2012; 7(3): e33952.

[http://dx.doi.org/10.1371/journal.pone.0033952] [PMID: 22439015]

[44] Zatovicova M, Sedlakova O, Svastova E, *et al.* Ectodomain shedding of the hypoxia-induced carbonic anhydrase IX is a metalloprotease-dependent process regulated by TACE/ADAM17. Br J Cancer 2005; 93(11): 1267-76.
[http://dx.doi.org/10.1038/sj.bjc.6602861] [PMID: 16278664]

[45] Závada J, Závadová Z, Zat'ovicová M, Hyrsl L, Kawaciuk I. Soluble form of carbonic anhydrase IX (CA IX) in the serum and urine of renal carcinoma patients. Br J Cancer 2003; 89(6): 1067-71.
[http://dx.doi.org/10.1038/sj.bjc.6601264] [PMID: 12966427]

[46] Brown-Glaberman U, Marron M, Chalasani P, *et al.* Circulating carbonic anhydrase IX and antiangiogenic therapy in breast cancer. Dis Markers 2016; 2016: 9810383.
[http://dx.doi.org/10.1155/2016/9810383]

[47] Carney WP. Circulating oncoproteins HER2/neu, EGFR and CAIX (MN) as novel cancer biomarkers. Expert Rev Mol Diagn 2007; 7(3): 309-19.
[http://dx.doi.org/10.1586/14737159.7.3.309] [PMID: 17489737]

[48] Woelber L, Kress K, Kersten JF, *et al.* Carbonic anhydrase IX in tumor tissue and sera of patients with primary cervical cancer. BMC Cancer 2011; 11: 12.
[http://dx.doi.org/10.1186/1471-2407-11-12] [PMID: 21223596]

[49] Rosenberg V, Pastorekova S, Zatovicova M, Vidlickova I, Jelenska L, Slezak P. High serum carbonic anhydrase IX predicts shorter survival in head and neck cancer. Bratisl Lek Listy (Tlacene Vyd) 2016; 117(4): 201-4.
[PMID: 27075382]

[50] Sadri N, Zhang PJ. Hypoxia-inducible factors: Mediators of cancer progression; prognostic and therapeutic targets in soft tissue sarcomas. Cancers (Basel) 2013; 5(2): 320-33.
[http://dx.doi.org/10.3390/cancers5020320] [PMID: 24216979]

[51] Wykoff CC, Beasley NJ, Watson PH, *et al.* Hypoxia-inducible expression of tumor-associated carbonic anhydrases. Cancer Res 2000; 60(24): 7075-83.
[PMID: 11156414]

[52] Li Y, Tu C, Wang H, Silverman DN, Frost SC. Catalysis and pH control by membrane-associated carbonic anhydrase IX in MDA-MB-231 breast cancer cells. J Biol Chem 2011; 286(18): 15789-96.
[http://dx.doi.org/10.1074/jbc.M110.188524] [PMID: 21454639]

[53] Yasinska IM, Gibbs BF, Lall GS, Sumbayev VV. The HIF-1 transcription complex is essential for translational control of myeloid hematopoietic cell function by maintaining mTOR phosphorylation. Cell Mol Life Sci 2014; 71(4): 699-710.
[http://dx.doi.org/10.1007/s00018-013-1421-2] [PMID: 23872956]

[54] Tannahill GM, Curtis AM, Adamik J, *et al.* Succinate is an inflammatory signal that induces IL-1β through HIF-1α. Nature 2013; 496(7444): 238-42.
[http://dx.doi.org/10.1038/nature11986] [PMID: 23535595]

[55] Maxwell PH, Wiesener MS, Chang GW, *et al.* The tumour suppressor protein VHL targets hypoxia-inducible factors for oxygen-dependent proteolysis. Nature 1999; 399(6733): 271-5.
[http://dx.doi.org/10.1038/20459] [PMID: 10353251]

[56] Salceda S, Caro J. Hypoxia-inducible factor 1alpha (HIF-1alpha) protein is rapidly degraded by the ubiquitin-proteasome system under normoxic conditions. Its stabilization by hypoxia depends on redox-induced changes. J Biol Chem 1997; 272(36): 22642-7. [http://dx.doi.org/10.1074/jbc.272.36.22642] [PMID: 9278421]

[57] Wykoff CC, Beasley NJ, Watson PH, *et al.* Hypoxia-inducible expression of tumor-associated carbonic anhydrases. Cancer Res 2000; 60(24): 7075-83. [PMID: 11156414]

[58] Semenza GL. Regulation of mammalian O_2 homeostasis by hypoxia-inducible factor 1. Annu Rev Cell Dev Biol 1999; 15: 551-78. [http://dx.doi.org/10.1146/annurev.cellbio.15.1.551] [PMID: 10611972]

[59] Ke Q, Costa M. Hypoxia-inducible factor-1 (HIF-1). Mol Pharmacol 2006; 70(5): 1469-80. [http://dx.doi.org/10.1124/mol.106.027029] [PMID: 16887934]

[60] Kallio PJ, Pongratz I, Gradin K, McGuire J, Poellinger L. Activation of hypoxia-inducible factor 1alpha: Posttranscriptional regulation and conformational change by recruitment of the Arnt transcription factor. Proc Natl Acad Sci USA 1997; 94(11): 5667-72. [http://dx.doi.org/10.1073/pnas.94.11.5667] [PMID: 9159130]

[61] Barnett DH, Sheng S, Charn TH, *et al.* Estrogen receptor regulation of carbonic anhydrase XII through a distal enhancer in breast cancer. Cancer Res 2008; 68(9): 3505-15. [http://dx.doi.org/10.1158/0008-5472.CAN-07-6151] [PMID: 18451179]

[62] Nilsson S, Gustafsson JA. Estrogen receptor action. Crit Rev Eukaryot Gene Expr 2002; 12(4): 237-57. [http://dx.doi.org/10.1615/CritRevEukaryotGeneExpr.v12.i4.10] [PMID: 12641394]

[63] Gruber CJ, Tschugguel W, Schneeberger C, Huber JC. Production and actions of estrogens. N Engl J Med 2002; 346(5): 340-52. [http://dx.doi.org/10.1056/NEJMra000471] [PMID: 11821512]

[64] Deroo BJ, Korach KS. Estrogen receptors and human disease. J Clin Invest 2006; 116(3): 561-70. [http://dx.doi.org/10.1172/JCI27987] [PMID: 16511588]

[65] Saarnio J, Parkkila S, Parkkila AK, *et al.* Immunohistochemistry of carbonic anhydrase isozyme IX (MN/CA IX) in human gut reveals polarized expression in the epithelial cells with the highest proliferative capacity. J Histochem Cytochem 1998; 46(4): 497-504. [http://dx.doi.org/10.1177/002215549804600409] [PMID: 9524195]

[66] Saarnio J, Parkkila S, Parkkila AK, *et al.* Immunohistochemical study of colorectal tumors for expression of a novel transmembrane carbonic anhydrase, MN/CA IX, with potential value as a marker of cell proliferation. Am J Pathol 1998; 153(1): 279-85. [http://dx.doi.org/10.1016/S0002-9440(10)65569-1] [PMID: 9665489]

[67] Liao SY, Lerman MI, Stanbridge EJ. Expression of transmembrane carbonic anhydrases, CAIX and CAXII, in human development. BMC Dev Biol 2009; 9: 22. [http://dx.doi.org/10.1186/1471-213X-9-22] [PMID: 19291313]

[68] Kummola L, Hämäläinen JM, Kivelä J, *et al.* Expression of a novel carbonic anhydrase, CA XIII, in normal and neoplastic colorectal mucosa. BMC Cancer 2005; 5: 41.

[http://dx.doi.org/10.1186/1471-2407-5-41] [PMID: 15836783]

[69] Kivelä AJ, Parkkila S, Saarnio J, *et al.* Expression of transmembrane carbonic anhydrase isoenzymes IX and XII in normal human pancreas and pancreatic tumours. Histochem Cell Biol 2000; 114(3): 197-204.
[PMID: 11083462]

[70] Ivanov S, Liao SY, Ivanova A, *et al.* Expression of hypoxia-inducible cell-surface transmembrane carbonic anhydrases in human cancer. Am J Pathol 2001; 158(3): 905-19.
[http://dx.doi.org/10.1016/S0002-9440(10)64038-2] [PMID: 11238039]

[71] Chen LQ, Howison CM, Spier C, *et al.* Assessment of carbonic anhydrase IX expression and extracellular pH in β-cell lymphoma cell line models. Leuk Lymphoma 2015; 56(5): 1432-9.
[http://dx.doi.org/10.3109/10428194.2014.933218] [PMID: 25130478]

[72] Lounnas N, Rosilio C, Nebout M, *et al.* Pharmacological inhibition of carbonic anhydrase XII interferes with cell proliferation and induces cell apoptosis in T-cell lymphomas. Cancer Lett 2013; 333(1): 76-88.
[http://dx.doi.org/10.1016/j.canlet.2013.01.020] [PMID: 23348702]

[73] Atkins M, Regan M, McDermott D, *et al.* Carbonic anhydrase IX expression predicts outcome of interleukin 2 therapy for renal cancer. Clin Cancer Res 2005; 11(10): 3714-21.
[http://dx.doi.org/10.1158/1078-0432.CCR-04-2019] [PMID: 15897568]

[74] Bui MH, Seligson D, Han KR, *et al.* Carbonic anhydrase IX is an independent predictor of survival in advanced renal clear cell carcinoma: Implications for prognosis and therapy. Clin Cancer Res 2003; 9(2): 802-11.
[PMID: 12576453]

[75] Leibovich BC, Sheinin Y, Lohse CM, *et al.* Carbonic anhydrase IX is not an independent predictor of outcome for patients with clear cell renal cell carcinoma. J Clin Oncol 2007; 25(30): 4757-64.
[http://dx.doi.org/10.1200/JCO.2007.12.1087] [PMID: 17947723]

[76] Yoo CW, Nam BH, Kim JY, *et al.* Carbonic anhydrase XII expression is associated with histologic grade of cervical cancer and superior radiotherapy outcome. Radiat Oncol 2010; 5: 101.
[http://dx.doi.org/10.1186/1748-717X-5-101] [PMID: 21040567]

[77] Griffiths JR. Are cancer cells acidic? Br J Cancer 1991; 64(3): 425-7.
[http://dx.doi.org/10.1038/bjc.1991.326] [PMID: 1911181]

[78] Creighton CJ, Cordero KE, Larios JM, *et al.* Genes regulated by estrogen in breast tumor cells *in vitro* are similarly regulated *in vivo* in tumor xenografts and human breast tumors. Genome Biol 2006; 7(4): R28.
[http://dx.doi.org/10.1186/gb-2006-7-4-r28] [PMID: 16606439]

[79] Wykoff CC, Beasley N, Watson PH, *et al.* Expression of the hypoxia-inducible and tumor-associated carbonic anhydrases in ductal carcinoma *in situ* of the breast. Am J Pathol 2001; 158(3): 1011-9.
[http://dx.doi.org/10.1016/S0002-9440(10)64048-5] [PMID: 11238049]

[80] Ilie MI, Hofman V, Ortholan C, *et al.* Overexpression of carbonic anhydrase XII in tissues from resectable non-small cell lung cancers is a biomarker of good prognosis. Int J Cancer 2011; 128(7): 1614-23.

[http://dx.doi.org/10.1002/ijc.25491] [PMID: 20521252]

[81] Kivelä A, Parkkila S, Saarnio J, *et al.* Expression of a novel transmembrane carbonic anhydrase isozyme XII in normal human gut and colorectal tumors. Am J Pathol 2000; 156(2): 577-84. [http://dx.doi.org/10.1016/S0002-9440(10)64762-1] [PMID: 10666387]

[82] Nordfors K, Haapasalo J, Korja M, *et al.* The tumour-associated carbonic anhydrases CA II, CA IX and CA XII in a group of medulloblastomas and supratentorial primitive neuroectodermal tumours: An association of CA IX with poor prognosis. BMC Cancer 2010; 10: 148. [http://dx.doi.org/10.1186/1471-2407-10-148] [PMID: 20398423]

[83] Kopecka J, Campia I, Jacobs A, *et al.* Carbonic anhydrase XII is a new therapeutic target to overcome chemoresistance in cancer cells. Oncotarget 2015; 6(9): 6776-93. [http://dx.doi.org/10.18632/oncotarget.2882] [PMID: 25686827]

[84] Lou Y, McDonald PC, Oloumi A, *et al.* Targeting tumor hypoxia: Suppression of breast tumor growth and metastasis by novel carbonic anhydrase IX inhibitors. Cancer Res 2011; 71(9): 3364-76. [http://dx.doi.org/10.1158/0008-5472.CAN-10-4261] [PMID: 21415165]

[85] McKenna R, Supuran CT. Carbonic anhydrase inhibitors drug design. Subcell Biochem 2014; 75: 291-323. [http://dx.doi.org/10.1007/978-94-007-7359-2_15] [PMID: 24146385]

[86] Aggarwal M, Kondeti B, McKenna R. Insights towards sulfonamide drug specificity in α-carbonic anhydrases. Bioorg Med Chem 2013; 21(6): 1526-33. [http://dx.doi.org/10.1016/j.bmc.2012.08.019] [PMID: 22985956]

[87] Alterio V, Di Fiore A, D'Ambrosio K, Supuran CT, De Simone G. Multiple binding modes of inhibitors to carbonic anhydrases: How to design specific drugs targeting 15 different isoforms? Chem Rev 2012; 112(8): 4421-68. [http://dx.doi.org/10.1021/cr200176r] [PMID: 22607219]

[88] Winum JY, Supuran CT. Recent advances in the discovery of zinc-binding motifs for the development of carbonic anhydrase inhibitors. J Enzyme Inhib Med Chem 2015; 30(2): 321-4. [http://dx.doi.org/10.3109/14756366.2014.913587] [PMID: 24939097]

[89] Wilkinson BL, Bornaghi LF, Houston TA, *et al.* Inhibition of membrane-associated carbonic anhydrase isozymes IX, XII and XIV with a library of glycoconjugate benzenesulfonamides. Bioorg Med Chem Lett 2007; 17(4): 987-92. [http://dx.doi.org/10.1016/j.bmcl.2006.11.046] [PMID: 17157501]

[90] Thiry A, Dogné JM, Supuran CT, Masereel B. Carbonic anhydrase inhibitors as anticonvulsant agents. Curr Top Med Chem 2007; 7(9): 855-64. [http://dx.doi.org/10.2174/156802607780636726] [PMID: 17504130]

[91] Pacchiano F, Carta F, McDonald PC, *et al.* Ureido-substituted benzenesulfonamides potently inhibit carbonic anhydrase IX and show antimetastatic activity in a model of breast cancer metastasis. J Med Chem 2011; 54(6): 1896-902. [http://dx.doi.org/10.1021/jm101541x] [PMID: 21361354]

[92] Ward C, Meehan J, Mullen P, *et al.* Evaluation of carbonic anhydrase IX as a therapeutic target for inhibition of breast cancer invasion and metastasis using a series of *in vitro* breast cancer models.

Oncotarget 2015; 6(28): 24856-70.
[http://dx.doi.org/10.18632/oncotarget.4498] [PMID: 26259239]

[93] Carradori S, Secci D, De Monte C, *et al.* A novel library of saccharin and acesulfame derivatives as potent and selective inhibitors of carbonic anhydrase IX and XII isoforms. Bioorg Med Chem 2016; 24(5): 1095-105.
[http://dx.doi.org/10.1016/j.bmc.2016.01.038] [PMID: 26810710]

[94] Scozzafava A, Briganti F, Ilies MA, Supuran CT. Carbonic anhydrase inhibitors: Synthesis of membrane-impermeant low molecular weight sulfonamides possessing *in vivo* selectivity for the membrane-bound versus cytosolic isozymes. J Med Chem 2000; 43(2): 292-300.
[http://dx.doi.org/10.1021/jm990479+] [PMID: 10649985]

[95] Mincione F, Menabuoni L, Briganti F, Mincione G, Scozzafava A, Supuran CT. Carbonic anhydrase inhibitors: Inhibition of isozymes I, II and IV with N-hydroxysulfonamides-a novel class of intraocular pressure lowering agents. J Enzyme Inhib 1998; 13(4): 267-84.
[http://dx.doi.org/10.3109/14756369809021475] [PMID: 9795865]

[96] Dubois L, Douma K, Supuran CT, *et al.* Imaging the hypoxia surrogate marker CA IX requires expression and catalytic activity for binding fluorescent sulfonamide inhibitors. Radiother Oncol 2007; 83(3): 367-73.
[http://dx.doi.org/10.1016/j.radonc.2007.04.018] [PMID: 17502120]

[97] Håkansson K, Carlsson M, Svensson LA, Liljas A. Structure of native and apo carbonic anhydrase II and structure of some of its anion-ligand complexes. J Mol Biol 1992; 227(4): 1192-204.
[http://dx.doi.org/10.1016/0022-2836(92)90531-N] [PMID: 1433293]

[98] Maresca A, Temperini C, Vu H, *et al.* Non-zinc mediated inhibition of carbonic anhydrases: Coumarins are a new class of suicide inhibitors. J Am Chem Soc 2009; 131(8): 3057-62.
[http://dx.doi.org/10.1021/ja809683v] [PMID: 19206230]

[99] Maresca A, Temperini C, Pochet L, Masereel B, Scozzafava A, Supuran CT. Deciphering the mechanism of carbonic anhydrase inhibition with coumarins and thiocoumarins. J Med Chem 2010; 53(1): 335-44.
[http://dx.doi.org/10.1021/jm901287j] [PMID: 19911821]

[100] Lopez M, Trajkovic J, Bornaghi LF, *et al.* Design, synthesis, and biological evaluation of novel carbohydrate-based sulfamates as carbonic anhydrase inhibitors. J Med Chem 2011; 54(5): 1481-9.
[http://dx.doi.org/10.1021/jm101525j] [PMID: 21314129]

[101] Carta F, Temperini C, Innocenti A, Scozzafava A, Kaila K, Supuran CT. Polyamines inhibit carbonic anhydrases by anchoring to the zinc-coordinated water molecule. J Med Chem 2010; 53(15): 5511-22.
[http://dx.doi.org/10.1021/jm1003667] [PMID: 20590092]

[102] Rodríguez OM, Maresca A, Témpera CA, Bravo RD, Colinas PA, Supuran CT. N-β-Glycosyl sulfamides are selective inhibitors of the cancer associated carbonic anhydrase isoforms IX and XII. Bioorg Med Chem Lett 2011; 21(15): 4447-50.
[http://dx.doi.org/10.1016/j.bmcl.2011.06.031] [PMID: 21723123]

[103] Lopez M, Paul B, Hofmann A, *et al.* S-Glycosyl primary sulfonamides-a new structural class for selective inhibition of cancer-associated carbonic anhydrases. J Med Chem 2009; 52(20): 6421-32.
[http://dx.doi.org/10.1021/jm900914e] [PMID: 19827837]

[104] Carta F, Aggarwal M, Maresca A, Scozzafava A, McKenna R, Supuran CT. Dithiocarbamates: A new class of carbonic anhydrase inhibitors. Crystallographic and kinetic investigations. Chem Commun (Camb) 2012; 48(13): 1868-70.
[http://dx.doi.org/10.1039/c2cc16395k] [PMID: 22218610]

[105] Morris JC, Chiche J, Grellier C, *et al.* Targeting hypoxic tumor cell viability with carbohydrate-based carbonic anhydrase IX and XII inhibitors. J Med Chem 2011; 54(19): 6905-18.
[http://dx.doi.org/10.1021/jm200892s] [PMID: 21851094]

[106] Winum JY, Colinas PA, Supuran CT. Glycosidic carbonic anhydrase IX inhibitors: A sweet approach against cancer. Bioorg Med Chem 2013; 21(6): 1419-26.
[http://dx.doi.org/10.1016/j.bmc.2012.10.043] [PMID: 23199483]

[107] Stander BA, Joubert F, Tu C, Sippel KH, McKenna R, Joubert AM. *In vitro* evaluation of ESE-15-ol, an estradiol analogue with nanomolar antimitotic and carbonic anhydrase inhibitory activity. PLoS One 2012; 7(12): e52205.
[http://dx.doi.org/10.1371/journal.pone.0052205] [PMID: 23300615]

[108] Lomelino CL, Supuran CT, McKenna R. Non-classical inhibition of carbonic anhydrase. Int J Med Mol Sci 2016; 17(7): 1150.
[http://dx.doi.org/10.3390/ijms17071150]

[109] Lomelino C, McKenna R. Carbonic anhydrase inhibitors: A review on the progress of patent literature (2011-2016). Expert Opin Ther Pat 2016; 26(8): 947-56.
[http://dx.doi.org/10.1080/13543776.2016.1203904] [PMID: 27387065]

[110] Oosterwijk E, Ruiter DJ, Hoedemaeker PJ, *et al.* Monoclonal antibody G 250 recognizes a determinant present in renal-cell carcinoma and absent from normal kidney. Int J Cancer 1986; 38(4): 489-94.
[http://dx.doi.org/10.1002/ijc.2910380406] [PMID: 2428759]

[111] Pryma DA, O'Donoghue JA, Humm JL, *et al.* Correlation of *in vivo* and *in vitro* measures of carbonic anhydrase IX antigen expression in renal masses using antibody 124I-cG250. J Nucl Med 2011; 52(4): 535-40.
[http://dx.doi.org/10.2967/jnumed.110.083295] [PMID: 21421715]

[112] Ahlskog JK, Schliemann C, Mårlind J, *et al.* Human monoclonal antibodies targeting carbonic anhydrase IX for the molecular imaging of hypoxic regions in solid tumours. Br J Cancer 2009; 101(4): 645-57.
[http://dx.doi.org/10.1038/sj.bjc.6605200] [PMID: 19623173]

[113] Gondi G, Mysliwietz J, Hulikova A, *et al.* Antitumor efficacy of a monoclonal antibody that inhibits the activity of cancer-associated carbonic anhydrase XII. Cancer Res 2013; 73(21): 6494-503.
[http://dx.doi.org/10.1158/0008-5472.CAN-13-1110] [PMID: 24030978]

[114] Krall N, Pretto F, Neri D. A bivalent small molecule-drug conjugate directed against carbonic anhydrase IX can elicit complete tumour regression in mice. Chem Sci (Camb) 2014; 5(9): 3640-4.
[http://dx.doi.org/10.1039/C4SC00685B]

[115] Muselaers CH, Boers-Sonderen MJ, van Oostenbrugge TJ, *et al.* Phase 2 study of lutetium 177-labeled anti-carbonic anhydrase IX monoclonal antibody girentuximab in patients with advanced renal cell carcinoma. Eur Urol 2016; 69(5): 767-70.

[http://dx.doi.org/10.1016/j.eururo.2015.11.033] [PMID: 26706103]

[116] Stillebroer AB, Boerman OC, Desar IM, *et al.* Phase 1 radioimmunotherapy study with lutetium 177-labeled anti-carbonic anhydrase IX monoclonal antibody girentuximab in patients with advanced renal cell carcinoma. Eur Urol 2013; 64(3): 478-85.
[http://dx.doi.org/10.1016/j.eururo.2012.08.024] [PMID: 22980441]

[117] Ahlskog JK, Schliemann C, Mårlind J, *et al.* Human monoclonal antibodies targeting carbonic anhydrase IX for the molecular imaging of hypoxic regions in solid tumours. Br J Cancer 2009; 101(4): 645-57.
[http://dx.doi.org/10.1038/sj.bjc.6605200] [PMID: 19623173]

[118] Murri-Plesko MT, Hulikova A, Oosterwijk E, *et al.* Antibody inhibiting enzymatic activity of tumour-associated carbonic anhydrase isoform IX. Eur J Pharmacol 2011; 657(1-3): 173-83.
[http://dx.doi.org/10.1016/j.ejphar.2011.01.063] [PMID: 21315712]

[119] Dekaminaviciute D, Kairys V, Zilnyte M, *et al.* Monoclonal antibodies raised against 167-180 aa sequence of human carbonic anhydrase XII inhibit its enzymatic activity. J Enzyme Inhib Med Chem 2014; 29(6): 804-10.
[http://dx.doi.org/10.3109/14756366.2013.856424] [PMID: 24400872]

[120] Dekaminaviciute D, Lasickiene R, Parkkila S, *et al.* Development and characterization of new monoclonal antibodies against human recombinant CA XII. Biomed Res Int 2014; 2014: 309307.
[http://dx.doi.org/10.1155/2014/309307]

[121] Lamers CH, Sleijfer S, van Steenbergen S, *et al.* Treatment of metastatic renal cell carcinoma with CAIX CAR-engineered T cells: Clinical evaluation and management of on-target toxicity. Mol Ther 2013; 21(4): 904-12.
[http://dx.doi.org/10.1038/mt.2013.17] [PMID: 23423337]

[122] Banerjee D, Slack F. Control of developmental timing by small temporal RNAs: A paradigm for RNA-mediated regulation of gene expression. BioEssays 2002; 24(2): 119-29.
[http://dx.doi.org/10.1002/bies.10046] [PMID: 11835276]

[123] Tiram G, Scomparin A, Ofek P, Satchi-Fainaro R. Interfering cancer with polymeric siRNA nanomedicines. J Biomed Nanotechnol 2014; 10(1): 50-66.
[http://dx.doi.org/10.1166/jbn.2014.1715] [PMID: 24724498]

[124] Ameres SL, Zamore PD. Diversifying microRNA sequence and function. Nat Rev Mol Cell Biol 2013; 14(8): 475-88.
[http://dx.doi.org/10.1038/nrm3611] [PMID: 23800994]

[125] Sakurai Y, Hatakeyama H, Sato Y, Hyodo M, Akita H, Harashima H. Gene silencing via RNAi and siRNA quantification in tumor tissue using MEND, a liposomal siRNA delivery system. Mol Ther 2013; 21(6): 1195-203.
[http://dx.doi.org/10.1038/mt.2013.57] [PMID: 23568259]

[126] Lock FE, McDonald PC, Lou Y, *et al.* Targeting carbonic anhydrase IX depletes breast cancer stem cells within the hypoxic niche. Oncogene 2013; 32(44): 5210-9.
[http://dx.doi.org/10.1038/onc.2012.550] [PMID: 23208505]

[127] Radvak P, Repic M, Svastova E, *et al.* Suppression of carbonic anhydrase IX leads to aberrant focal

adhesion and decreased invasion of tumor cells. Oncol Rep 2013; 29(3): 1147-53.
[PMID: 23291973]

[128] Yu SJ, Yoon JH, Lee JH, *et al.* Inhibition of hypoxia-inducible carbonic anhydrase-IX enhances hexokinase II inhibitor-induced hepatocellular carcinoma cell apoptosis. Acta Pharmacol Sin 2011; 32(7): 912-20.
[http://dx.doi.org/10.1038/aps.2011.24] [PMID: 21666701]

[129] Bryna J, Cigler P, Gruner B, *et al.* Carbonic anhydrase inhibitors and method of their production. World Patent WO2013060307, 2013.

[130] Cianchi F, Vinci MC, Supuran CT, *et al.* Selective inhibition of carbonic anhydrase IX decreases cell proliferation and induces ceramide-mediated apoptosis in human cancer cells. J Pharmacol Exp Ther 2010; 334(3): 710-9.
[http://dx.doi.org/10.1124/jpet.110.167270] [PMID: 20519553]

[131] Lee CH, Jin GF, Kim HS, Nakamura H, Chung Y, Lee JD. Preparation of boronated heterocyclic compounds using intramolecular cyclization reaction. Bull Korean Chem Soc 2008; 29(2): 357-62.
[http://dx.doi.org/10.5012/bkcs.2008.29.2.357]

[132] Lee JD, Lee CH, Nakamura H, Ko JJ, Kang SO. A convenient synthesis of the novel carboranyl-substituted tetrahydroisoquinoline-s: Application to the biologically active agent for BNCT. Tetrahedron Lett 2002; 43(31): 5483-6.
[http://dx.doi.org/10.1016/S0040-4039(02)01034-1]

[133] Babich JW, Zimmerman C, Joyal J, *et al.* Metal complexes of poly(carboxyl)amine-containing ligands having an affinity for carbonic anhydrase IX. World Patent WO2013103813, 2013.

[134] Zimmerman C, Babich JW, Joyal JL, Lu G, Maresca KP, Barone C. Inhibitors of carbonic anhydrase IX. European patent EP2823826A3, 2015.

[135] Liu G, Dou S, He J, Vanderheyden JL, Rusckowski M, Hnatowich DJ. Preparation and properties of 99mTc$(CO)_3$+-labeled N,N-bis(2-pyridylmethyl)-4-aminobutyric acid. Bioconjug Chem 2004; 15(6): 1441-6.
[http://dx.doi.org/10.1021/bc049866a] [PMID: 15546213]

[136] Dubois L, Peeters SG, van Kuijk SJ, *et al.* Targeting carbonic anhydrase IX by nitroimidazole based sulfamides enhances the therapeutic effect of tumor irradiation: A new concept of dual targeting drugs. Radiother Oncol 2013; 108(3): 523-8.
[http://dx.doi.org/10.1016/j.radonc.2013.06.018] [PMID: 23849171]

[137] Hay M, Wang J, Pruijn FB, Bonnet M, Hicks K. Nitroimidazole compounds and their use in cancer therapy. World Patent WO2014030142, 2014.

[138] Doyen J, Parks SK, Marcié S, Pouysségur J, Chiche J. Knock-down of hypoxia-induced carbonic anhydrases IX and XII radiosensitizes tumor cells by increasing intracellular acidosis. Front Oncol 2012; 2: 199.
[PMID: 23316475]

[139] Dubois LJ, Niemans R, van Kuijk SJ, *et al.* New ways to image and target tumour hypoxia and its molecular responses. Radiother Oncol 2015; 116(3): 352-7.
[http://dx.doi.org/10.1016/j.radonc.2015.08.022] [PMID: 26324018]

[140] Rami M, Dubois L, Parvathaneni NK, *et al.* Hypoxia-targeting carbonic anhydrase IX inhibitors by a new series of nitroimidazole-sulfonamides/sulfamides/sulfamates. J Med Chem 2013; 56(21): 8512-20.
[http://dx.doi.org/10.1021/jm4009532] [PMID: 24128000]

[141] Supuran C, Dedhar S, McDonald PC, Carta F. Novel sulfonamide compounds for inhibition of metastatic tumor growth. World Patent WO2012021963, 2012.

[142] Pastorekova S, Vullo D, Casini A, *et al.* Carbonic anhydrase inhibitors: Inhibition of the tumor-associated isozymes IX and XII with polyfluorinated aromatic/heterocyclic sulfonamides. J Enzyme Inhib Med Chem 2005; 20(3): 211-7.
[http://dx.doi.org/10.1080/14756360400028101] [PMID: 16119190]

[143] Gieling RG, Babur M, Mamnani L, *et al.* Antimetastatic effect of sulfamate carbonic anhydrase IX inhibitors in breast carcinoma xenografts. J Med Chem 2012; 55(11): 5591-600.
[http://dx.doi.org/10.1021/jm300529u] [PMID: 22621623]

[144] Supuran C, Dedhar S, Carta F, Winum JY, McDonald PC. Carbonic anhydrase inhibitors with antimetastatic activity. World Patent WO2012070024, 2012.

[145] Carradori S. Selective carbonic anhydrase IX inhibitors based on coumarin scaffold as promising antimetastatic agents: WO2012070024. Expert Opin Ther Pat 2013; 23(6): 751-6.
[http://dx.doi.org/10.1517/13543776.2013.769523] [PMID: 23387899]

[146] Sippel KH, Stander A, Tu C, Venkatakrishnan B, Robbins AH, Agbandje-McKenna M, *et al.* Characterization of carbonic anhydrase isozyme specific inhibition by sulfamated 2-ethylestra compounds. Lett Drug Des Discov 2011; 8(8): 678-84.
[http://dx.doi.org/10.2174/157018011796576105]

[147] Touisni N, Maresca A, McDonald PC, *et al.* Glycosyl coumarin carbonic anhydrase IX and XII inhibitors strongly attenuate the growth of primary breast tumors. J Med Chem 2011; 54(24): 8271-7.
[http://dx.doi.org/10.1021/jm200983e] [PMID: 22077347]

[148] Marasco WA, Lo A, Xu C. Carbonic anhydrase IX (G250) antibodies and methods of use thereof. World Patent WO2012070024, 2007.

[149] Davis ID, Wiseman GA, Lee FT, *et al.* A phase I multiple dose, dose escalation study of cG250 monoclonal antibody in patients with advanced renal cell carcinoma. Cancer Immun 2007; 7: 13-20.
[PMID: 17705349]

[150] Mulders P, Bleumer I, Debruyne F, Oosterwijk E. Specific monoclonal antibody-based immunotherapy by targeting the RCC-associated antigen carbonic anhydrase-IX(G250/MN). Urologe A 2004; 43(3) (Suppl. 3): S146-7.
[http://dx.doi.org/10.1007/s00120-004-0609-3] [PMID: 15164181]

[151] Bleumer I, Oosterwijk E, Oosterwijk-Wakka JC, *et al.* A clinical trial with chimeric monoclonal antibody WX-G250 and low dose interleukin-2 pulsing scheme for advanced renal cell carcinoma. J Urol 2006; 175(1): 57-62.
[http://dx.doi.org/10.1016/S0022-5347(05)00040-6] [PMID: 16406869]

[152] Siebels M, Rohrmann K, Oberneder R, *et al.* A clinical Phase I/II trial with the monoclonal antibody cG250 (RENCAREX®) and interferon-alpha-2a in metastatic renal cell carcinoma patients. World J

Urol 2011; 29(1): 121-6.
[http://dx.doi.org/10.1007/s00345-010-0570-2] [PMID: 20512580]

[153] Li Z, Belldegrun A. Fusion molecule based on novel taa variant. US Patent US20130230483, 2013.

[154] Kim BR, Yang EK, Kim DY, *et al.* Generation of anti-tumour immune response using dendritic cells pulsed with carbonic anhydrase IX-*Acinetobacter baumannii* outer membrane protein A fusion proteins against renal cell carcinoma. Clin Exp Immunol 2012; 167(1): 73-83.
[http://dx.doi.org/10.1111/j.1365-2249.2011.04489.x] [PMID: 22132887]

[155] Hernández JM, Bui MH, Han KR, *et al.* Novel kidney cancer immunotherapy based on the granulocyte-macrophage colony-stimulating factor and carbonic anhydrase IX fusion gene. Clin Cancer Res 2003; 9(5): 1906-16.
[PMID: 12738749]

[156] Zeidler R, Battke C, Kremmer E, Flatley A, Supuran C. Novel antibody to a carbonic anhydrase. World Patent WO2011138279, 2011.

[157] Battke C, Kremmer E, Mysliwietz J, *et al.* Generation and characterization of the first inhibitory antibody targeting tumour-associated carbonic anhydrase XII. Cancer Immunol Immunother 2011; 60(5): 649-58.
[http://dx.doi.org/10.1007/s00262-011-0980-z] [PMID: 21298264]

Topics in Anti-Cancer Research, 2015, *Vol. 5*, 43-86

CHAPTER 2

Tumor Homing Peptides: Promising Futuristic Hope for Cancer Therapy

Rekha Khandia[1], Swati Sachan[2], Ashok K. Munjal[1], Ruchi Tiwari[3] and Kuldeep Dhama[4,*]

[1] Department of Biochemistry & Genetics, Barkatullah University, Bhopal-462 026, Madhya Pradesh, India

[2] Immunology Section, ICAR-Indian Veterinary Research Institute, Izatnagar, Bareilly- 243 122, Uttar Pradesh, India

[3] Department of Veterinary Microbiology and Immunology, College of Veterinary Sciences, UP Pandit Deen Dayal Upadhayay Pashu Chikitsa Vigyan Vishwavidyalay Evum Go-Anusandhan Sansthan (DUVASU), Mathura-281001, Uttar Pradesh, India

[4] Division of Pathology, ICAR-Indian Veterinary Research Institute, Izatnagar, Bareilly- 243 122, Uttar Pradesh, India

Abstract: Tumor homing peptides (THPs) are cyclic or linear peptides of few amino acids having inherent property to recognize the tumor cells, which specifically bind to the receptors present on the tumor cells, tumor blood vessels or tumor lymphatic vessels. These can be utilized as major tool for targeted drug delivery particularly to cancerous cells, hence these are important for efficient cancer treatment. The present chapter summarizes the recent progression in the researches, databases and patents available in the field of cancer therapies utilizing THPs. It elucidates details about THPs; their modes of functioning, the molecules these may translocate; different methods of entry into the cells as well as diverse uses like gene correction and targeting of various tissues. Screening of THPs from phage library, natural occurrence of THPs in bacteria like *Salmonella*, *Pseudomonas* and engineered baculovirus have also been explicated. The specificity of THPs can be further enhanced by blending these with amphipathic conjugates, whereas the penetrability may be improved by adding cysteine or maleimidohexanoic acid to their N-terminal. Their half-life can also be increased by

* **Corresponding author Kuldeep Dhama**: Division of Pathology, ICAR-Indian Veterinary Research Institute (IVRI), Izatnagar, Bareilly-243 122, Uttar Pradesh, India; Tel. +91 9837654996; E-mail: kdhama@rediffmail.com

Atta-ur-Rahman and Khurshid Zaman (Eds.)

adding unnatural amino acids and modifying backbone or cyclization of THPs. For diagnostic and therapeutic purposes, several THPs have already been entered in different stages of clinical trials. THPs could serve as an ideal futuristic approach for targeting tumors based on their higher specificity, improved penetrability and half-life, acting as efficient delivery cargos for anticancer drugs and large therapeutic molecules.

Keywords: Angiogenesis, anticancer therapy, barrel stave pore, cancer therapies, CendR pathway, cell-penetrating peptides, clinical trials, inverted micelle, nanoparticles, phage display, RGD domain, toroidal pore, THP receptors, tumors, tumor homing peptides, vascular supply.

INTRODUCTION

'Cancer' is amongst the frightening diseases which is inexorably seeking attention for the search of its cure, as its occurrence is dynamically increasing in living beings. This disease has become a challenge to both developed and developing countries of the world. It is no more amongst the rare diseases now, since it has got a greater frequent incidence rate among the masses. One of the challenges in designing drugs for treating cancer is the necessity of focused medication towards cancerous cells pardoning normal body cells from its lethal effects. Many treatment options such as radiation therapy, chemotherapy, surgery, photodynamic therapy etc. have been explored for this deadly disease but none has been effective to provide absolute cure without ill effects [1, 2]. Drugs often have issues like non-specificity, residual toxicity and poor efficacy within the *in vivo* system [3]. Designing cancer therapeutics in such a way that they can smartly differentiate between normal and altered cells will definitely reduce the systemic toxicity of present anti-tumor agents. Tumor cells and tumor vasculature have shown to express significantly different molecules on their surface than the normal ones. Drug resistance is also one of the bottlenecks of cancer treatment that usually arises due to many drug and host related factors. Monoclonal antibodies are one of the options available in case of targeted therapeutics but they suffer from many shortcomings such as low tissue penetration owing to their large size and toxicity due to non-specific trapping in the liver/reticuloendothelial system (RES).

In this direction, one amongst the pioneering innovative initiatives is the identification of certain peptides termed as "tumor homing peptides", which are specific to certain receptors on cancerous cells or cancer vasculature [4, 5]. It has increased the efficacy of targeted delivery since these functioning in conjunction with therapeutic molecules/ drugs are able to minimize the side effects of the drugs. Tumors have low blood vessel perfusion and high interstitial pressure due to dysfunctional lymph vessels that result in low drug absorption [6]. This problem of low absorption of anti-cancerous agents can be overcome by employing such delivery agents that are smaller in size with no binding to RES and it can further reduce the cost of cancer treatment as well [7].

Cancer is just one dimension, where these peptides find useful applications, but their use is not limited up to here. Even, these can be used to design placenta based therapeutics to treat any condition in foetus [8]. Certainly, these are one amongst the most wonderful findings in the field of medical science for the benefit of the mankind and animal kingdom and definitely in providing the relief from many deadly conditions. These can be used in different ways to treat cancer such as they themselves acting as drugs or carriers of the drug, hormone etc. at the site of action. Seeing the potential of these tumor targeting peptides, it is required to increase the pace of their identification using computer aided approach so that we get a collection of these in our hands readily available for present and futuristic therapeutics.

TUMOR HOMING PEPTIDES (THPS)

Tumor homing peptides (THPs) are short peptide sequences, generally having 3 to 15 amino acids; however Porkka *et al.* derived a 31-aa synthetic peptide [9], and possessing certain common motifs in them can target specific tumor [10 - 12] on its surface or tumor vasculature after their delivery. Homing peptides can be grouped into three classes (i) peptides that home to specific target site recognizing cell surface molecules without internalization, (ii) peptides that recognize the cell surface molecules and are internalized; and (iii) peptides capable of targeting, internalization and destruction [13, 14].

Tumor-specific internalizing peptides' (TSIPs) are capable of translocating on the plasma membrane of the cell. TSIPs have target specificity as well as penetration properties. However, several THPs show reduced applicability due to their limited cell penetrating properties [15] and these are unable to carry drug molecules with them. Contrarily, cell-penetrating peptides (CPPs) have ability to penetrate the cells [16], but lack specificity, hence chimeric peptides of CPP and THP may be created with improved penetration and specificity (Table **1**) [17 - 52]. In fact, linear breast tumor homing peptide CREKA (Table **2**) [53 - 77], which recognizes clotted plasma proteins and specifically homes to blood vessels of tumor but fails to traffic inside the tumor cell [53] has been fused with CPP pVEC [54]. Shadidi and Sioud revealed that LTVSPWY peptide, linked with antisense phosphorothioate oligonucleotide, exhibited specific delivery to the breast caricinoma through ErbB2 receptors [55]. Cell penetrating capacity can be further increased by addition of fatty acids [56]. CPP can be made specific by attaching or conjugating it with homing peptides. CPP like TAT peptide has been successfully implicated for delivering the diverse nanopharmaceutical cargos including liposomes, micelles, nanoparticles and DNA molecules [57].

Table 1. Patents involving development of tumor homing peptides.

S. No.	Patent's Title	Patent Number	Inventor(s)	Year	Reference
1.	Cell-killing peptide	WO2006001582	Kim, T.H.	2006	[6]
2.	Targeting peptides	WO2001057069	Schugart, K., Rassmussen, U., Schreiber, V.	2001	[10]
3.	Tumor targeting peptides, therapeutic and diagnostic compositions comprising the peptides	WO2010114539	Wolf, I.S., Messmer, D.	2010	[11]
4.	Cancer targeting peptides for enhancing anti-cancer drug delivery and therapeutic efficiencies	EP2896403	Wu, H.-C., Wu, C.-H.	2015	[12]
5.	Tumor cell-killing peptides	US8877889	Kim, T.-H.	2014	[14]
6.	Cell penetrating peptides	WO2003106491	Hällbrink, M., Pooga, M., Metsis, M., *et al.*	2003	[16]
7.	Chimeric constructs between cancer-homing peptides and cell-penetrating peptides coupled to anticancer drugs and/or diagnostic agent/agents	EP1991586	Langel, U., Maarja, M.Ä.E., Myrberg, H., Ruoslahti, E., Zhang, L.	2011	[17]

(Table 1) contd.....

S. No.	Patent's Title	Patent Number	Inventor(s)	Year	Reference
8.	Chimeric constructs between glioma-homing peptide and cell-penetrating peptides, gHoPe2	EP2671597	Kurrikoff, K., Eriste, E., Oskolkov, N., *et al.*	2013	[18]
9.	Peptide-conjugates that bind to VEGF-stimulated or tumor vasculature and methods of treatment	US8088887	Wu, H.C., Lin, C.T., Lee, T.Y., Kuo, S.	2012	[19]
10.	Continuous administration of cilengitide in cancer treatments	WO2010136168	Picard, M.A., Bethe, U., Dotzaeur, M., Moyal, E.C.J.	2010	[20]
11.	Peptides that home to tumor lymphatic vasculature and methods of using same	US7671021	Laakkonen, P., Porkka, K., Hoffman, J.A., Ruoslahti, E.	2010	[21]
12.	Peptide homing to brain tumors	US8188221	Laakkonen, P., Ruoslahti, E., Bergers, G.	2012	[22]
13.	Methods and compositions for enhanced delivery of compounds	EP2555802	Ruoslahti, E., Agemy, L., Friedmann-Morvinski, D., Kotamraju, V.R., Sugahara, K., Verma, I.	2013	[23]
14.	Methods for targeting and killing glioma cells	US7642063	Samoylova, T.I., Baker, H.J., Cox, N.R., Globa, L.P., Morrison, N.E.	2010	[24]
15.	Nanoparticular tumor targeting and therapy	US20050008572	Prokop, A., Davidson, J., Carlesso, G., Roberts, D.	2005	[25]
16.	Nanoworms for *in vivo* tumor targeting	US20100254914	Park, J.-H., Zhang, L., Derfus, A.M., Sailor, M.J., *et al.*	2010	[26]
17.	Peptide-bound gold metal nano-clusters as cancer cell killing agents	US9090660	Gao, X.	2015	[27]
18.	Treatment of tumors using conjugates	WO2016041014	Ganss, R., Anna Johansson, A.	2016	[28]
19.	Therapeutic and diagnostic targeting of cancers cells with tumor homing peptides	US20030232013	Sieckman, G., Volkert, W., Forte, L., Hoffman, T., Gali, H.	2003	[29]
20.	Human and mouse targeting peptides identified by phage display	WO2002020769	Arap, W., Pasqualini, R.	2002	[30]
21.	Truncated LyP-1 peptide and methods and compositions using truncated lyp-1 peptides	US20150259380	Ruoslahti, E., Teesalu, T., Sugahara, K., Roth, L.	2015	[31]

(Table 1) contd.....

S. No.	Patent's Title	Patent Number	Inventor(s)	Year	Reference
22.	Molecules for targeting compounds to various selected organs, tissues or tumor cells	US8609065	Van Kuik-Romeijn, P., Platenburg, G.J.	2013	[32]
23.	Serum albumin binding peptides for tumor targeting	US20050287153	Dennis, M.	2005	[33]
24.	Lung cancer targeted peptides and applications thereof	US20080193375	Wu, H.C., Lin, C.T., Lee, T.Y., Kuo, S.	2008	[34]
25.	Carcinoma Homing Peptide (CHP), its analogs, and methods of using	US20120208770	Li, S., Cutrera, J., Xia, X.	2012	[35]
26.	Homing peptide for tumor vasculature	US8247378	Cho, C.H., Li, Z.J	2012	[36]
27.	Brain tumor targeting peptides and methods	US8530429	Robbins, S.M., Rahn, J., Senger, D.L.	2013	[37]
28.	Compositions and methods of use of targeting peptides for diagnosis and therapy of human cancer	US8507445	Arap, W., Kolonin, M.G., Mintz, P.J., Pasqualini, R., Zurita, A.J.	2013	[38]
29.	LY75 as cancer therapeutic and diagnostic target	WO2014072700	Ackroyd, J.E.	2014	[39]
30.	Target peptides for colorectal cancer therapy and diagnostics	US20150328297	Hunt, D.F., Shabanowitz, J., Abelin, J.G., Cobbold, M., Penny, S.A.	2014	[40]
31.	Target peptides for ovarian cancer therapy and diagnostics	EP2931312	Hunt, D.F., Shabanowitz, J., Malaker, S.A., *et al.*	2015	[41]
32.	Target peptides for immunotherapy and diagnostics	WO2014036562	Hunt, D.F., Shabanowitz, J., Abelin, J.G., Hildebrand, W.H.	2014	[42]
33.	Cancer targeting peptides for enhancing anti-cancer drug delivery and therapeutic efficiencies	EP2896403	Wu, H.-C., Wu, C.-H.	2015	[43]
34.	Peptide antiestrogen compositions and methods for treating breast cancer	US6306832	Pietras, R.J.	2001	[44]
35.	Hunter killer peptides and methods of use	WO2005094383	Bredesen, D.E., Ellerby, M., Ellerby, L.	2005	[45]
36.	Peptides and methods for inducing cell death	US8492333	Yeaman, M.R., Yount, N.Y., Brass, E.P.	2013	[46]
37.	Multilevel specific targeting of cancer cells with IL13	US8362207	Debinski, W., Pandya, H., Gibo, D.	2013	[47]

(Table 1) contd.....

S. No.	Patent's Title	Patent Number	Inventor(s)	Year	Reference
38.	HMGN2 peptides and related molecules that selectively home to tumor blood vessels and tumor cells	US8598112	Ruoslahti, E., Porkka, K., Christian, S.	2013	[48]
39.	HYD1 peptides for relapsed cancer	US20140080762	Hazlehurst, L.A., Dalton, W.S., Emmons, M., Gebhard, A.W.	2014	[49]
40.	Interleukin -13 receptor alpha2 peptide brain cancer vaccine	JP2013536240	Okada, H.	2014	[50]
41.	Membrane resident peptide in anti-cancer peptides causes tumor cell necrosis rather than apoptosis of cancer cells	US8822419	Pincus, M.R., Michl, J., Yazdi, E.S.	2014	[51]
42.	Bladder cancer specific ligand peptides	US8946379	Pan, C.-X., Zhang, H., Lam, K.S., Aina, O.H.	2015	[52]

Receptors for THPs are very precisely present on different tissues. These particular receptors may be those expressed by metastatic tumors which assist their migration to various body organs or those present on blood and lymph vessels for trafficking of various migrating cells like lymphoid cells [58]. Aminopeptidase N (APN or CD13) is over-expressed by many cancer cells and imparts role in motility and metastasis of tumor cell. Also, it serves the role of a receptor for many THPs, and can be targeted by cyclic peptides like CNGRC [59]. APN binds NGR motifs but does not degrade them due to the distorted scissile peptide bond [60]. On binding to the specific receptors, THPs undergo receptor mediated endocytosis, which is dissimilar to macropinocytosis and can act as drug delivery cargos [61, 62]. This process is quite complex involving many steps: first binding to receptor on tumor through tumor homing motif present on THPs, then undergoing proteolytic cleavage, followed by binding with secondary receptor that activates the transport pathway [62]. The prototype peptide of this class is iRGD which contains the RGD motif, specifically bound to αv integrin receptors, and is over-expressed on various tumors including tumor vasculature. These contain three independent modules; a homing domain, a protease recognition site, and an R/KXXR/K penetration motif. R/KXXR/K motif is also called C-end motif or C-end Rule (CendR) as the C terminal exposure of peptide is essential for the activity [62]. Through the homing RGD motif, the THPs bind to the integrin receptors, which are the primary receptors. Followed by binding, the protease recognition site is identified by protease and cleaved to expose the R/KXXR/K or CendR motif. This exposed CendR motif interacts with secondary receptor neuropilin-1 (NRP-1) and initiates CendR pathway through receptor mediated endocytosis [15]. To THPs, drug molecules may be conjugated to deliver them inside the cytosol. During the CendR pathway, other co-administered macromolecules may also be co-translocated inside the cell though energy incurring but receptor independent mechanism [13]. The detailed mechanism of CendR pathway is given in Fig. (**1**).

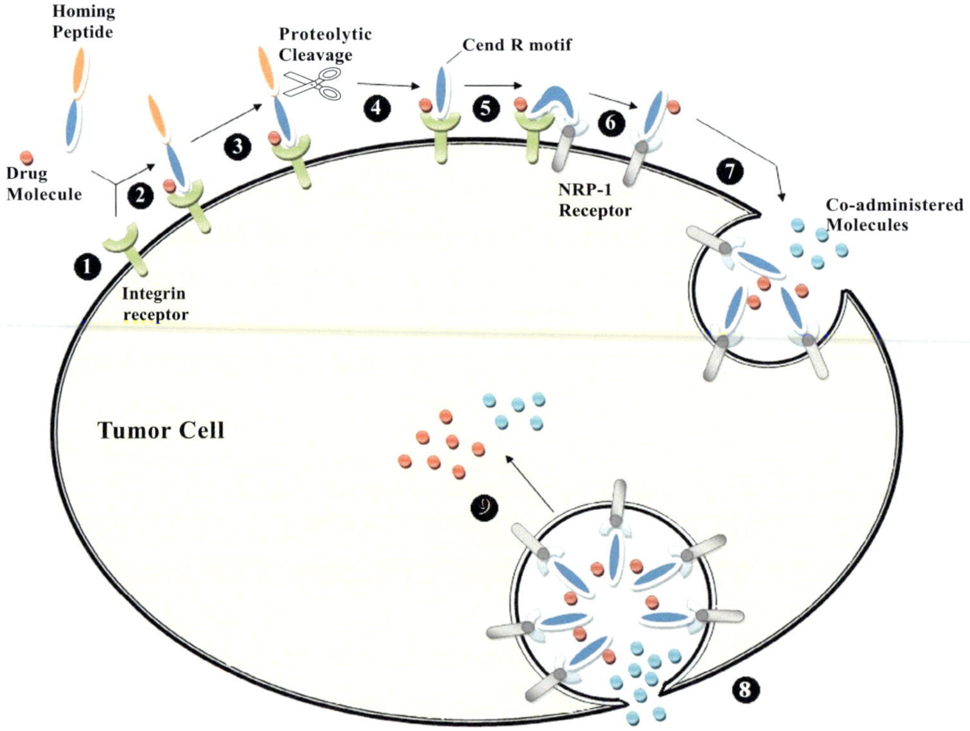

Fig. (1). Drug delivery to cancerous cell through homing peptide (1) Integrin receptors over expressed on tumor cells (2) Tumor homing peptides encompassing RGD domain along with tumor targeting drug specifically binds to integrin receptors (3 and 4) Upon binding, proteolytic cleavage of tumor homing peptides occurs exposing RXXR/Cend R motif (5 and 6) Exposed Cend R motif interact with secondary receptor NRP-1 (7) Cend R pathway is activated and initiate energy incurring bulk transport of (8) Along with homing peptide, drug and co-administered molecules are trafficked (9) Drug and co-administered molecules are released inside the tumor cell cytosol.

This is an active process involving expenditure of energy and is not based on diffusion simply. Since it is an active process, it activates bulk transport pathway so that the agents administered along with it can be helped in entering the activated target tumor tissue [63]. NRP-1 is a vascular endothelial growth factor co-expressed on vascular and tumor cells [64]. Therefore, these can be used as targeted delivery agents or vehicles for anti-cancerous agents in the form of payload sometimes even not attached with the peptide such as Paclitaxel, anti-cancerous bacteria etc. [63, 65, 66].

Studies carried out on protypic CendR peptide, RPARPAR, indicated that binding takes place in presence of L-amino acids only. NRP-1 has a major role in cell migration and endothelial cell sprouting in blood vessels and is a co-receptor for VEGF, semaphorins and TGFβ, all known to contain C-terminal CendR motifs [67]. CendR motif is being used by several pathogens like Human T-lymphotropic virus-2, tick-born encephalitis virus, Crimean-Congo hemorrhagic fever virus and Ebola virus, and is also present in snakes and bee venoms and possibly contributes in toxin spread in the tissue [63]. THPs can be designed with more desirable features for killing cancer cells by using computational methods [68]. Administration of THP with anticancer agents such as doxorubicin increases their activity without further enhancing the toxicity to normal body cells [69].

Table 2. Tumor Homing Peptides with their Tumor Targets.

S. No.	Tumor Homing Peptide Name	Receptor(s)	Homing Peptide Target(s)	Reference(s)
1.	CREKA (Linear five amino acid long peptide)	Integrins	Breast tumors in MMTV-PyMT transgenic mice	Simberg *et al.*, 2007 [53]
2.	LTVXPWY	ErbB2 receptor	Breast cancer cells	Shadidi and Sioud, 2003 [55]
3.	CRGDKGPDC	Integrin and neurophilin-1 receptors	MDA-MB-435 cells	Teesalu *et al.*, 2013 [63]
4.	RGD (Displayed as looped region of *Salmonella* outer membrane protein)	αvβ3 and αvβ5 integrin	Human melanoma (MDA-MB-435)	Park *et al.*, 2016 [66]

(Table 2) contd.....

S. No.	Tumor Homing Peptide Name	Receptor(s)	Homing Peptide Target(s)	Reference(s)
5.	LyP-1 (CGNKRTRGC)	p32 (p32/gC1q-R/HABP1)	Tumor lymphatics, tumor cells.	Fogal *et al.*, 2008 [70]
6.	CRGRRST (RGR)	PDGFR-beta	Pericytes and endothelial cells	Joyce *et al.*, 2003 [71]
7.	Interleukin-13	Interleukin 13 receptor α 2 (IL-13Rα2)	GBM cells	Gao *et al.*, 2014 [20]
8.	CooP	MDGI, also known as the fatty-acid binding protein 3 (FABP3) receptor	HIFko, U87MG, and BT4C tumors	Hyvönen *et al.*, 2014 [72]
9.	CGKRK delivering iron oxide nanoworm and D(KLAKLAK)2	p32/gC1qR/HABP	U87 human GBM cells	Wang and Huang (2012) [73]; Agemy *et al.*, 2013 [24]
10.	TT1 peptide (CKRGARST)	p32/gC1qR/HABP	WT GBM and P13 gliomas	Säälik *et al.*, 2016 [74]
11.	F3 (CKDEPQRRSARLSAKPAPPKPEPKPKKAPAKK)	Nucleolin receptor	Glioma cell line 9L and the breast cancer cell line MCF-7	Porkka *et al.*, 2002 [9]; Qin *et al.*, 2014 [75]
12.	Chlorotoxin (CTX) [scorpion-derived peptide]	Small conductance epithelial chloride channels, αvβ3 integrin, MMP-2 and annexin-2	GBM cells	Fang *et al.*, 2015 [28]; Dardevet *et al.*, 2015 [29]
13.	YHWYGYTPQNVI (GE11)	Human EGF receptor (hEGFR)	Human hepatocarcinoma cell line SMMC-7721	Krumpe and Mori, 2007 [76]
14.	NGR	Aminopeptidase N (APN)	Angiogenic blood vessel of human breast cancer xenografts	Laakkonen and Vuorinen, 2010 [77]

DESIGNING OF HOMING PEPTIDE

Many THPs have been identified since the dawn of the concept of homing peptide. THPs have some very common motifs like RGD, NGR etc. These bind to the tumor cell surface expressed antigens and tumor vasculature and the results are so promising that few of them have been entered in clinical trial phase [78]. Computer aided designing and efficacy prediction may be useful in saving time as well as labor for searching new THPS. An attempt has been made for the making of a highly accurate support vector machine (SVM)-based model. Computational analysis of THPs revealed the dominance of certain residues like C, R, G, W, P, L and S in THPs with dominance of C, G, L, P at most of the positions. TumorHPD (http://crdd.osdd.net/raghava/tumorhpd/) is an *in silico* tool for predicting the THPs [79]. Wide variety of THPs are cyclic peptides with start and end residue as cysteine. The latter is unusually highly occupied in THPs, where it is rare in other natural peptides and proteins.

CELL PENETRATING PEPTIDES (CPPS)

The first cell-penetrating peptide was described by Derossi *et al.* [80]. All CPPs possess diverse characteristics excluding few common features like having net positive charge and ability to translocate molecules across the cell membrane [81]. The cellular internalization process of course depends on secondary structure acquired by these peptides typically after interacting with plasma membrane, whereas acquiring secondary structure is dependent on hydrogen bonds, non-ionic interactions and net charge. Interaction between the plasma membrane and CPPs, determines the uptake efficiency. The mechanism of cellular uptake of CPPs is dependent upon the cargo molecule attached with these. Exact mechanism of CPPs transport is still to be resolved [82, 83]. THPs can enter inside the cell through endocytosis or directly.

When CPPs are coupled with larger molecules like proteins, oligonucleotides, small interfering RNA (siRNA), microRNA (miRNA), plasmid DNA (pDNA) etc., the transportation is through endocytosis. The process of endocytosis starts with the coupling of CPPs with cargo molecule, through covalent or non-covalent interactions. Covalent conjugation is always via disulfide bond, amide bond, or specific linkers. Non-covalent conjugation involves positive charged CPPs and negatively charged nucleic acid molecules like pDNA, siRNA, miRNA etc. It is a highly regulated process, and occurs via clathrin mediated [84], caveolin mediated [85] or clathrin and caveolin independent pathways. Since CPPs are generally positively charged, these interact with negatively charged glycosaminoglycans (GAGs) [N-linked GAG-Sialic acid and O-linked GAG-Heparansulfate] and negatively charged lipids. Followed by binding, selective activation of the small GTPase occurs [86]. The second step involves process of endocytosis and release of cargo inside the cell. The possible proposed method of release of cargo is:

a. interaction between the trafficked nanomolecule (CPP-cargo) and membrane of endosome, causing disruption of endosome.
b. proton sponge theory into which the endosome bursts [87] due to osmotic shock.
c. fusion of endosome with lysosome [88].

Independent endocytosis i.e. direct entry of CPPs also occurs through several mechanisms. Positively charged CPPs cover extensively the lipid membrane. Electro-statistically, hydrophobic group of peptide faces the membrane [89] and after increasing local concentration of peptides, lipid packing of the membrane is disturbed and micelle formation takes place [90]. Often the bilayer is disturbed in a detergent like manner [91] and this process is called detergent-like mechanism [92, 93]. The inverted micelle model of internalization was projected on the basis of NMR studies by Alain Prochiantz's group [80], which is endocytosis and energy independent method of peptide penetration through lipid bilayer [94]; by forming an inverted micelle, a cavity occurs in between two cell membrane bilayers, where CPP is surrounded by hydrophilic environment. The most common way of CPP trafficking is through barrel stave mechanism by forming transmembrane pores of amphipathic α-helices. The formed pores are less than 10nm in size [92, 93]. Such pores are lined by peptide.

DESIGNER HOMING PEPTIDE FOR CENDR ACTIVATION

Two imperative motifs of any homing peptide determine the CendR activity. The first motif is required to bind to the receptors and is generally over-expressed on tumor cells; the second motif binds to NRP-1 and commence CendR pathway. Sometimes proteolytic cleavage of peptide, upon binding to the receptor, may expose the CendR motifs. Alberici *et al.* [95] in an attempt added one extra base to the NGR motif (RNGR) to make CendR motif and it was embedded in iRGD frame. The resultant iNGR revealed all the properties of iRGD; but it was recruited to tumor tissues via aminopeptidase N and not through integrins. More designer THPs may be synthesized by fusing CendR motif with a proteolytic cleavage site, cleavable through tumor associated proteases and a motif having tumor homing capability.

BACTERIAL HOMING PEPTIDES

Bacteria have been known for their advantages, apart from posing nuisance and harmful effects to humans and animals' health. One such implication is their use as an anticancer agent [96]. They can act as an important player in anticancer therapy as evident by poor response to therapeutic agents in the absence of gut commensal microbiota [97]. Attenuated strain of *Salmonella typhimurium* has been shown to possess cancer tissue tropism, owing to its RGD domain (ACDCRGDCFCG) in external loop of outer membrane protein A (OmpA). Such *Salmonella* strains bind with great affinity to tumor expressing integrins such as $\alpha v\beta 3$ and thus this bacterium can act against tumor cells employing elevating cytokine (TNFα and IL-1β) secretion and providing longer survival rate in mice models of human breast cancer and human melanoma [66] [Fig. (**2**)]. *Pseudomonas aeruginosa* is yet another bacterium with anticancer properties. *P. aeruginosa* is an opportunistic pathogen having PilY1, a type IV pilus (tfp)-associated protein. PilY1 protein is reported to contain RGD motif at residues 619-621, which bind to $\alpha V\beta 3$ integrin over-expressed on cancer cells [98]. This property may also be attributed to the bacteriocin such as azurin [99].

BACULOVIRAL HOMING PEPTIDES

Baculovirus, an insect pathogen, has been utilized as multifunctional, biotechnological tool with the potential for biomedical applications. It offers excellent molecular flexibility to not only accommodate foreign genes but also allows modifying its phenotype for target tissue specificity. Further, this is freed from innate immunity [100]. It is also considered safer due to having negligible pathogenecity in human. It can be grown up to very high titers, induces no cytotoxicity and is able to mediate stable or transient expression. The exact mechanism for entry of baculovirus in mammalian cell is not precisely known, but use of some ubiquitous molecules, heparansulphate proteoglycans or phospholipids, for binding to cells [101] and clathrin mediated endocytosis along with macropinocytosis [102] for its entry has been speculated.

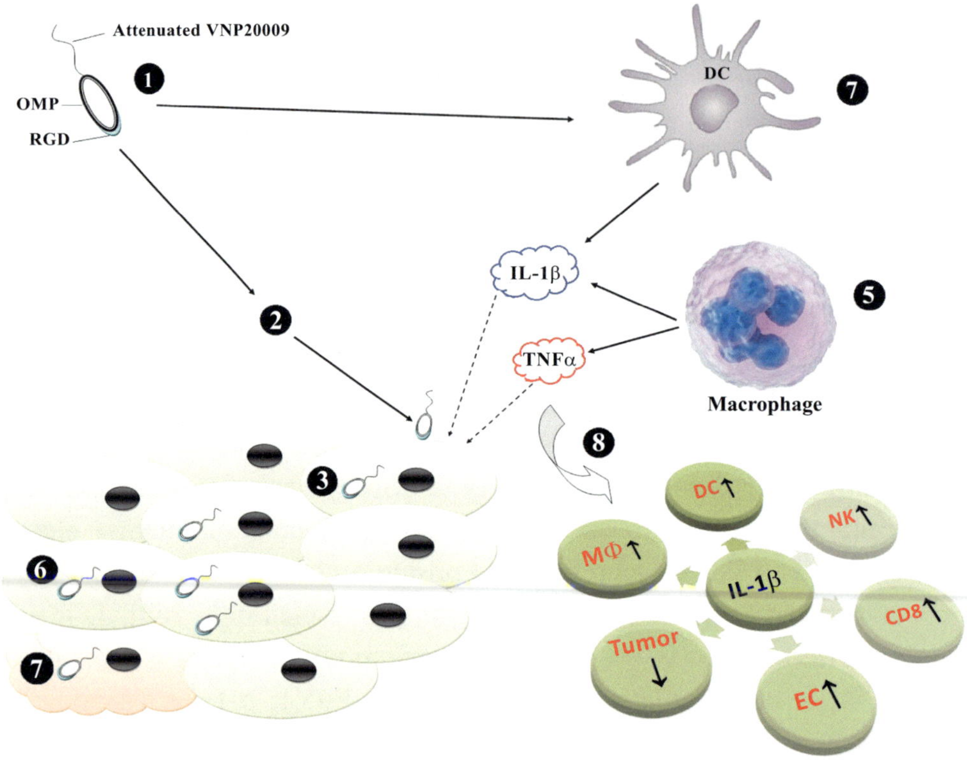

Fig. (2). *Salmonella* homing to cancer cells through inherent homing peptide RGD (1) On outer membrane protein (OMP) of attenuated *Salmonella* VNP20009 strain, RGD domain is present (2) Tumor cells over express αvβ3 integrins, through RGD domain *Salmonella* binds to integrin receptors; (3) LPS, lipoteichoic acid and flagillin of bacterium activates dendrite cell and macrophage cells (4) Infection cause dendritic cells to release IL-1β (5) Macrophages secrete IL-1β and TNFα (6) in infected cells Akt/mTOR/p70S6K is reduced leading to autophagy of infected cell (7) Caspase 3 mediated cell death of infected tumor cell (8) IL-1β secretion chemoattracts dendritic cells, macrophages, CD8 cells, NK cells etc. and reduce tumor mass.

THPS TARGETING TUMOR ANGIOGENESIS

Tumor growth is enhanced through the nutrients supplied by the blood vessels entering into them. It leaves no or very less nutrients for normal blood cells owing to their starvation and death. Tumor blood vessels are different from normal blood vessels in many aspects viz. being more tortuous, leaky and expressing unique receptors [103]. Thus, identification of specific and unique receptors on tumor blood vessels can also be utilized in cancer treatment [70]. These receptors on tumor blood vessels are advantageous to target than those on tumor cells themselves due to their genetic stability and penetrability to drugs [104]. Because of this, it is possible to avoid multi-drug resistance to chemotherapeutic agents by tumor cells by making drug available in a desirable quantity to act. These receptors can be identified by certain techniques such as cloning, *in vivo* biotinylation, screening based on phage displaying peptide libraries and antibodies [6]. Some of these receptors are either absent or expressed at a very low level on normal blood vessels but over-expressed on the tumor cells blood vessels for e.g. some integrins, certain growth factor receptors, matrix metalloproteinases, etc. [105]. These receptors are important for the growth and development of these vessels [106]. While others are adhesion receptors such as integrins which are important for entry of blood cells [71]. THPs targeting blood vessels [19] have entered the phase of clinical trial to treat various tumors, cardiovascular and neurological disease conditions. Vascular homing peptides have been identified by using *in vivo* phage display technique [71, 107]. Two of the most important first generation peptides that target the tumor vasculature are Arginine-glycin--aspartic acid (RGD) [108, 109] and asparagine-glycine-arginine (NGR) [110] whose receptors are significantly upregulated at the time of angiogenesis [111]. RGD is the first peptide discovered with internalization property. It has affinity towards integrins ($\alpha_v\beta_3$ and $\alpha_v\beta_5$), which are utilized by adenoviruses to enter the cell explaining the possible mechanism of internalization of RGD [112]. $\alpha_v\beta3$ and $\alpha_v\beta5$ receptors are also present on surface of tumor angiogeneic blood vessels. NGR is having affinity to aminopeptidase N, embracing the role in tumor angiogenesis [71]. One of the derivatives of RGD termed as Cilengitide (Merck) [20], has already entered in its Phase II of clinical trials [113]. Further, it has also been evaluated that on reversing the sequence of RGD, a retro-inverso peptide (dGR) created is equally potent to target any new blood vessel formation to tumor [114]. Micelles system consisting of paclitaxel as anti-tumor agent along with THP targeting angiogenic vessel can effectively reduce the tumor growth [115]. Coupling of THPs that home the neoangiogenic blood vessels with TNF-α was found to significantly limit the tumor metastasis [116]. Despite the therapeutic potential of THPs targeting tumor vessels, one needs to be careful in selecting the markers as angiogenesis is not a phenomenon unique to cancer progression. It also occurs in case of tissue regeneration or inflammation. Many of such conditions that require angiogenesis for repair such as myocardial infarction, stroke etc. are associated with cancers due to cancer emboli [117, 118]. Targeting them may not only hamper the repair, but also the effect can be reversed. Thus, this complicates the use of THPs targeting angiogenesis and raises the need to detect tumor specific angiogenesis markers in place of all common markers [6].

RLW (RLWMRWYSPRTRAYG) is among the cell penetrating peptides, which specifically targets non-small cell lung cancer A549 cells. RLW peptide, along with nanoparticles and docetaxel (a microtubule depolymerization inhibitor, commonly used for treating wide variety of cancers) offers an improved cell selectivity and cell penetrating capability [115].

THPS TARGETING LYMPHATIC VESSELS

Another vascular supply apart from blood vessels to the tumor mass is of lymphatic vessels. It is a network of vessels collecting interstitial fluid from tissue to blood vessels. It also helps in tumor metastasis and it has been found that while inhibiting lymph-angiogenesis, tumor metastasis can also be significantly reduced [119, 120]. Using *in vivo* phage display technology, lymphatic system targeting phages have been screened, which not only provide lymphatic system specificity but also enable differentiation between different stages of tumors [119, 121]. AGR are some of the peptides, which specifically home to lymphatic system [21], and few among these include LSD, LyP-1, LyP-2, REA etc. [122].

Several peptides such as LyP-1 (cyclic 9 amino acid peptide, CGNKRTRGC) are specific for lymphatic endothelial markers along with some tumor such as prostate cancer, breast cancer and can act on lymph vessels supplying tumor mass [119, 122]. LyP-1 is a cytolytic cell penetrating peptide (CPP); it is internalized after binding with its receptor and gets accumulated in the nucleus of the cell leading to apoptosis [123]. These lymph vessel specific peptides are specific only to certain tumor types and do not home to all the lymphatic vessels of the tumors [124]. Another THP showing affinity to lymphatic vessels and not to blood vessels is again a cyclic 9 amino acid peptide specific to C8161 melanoma lymphatics [111]. Conjugating lymph vessel specific THPs with apoptosis initiating peptides helps in significant reduction of the tumor mass [125]. When these peptides are conjugated with apoptosis-inducing peptide D(KLAKLAK)2, a significant reduction in tumor lymphatic vessels is observed, while the blood vessels remain unaffected.

THPS TARGETING EXTRACELLULAR MATRIX PROTEIN (ECM)

ECM holds an important place in tumor growth and dissemination opposed to the older concept of presenting them as a hurdle in the way of tumor [125 - 128]. Vitronectin is one of the ECM proteins that protect apoptosis of tumor cells thus permitting its uncontrolled growth [129]. As tumor development is assisted by stromal cells and tumor microenvironment, thus it can be thought of as an alternate target in tumor therapeutics. They could serve as potential target as they are more stable genetically than the tumor cells, which keep on undergoing mutation [130, 131]. Some of the ECM proteins are also expressed in large amount by solid tumors such as Tenacin-C that can be targeted by its specific peptides PL1-3 and can deliver anticancer agents to tumor stroma [132]. On being expressed on tumor cells, Tenacin-C assists in tumor metastasis [133].

THPS USED AS GENE CORRECTION AGENTS TO TREAT CANCER

Gene therapy aims at treating many conditions by opposing or replacing any defective gene in the body thus, acting at the root cause of the disease and completely eradicating it [134]. This technique is not new and has shown promising results in laboratories but has not been able to cure the patients suffering from deadly cancers. This certainly indicates that still more optimizations are needed to bring gene therapy into the real practice. One challenge could be targeted delivery of corrective gene to its appropriate place in the body of the sufferer. THPs can be used to carry DNA or RNA lipoplexes to the cancerous cells developed due to mutation or to treat any other genetic disorder [135]. In gene therapy, cDNA encoding fusion protein consisting of THP and TNF-α can be used for targeting tumor tissue with TNF-α, which can further cause destruction of cancer cells selectively [136]. RNA interference (RNAi) is also a novel technique, which provides cure from cancer by inhibiting oncogene of interest [137]. RNAi used to treat cancers suffering from limitations, such as lesser half-life of RNA and non-specific accumulation in the tissue after administration. To make them focused to the target sites, complexing them with THPs is also of great advantage so that these can specifically down-regulate the gene of interest only amongst the tumor cells [138]. Further, THPs also enhance the transduction potential of baculovirus mediated gene delivery to cancer mass as a corrective option for tumor cells [100]. Gene therapy for selective toxicity to tumor mass can be made more effective by forming nano-complexes consisting of THPs, modified silk polymer that interacts with plasmid DNA to yield stable complex for targeted delivery [139]. Other hurdles of gene silencing technique such as poor penetration in the cell, low stability, non-specific immune stimulation etc. can also be overcome by this targeted approach [140].

THPS TARGETING BRAIN TUMORS

Nervous system has selective entry of chemicals through its blood vessels. Therefore, it is quite difficult to eradicate any cancerous cells developed as in case of glioblastoma multiforme (GBM) by chemotherapy. GBM is the most aggressive brain tumor seen among adults and comprise 60-70% of all gliomas, and the survival rate of affected individual is less than 25% in case of reoccurrence. Due to infiltrative growth, gliomas are mostly malignant in nature. Only grade I tumors are benign which eventually can be surgically removed. A novel homing peptide, CooP(CGLSGLGVA), has been identified through phage display library [22], which interacts with mammary-derived growth inhibitor (MDGI), also known as fatty-acid binding protein 3 (FABP3) receptors. It is a receptor preferentially expressed only on human glioblastomas. This homing peptide has tremendous potential to be used as a therapeutic against brain tumors, since it accumulates in negligible quantities in liver, kidney, lung and normal brain [141]. To treat GBM, a tumor-homing peptide CGKRK is linked to iron oxide nano-worm (NW) [23] and a cytotoxic proapoptotic peptide, D(KLAKLAK)2 through 5K–polyethylene glycol linker [142]. After internalization, the peptide destabilizes mitochondrial membrane and induces mitochondria-dependent apoptosis leading to cell death [72, 143]. Some of the glioma specific peptides coupled to nanoparticles can be utilized for this purpose [73, 144] or for targeting drug on the basis of molecular profiles of individual tumors [24]. Conjugation of p16(INK4a) to GBM specific THP gives good result in tumor regression by inducing GBM specific apoptosis [64]. One such peptide is TT1 that has capability for targeting glioma. TT1 peptide (CKRGARST) linked with PEGylated with iron oxide nanoworms, using P32 receptor, a mitochondrial chaperone aberrantly expressed in activated malignant tumor cells, is capable of targeting GBM (Table **2**) [145].

THPS TARGETING NORMAL MESENCHYMAL CELLS

Certain THPs target mesenchymal cells, which infiltrate the cancerous growth and further support its progression. Such THPs are able to inhibit the tumors appreciated by such normal cells such as adipose stromal cells [146]. Targeting of tumor mass can be carried out by two ways; by targeted delivery of therapeutic agents to the tumor cells, and by further targeting mesenchymal cells that selectively migrate to the primary tumor cells as well as to the metastases [147]. Loading them with the drug can further increase the concentration of anti-cancer agent to the tumor site [74].

THPS CONJUGATED WITH NANOPARTICLES TO TARGET CANCER CELLS

Nanoparticles in cancer therapy hold an important place (Table **1**) [25 - 27] by acting as drug reservoirs, protectors of the drug from inactivation and enhancing anticancer activities of the drugs within them [148, 149]. Conjugating THPs with nanoparticles yield nanomaterial toxic to various cancerous cells and can treat many cancers such as breast cancer [150, 151]. While administering THP conjugated nanoparticles as therapeutics to cancer, proper care must be taken that these should be devoid of any free THP, since it competitively inhibits the activity of conjugated nanoparticle [152]. Though smaller in size, these are still larger than the molecules traversing through the cells via blood vessels. But this is not an issue with the blood vessels supplying to the tumor cells as these are more accessible being leaky. Still drug accumulation by way of nano-carriers can be further improved by targeting them to dual receptors such as integrins and nucleolins via THPs. This strategy to identify the receptors present both on tumor blood vessel and tumor cells can certainly solve the problem of lower drug adsorption at the target site [6]. Administration of anti-tumor agent such as TNF-α with gold nanoparticles increases their therapeutic efficacy than when used alone. Tagging such drug carriers with vascular receptor targeting THPs leads to improvisation in the anti-cancer response by enhancing drug penetration [153]. This can be due to the increased stability, decreased immunogenicity and ease of administration by THP tagging [75]. Temozolomide (TMZ) is a DNA-alkylating agent causing methylation of adenine and guanine residues of DNA, resulting in double stranded nicks and breaks in DNA, arrest of cell cycle and finally cell death. Though, TMZ indiscriminately causes nicks in DNA amongst all the cells; however hematopoietic stem cells are the severely affected ones. Under normal physiological conditions, it rapidly degrades which limits its utility. The TMZ is attached with biotin-functionalized chitosan nanopartcle core, further attached to tumor targeting peptide chlorotoxin (CTX; Table **2**) [154, 155], which recognizes and targets a variety of tumors having neuro-ectodermal origin, while sparing the normal cell [78, 156]. The said complex has capability to cross blood brain barrier and it can transport the TMZ into avascular region of brain too.

THPS ASSISTED RADIOTHERAPY

Radiotherapy is used to get rid of any kind of tumor mass developed in the body. Researchers have invented the uses of protein conjugated with THPs adjunct to immunotherapy, chemotherapy and radiotherapy [28] or coupled with radiolabel diagnostic agents; hence this can be used for therapeutic and diagnostic targeting of cancer cells [29]. Its efficiency can be increased by certain peptides such as wild type NBS1 inhibitory peptide by certain mechanism. Conjugating such inhibitory peptides with THP such as NGR improves their localization and internalization to tumor cells [157]. This is referred to as 'Peptide Receptor Radionuclide Therapy' (PRRT). Isotopes emitting α particle have immense potential to kill tumor cells by breaking double strand bond in DNA, but to execute this, it is essential that it must be delivered carefully to the altered cell that ultimately needs to be destroyed. For this coupling, such isotopes emitting α particle with THPs can provide a good solution [158]. Somatostatin receptor density is comparatively higher on tumor cells than the normal cells. Radiolabeled somatostatin analogs available in the market are Octreotide and NeoTect which can bind the cancer cells and kill them with radiations emitted by them [159].

HOMING PEPTIDE FOR PLACENTAL TARGETING

The villous placenta has some common physiological and biochemical characteristics with solid tumors; like ability to undergo rapid proliferation, production of variety of growth factors and cytokines, and ability to evade immune surveillance [160]. Also, a distinctive population of extravillous trophoblast (EVT) cell egress from placental villi, intrude into uterine wall and remodel the uterine spiral arteries [161]. Hence, it could be considered that placenta behaves like tumor, and therefore binding of THP on placental receptors can be speculated. In fact, calreticulin is highly expressed over the surface of spiral arteries of the mouse placenta and acts as a receptor for pentapeptide CGKRK [8]. Intravenously administered CGKRK or CRGDKGPDC (iRGD) into pregnant mice, accumulated in placental tissue and IGF-2 containing liposomes targeted with iRGD, improve placental weight and foetal weight distribution in mice model and do not show adverse effect on foetal or maternal health, if administered repeatedly [8].

POTENTIATING THE EFFECT OF DRUG THROUGH HOMING PEPTIDE

Mapsin is a serine protease non-inhibitor protein and its expression is reduced in case of numerous cancers including breast, prostate, gastric, and melanomas and its over-expression has been reported to reduce the growth and metastasis in breast tumors [162]. Exogenously administered mapsin or its fragments have moderate dose dependent tumor suppressor activity [163]. Mapsin conjugated with RGD and poly-histidine peptide as hinge, shows improved antitumor activity than mapsin alone [164]. CREKA tumor homing peptide conjugated PEG hydrogel has been found more effective in inducing doxorubicin mediated apoptosis of cancer cells, when compared with the conjugation involving laminin peptide IKVAV [75].

DATABASES PROVIDING INFORMATION ABOUT THPS

THPs specific for particular cancer can be traced from various databases available on the web, such as 'TumorHoPe: A database of tumor homing peptides', which contain information generated by identifying THPs targeting tumor and tumor environment, and all the information is derived from the published research work, databases or patents [165]. 'SATPdb', a database of therapeutic peptides, also possesses information about anticancer peptides apart from other peptides having other treatment potential [166]. Yet another comprehensive database for THPs is 'CPPsite' that provides information about cell penetrating peptides along with their ID, PubMed ID, peptide name, sequence, origin etc. [107].

PHAGE DISPLAY SCREENING OF NEW THPS

New THPs are generally identified by employing *in vivo* phage display technique [30, 167 - 169]. The technique is based on the ability of phages to express unique peptides as fusion proteins on their capsids [170]. Next step involves injecting these libraries in the tail vein of mouse, allowing it to circulate in the body for 5-10 minutes and then obtaining phage from the target organs. After much amplification, this phage can be enriched while displaying the homing peptide with which it has high affinity. In the absence of tumor mice model, the THPs screening from phage library can also be carried out using cancer cell line. The phage library is subjected to binding with cancer cells and adherent and penetrating phages are recovered and amplified by infecting them in *E. coli* separately. Both kinds of phages are selectively amplified through repeated rounds of panning. DNA of phage preparation is sequenced and amino acids sequence deduced is aligned for consensus sequence. Consensus peptide motif is selected and further utilized for tumor homing. Detailed mechanism is shown in Fig. (**3**). This screening procedure is based on both the positive and negative selection where peptide entering target tissue is included whereas the one reaching the other organs is excluded. *Ex vivo* step where peptides have affinity to target are selected by incubating with the cells derived from such tissues before injecting into the tail vein of mouse has increased the efficiency of peptide recovery [76].

While biopanning of phage display libraries, several peptides have been identified, which selectively target tumor blood vessel or lymphatic vessels [112]. LyP-1 is a nine amino-acid cyclic peptide, obtained during screening of phage display libraries using human MDA-MB-435 carcinoma xenografts [171]. The peptide specifically homes to the tumor lymphatic vessels and is able to internalize inside tumor and lymphatic endothelial cells. While the process of

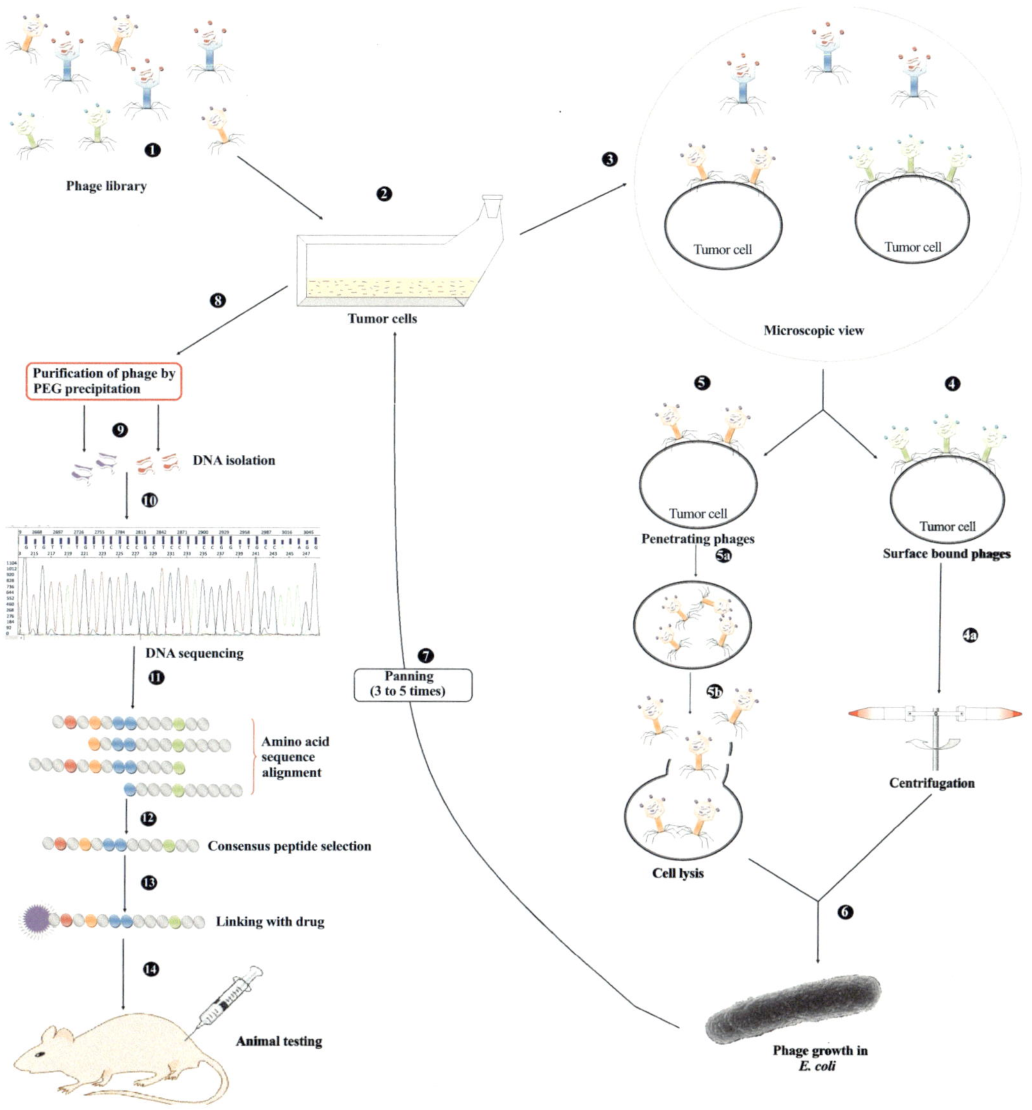

Fig. (3). Strategy of screening tumor homing peptides using phages (Phage display) (1) a phage library, displaying unique peptides on its major coat protein pIII (2) incubation of phage library with cancer cells (3-5) Inset: upon incubation some phage may remain unbound to cancer cell, while few binds on the surface of cancer cell and (5a) some penetrate cancer cell; (4a) Surface bound phages are recovered by centrifugation, whereas (5b) penetrating phages are recovered by cell lysis; (6) Phages are replicated by infection to *E. coli* (7) Several rounds of panning (8) Purification of phage by PEG precipitation (9) Genomic DNA isolation (10) Sequencing of DNA (11) Nucleotide sequence is converted into amino acids sequence and different sequences are aligned (12) Common motif is identified (13) Tumor target drug is conjugated with consensus motif (14) Validation through animal testing.

internalization, it may carry some therapeutic payloads like fluorescein and quantum dots inside the target cells [31, 171]. Soluble LyP-1 peptide has been shown to inhibit tumor growth in xenograft-bearing mice and cause concentration dependent cell death in cultured MDA-MB-435 cells [77].

Other method to identify THPs among phage displayed peptide library (PDPL) is *in vitro* phage display. In this method, PDPL is identified by using whole tumor cell or protein/target isolated from the tumor cells. Selection of target specific phage involves same procedure of negative and positive screening as carried out in case of *in vivo* phage display technique to eliminate peptide targeting normal cell receptors and selecting the one with specificity towards tumor cell receptors. Identified phages, which have been internalized or have bound to the target, are rescued. This step is followed three to four times for enrichment of desirable product. Later, phage sequences can be identified and aligned to identify common motifs which are labeled by flourophore. These labeled motifs are then evaluated *in vivo* in mice to confirm the tumor homing property [172]. One bead one compound (OBOC) combinatorial library can also be used to identify new THPs in less time and with a smaller amount of expenditure [173]. This is based on the expression of one peptide on one bead surface and there are millions of beads which are created by split and mix synthesis method. These large numbers of libraries can be screened in multiple stages for particular peptide by magnetic sorting, on-bead enzyme linkage and fluorescence based assays [174]. By the use of OBOC, even peptides with non-natural amino acids can be traced which is advantageous as they are not prone to proteolysis. Thus, THPs which are specific and also stable in the body can be traced and used for cancer therapeutics [175, 176].

Now-a-days, importance of THPs is being realized. It has become mandatory to come up with many new such peptides developed within a short span of time. Computational approach has made it easy to design and develop new THPs in less time and with minimum efforts. Web service named as Tumor-HPD has been generated based on various computational approaches such as support vector machine (SVM) model that provides prediction of THPs [79]. With this web service, we can even design analogues of THPs which have been created by introducing mutation in them and then comparing their tumor homing ability from parent peptide. This gives an opportunity to find out better design of THP, if originating from mutation to serve our purpose. Designing THPs involves a lot of efforts. Amino acid composition of THPs and non-THPs varies considerably with THPs having comparatively higher percentage of C, R, G, W, P, L and S. But no difference has been noticed at both the terminals among THP and non-THPs. This can be very well determined by amino acid composition (AAC) model, where THPs and non-THPs can be discriminated by analyzing their amino acid composition and then THPs can be easily designed. Other models, such as dipeptide composition (DPC) and binary profile pattern (BPP) model are also performing well with BPP having highest overall efficiency in predicting THPs for use in therapy and diagnosis [79].

ADVANTAGES OF THPS OVER OTHER DELIVERY VEHICLES

Owing to their smaller size, these penetrate easily in to the target sites and can be synthesized very easily by automation, thus being quite economical in terms of production [30]. This is the drawback of the use of monoclonal antibodies (mAbs), which are larger in size and tend to cause toxicity in various organs (liver, bone marrow etc.). THPs, on the other hand, possess good biocompatibility, thus are safer to use [116]. Also, many modifications can be made in THPs for making them more specific only to the tumor cells. Some may point out the low stability and half-life of peptides which can be easily increased by several ways such as inserting D-amino acids or unnatural amino acids in its sequence, modifying back bone or both the terminals, cyclization of peptides, adding cysteine etc. [175, 177]. Specificity may be further enhanced by incorporating tumor environment specific motifs to THPs; such as proteolytic cleavage site, which is cleaved by proteases expressed only on the surface of cancer cell. One example of such protease is urokinase [178]. These cause very less or no tissue damage by their selective toxicity to cancer cells as they are highly specific to their target of action [62, 179]. Along with better penetration to the tumor cells, THPs provide circulation independent targeting to tumor in peritoneal area thereby increasing the therapeutic index of intraperitoneal chemotherapy [180]. Some of the anticancer agents that have shown major improvement in their efficacy are platinum drugs viz. cisplatin and carboplatin by linking them with THP such as CNGRC [181, 182]. These drugs crosslink the cellular DNA and initiate apoptosis of the cell. By conjugating them with THPs, toxicity of these agents is reduced considerably. If some of the receptors are expressed by tumor and the blood neovasculature, then by designing THPs, targeting of it can be used to simultaneously inhibit both the tumor mass and the new vessels developed to support such mass. One such target of homing peptide YSA that binds EphA2 expressed on both tumor cells and new blood vessels developed in cancerogenesis [183], acts from both the sides to tackle any tumor mass. Targeted delivery increases bioavailability of anti-cancer agents, which further reduces their dose; hence their toxic effects on body cells e.g. podophyllotoxin is used for treating lung cancer, genital tumors, etc. [32, 184 - 186].

Moreover, penetrability to tumor can be further enhanced by linking them with amphipathic conjugates such as hyaluronic acid [187]. Penetrability can also be improved of certain THPs such as Lyp-1, iRGD by adding cysteine or maleimidohexanoic acid to their N-terminal [188]. Cytolytic peptides can be made more specific by linking them with pro-apoptotic system which is activated on entering tumor cells to be expressed by cathepsin mediated proteolysis generated by cellular death pathways [189]. This reduces both the tumor growth as well as tumor metastasis [190]. Further, they can increase the tumor inhibiting property of anti-tumor agents such as Maspin, thymosin-α1 etc. apart from acting just as delivery vehicle to them [76, 191]. Though these THPs suffer from low half-life but due to their easy modifications, such obstacle which reduces their half-life can also be crossed by linking them to other proteins such as serum albumin [192]. In turn, THPs can also increase the half-life of certain metabolizable anticancer agents such as Epigallocatechin-3-gallate derived from green tea [193]. Thus, health benefits of natural anticancer agents can be successfully employed in anticancer regimen without worrying about their stability inside the body. RGD conjugated with doxorubicin (DOX) inhibits tumor growth and increased life span of experimental animals in comparison to doxorubicin alone or conjugated with control peptide [194]. Long-circulating liposomes (LCL) coated with PEG are having superior circulating half-life. RGD-LCL-DOX is found effective against DOX-insensitive murine C26 colon carcinoma model [195]. RGD and NRG peptides, when fused to $(KLAKLAK)_2$, result in reduction in tumor size and prolonged survival. $(KLAKLAK)_2$ is an antimicrobial, apoptosis inducing peptide, which leads to mitochondrial membrane disruption and apoptosis [144]. $(KLAKLAK)_2$ coupled to CKGGRAKDC, a white fat vasculature homing peptide lowers white fat [196].

THPS IN DIAGNOSTICS

Proper diagnosis, particular in an early stage, is the most important aspect of the cancer therapeutics. Generally, antitumor antibodies are being used as targeting agents for molecular imaging. Numerous monoclonal antibodies viz. Trastuzumab, Bevacizumab, Cetuximab, Ibritumomabtiuxetan etc. are being used against the therapy of breast cancer, colorectal cancer, head and neck cancer and Non-Hodgkin lymphoma, respectively [197]. However, their bulky size, low penetrance and phagocytosis by immune cells make them ineffective.

To overcome such shortcomings, various THPs have been identified and validated by the scientists throughout the globe using various models and different carcinomas, further increasing the scope of cancer diagnosis and treatment (Table **1**). For example, to diagnose a special subset of brain tumor cells of human glioblastomamultiforme (GBM) cells, having stem cell like characters of self-renewal, generating spheres and *in vivo* tumor formation even in absence of external mitogens and growth factors, a peptide has been identified through the phage display screening method. These peptides may be fused to a biologically active molecule to exhibit altered pharmacokinetic properties, which can be explored in diagnostics as well as in therapy [33]. The peptide PC5-2 identified by phage display and synthetic peptide SP5-2 are able to differentiate human pulmonary tumor, and when coupled to liposomes containing vinorelbine or doxorubicin, improve the drug anticancer efficacy [34]. These THPs are useful in detecting and treating carcinomas, lung, brain, colorectal, and ovarian tumors [33 - 43]. Due to their high specificity for tumor cells, these not only can deliver drugs efficiently to treat cancerous cells as therapeutics agents, but also can be utilized as novel diagnostic tools and imaging agents to tumor sites.

THPS IN CLINICAL TRIAL PHASE

Many of the THPs have entered the phase of clinical trials. RGD and NGR are the most important ones that have already entered the various stages of clinical trials [198, 199]. Cilengitide is an anti-angiogenic agent (EMD 121974, Merck) and a cyclic derivative of RGD peptide [200]. In phase I/IIa trial, 52 GBM patients underwent combined cilengitide, radiotherapy and Temozolomide treatment, and one year total survival percentage of 67% was achieved [77]. In a Phase I study conducted on living cancer patients, they received phage library infusions followed by phage recovery and reinfusion of tumor binding phages. Patients having different kinds of cancers viz. breast cancer, malignant melanoma, and pancreatic cancer were included in the study and no prominent toxicity against infused phage was observed in the preliminary study. A lot of tumor homing peptides (Table **1**), their targets and applications in diagnostics have already been identified [44 - 52] and many more are to divulge in future epoch.

CURRENT & FUTURE DEVELOPMENTS

THPs have evolved as potent therapeutic agents for many diseases such as cancer, cardiovascular disease, etc. After many clinical trials, these have appeared in the market. The amazing property of these peptides is their specificity towards the altered cells. This targeted approach can certainly minimize the shortcomings of conventional cancer therapies like toxicity and relieve the patients from painful unpleasing experiences with chemotherapy. Improvement in knowledge pertaining to the mechanism of THP entry and the knowledge about fusion homing peptides having tumor homing domain fused with apoptotic peptide or anticancer drug like doxorubicin may help further in better utilization of their properties in clinical practice. As more and more such peptides will come up successfully in the near future, then this treatment will become more affordable to the general public due to their large scale production and will be available as personalized medicine too. However, computational analysis has made the screening of homing peptide easier, time and cost effective. *In silico* screening has provided the insight for efficient usage of synthetic homing peptides. Such homing peptides are not only directly involved in binding to the tumor cells through specific receptors, but also help in trafficking the therapeutic macromolecules as payload. Much progress in this field has already been made, as evident from many such THPs undergoing clinical trials. However, the possibility of improvement still exists. There are many issues, such as tumor penetrability of

THPs, their optimum concentration to be used, which particular receptor to be targeted etc., that need to be figured out precisely. This is possible simply by learning more about the biochemical nature, mechanism of THP entry into the cell and the modes of action of THPs. It will be wise to explore this area, when the number of cancer patients is rising at a high alacrity, and in such scenario, tumor homing peptide appears as a ray of hope.

CONFLICT OF INTEREST

The authors confirm that they have no conflict of interest to declare for this publication.

ACKNOWLEDGEMENTS

Authors of the article thank and acknowledge their respective Universities/ Institutes.

REFERENCES

[1] Schnipper LE, Davidson NE, Wollins DS, *et al.* American Society of Clinical Oncology Statement: A conceptual framework to assess the value of cancer treatment options. J Clin Oncol 2015; 33(23): 2563-77.
[http://dx.doi.org/10.1200/JCO.2015.61.6706] [PMID: 26101248]

[2] Brown SB, Brown EA, Walker I. The present and future role of photodynamic therapy in cancer treatment. Lancet Oncol 2004; 5(8): 497-508.
[http://dx.doi.org/10.1016/S1470-2045(04)01529-3] [PMID: 15288239]

[3] Cook KM, Figg WD. Angiogenesis inhibitors: Current strategies and future prospects. CA Cancer J Clin 2010; 60(4): 222-43.
[http://dx.doi.org/10.3322/caac.20075] [PMID: 20554717]

[4] Aina OH, Sroka TC, Chen ML, Lam KS. Therapeutic cancer targeting peptides. Biopolymers 2002; 66(3): 184-99.
[http://dx.doi.org/10.1002/bip.10257] [PMID: 12385037]

[5] Ruoslahti E, Bhatia SN, Sailor MJ. Targeting of drugs and nanoparticles to tumors. J Cell Biol 2010; 188(6): 759-68.
[http://dx.doi.org/10.1083/jcb.200910104] [PMID: 20231381]

[6] Kim TH. Cell-killing peptide. World Patent WO2006001582, 2006.

[7] Lu L, Li ZJ, Li LF, *et al.* Vascular-targeted TNFα improves tumor blood vessel function and enhances antitumor immunity and chemotherapy in colorectal cancer. J Control Release 2015; 210: 134-46.
[http://dx.doi.org/10.1016/j.jconrel.2015.05.282] [PMID: 26003042]

[8] King A, Ndifon C, Lui S, *et al.* Tumor-homing peptides as tools for targeted delivery of payloads to the placenta. Sci Adv 2016; 2(5): e1600349.
[http://dx.doi.org/10.1126/sciadv.1600349] [PMID: 27386551]

[9] Porkka K, Laakkonen P, Hoffman JA, Bernasconi M, Ruoslahti E. A fragment of the HMGN2 protein homes to the nuclei of tumor cells and tumor endothelial cells *in vivo.* Proc Natl Acad Sci USA 2002; 99(11): 7444-9.
[http://dx.doi.org/10.1073/pnas.062189599] [PMID: 12032302]

[10] Schugart K, Rassmussen U, Schreiber V. Targeting peptides. US Patent Application WO2001057069, 2001.

[11] Wolf IS, Messmer D. Tumor targeting peptides, therapeutic and diagnostic compositions comprising the peptides. WO2010114539, 2010.

[12] Wu HC, Wu CH. Cancer targeting peptides for enhancing anti-cancer drug delivery and therapeutic efficiencies. EP2896403, 2015.

[13] Enbäck J, Laakkonen P. Tumour-homing peptides: Tools for targeting, imaging and destruction. Biochem Soc Trans 2007; 35(Pt 4): 780-3.
[http://dx.doi.org/10.1042/BST0350780] [PMID: 17635147]

[14] Kim TH. Tumor cell-killing peptides. US8877889, 2014.

[15] Mäe M, Myrberg H, El-Andaloussi S, Langel U. Design of a tumor homing cell-penetrating peptide for drug delivery. Int J Pept Res Ther 2009; 15: 11-5.
[http://dx.doi.org/10.1007/s10989-008-9156-x]

[16] Hällbrink M, Pooga M, Metsis M, *et al.* Cell penetrating peptides. US Patent Application PCT/IB2003/003163, 2003.

[17] Langel U, Maarja MÄE, Myrberg H, Ruoslahti E, Lianglin Zhang L. Chimeric constructs between cancer-homing peptides and cell-penetrating peptides coupled to anticancer drugs and/or diagnostic agent/agents. EP1991586, 2011.

[18] Kurrikoff K, Eriste E, Oskolkov N, *et al.* Chimeric constructs between glioma-homing peptide and cell-penetrating peptides, gHoPe2. EP2671597, 2013.

[19] Wu HC, Lin CT, Lee TY, Kuo S. Peptide-conjugates that bind to VEGF-stimulated or tumor vasculature and methods of treatment. US8088887 B2, 2012.

[20] Picard MA, Bethe U, Dotzaeur M, Moyal ECJ. Continuous administration of cilengitide in cancer treatments. WO2010136168, 2010.

[21] Laakkonen P, Porkka K, Hoffman JA, Ruoslahti E. Peptides that home to tumor lymphatic vasculature and methods of using same. US 7671021 B2, 2010.

[22] Laakkonen P, Ruoslahti E, Bergers G. Peptide homing to brain tumors. US8188221, 2012.

[23] Ruoslahti E, Agemy L, Friedmann-Morvinski D, Kotamraju VR, Sugahara K, Verma I. Methods and compositions for enhanced delivery of compounds. EP2555802, 2013.

[24] Samoylova TI, Baker HJ, Cox NR, Globa LP, Morrison NE. Methods for targeting and killing glioma cells. US7642063, 2010.

[25] Prokop A, Davidson J, Carlesso G, Roberts D. Nanoparticular tumor targeting and therapy. US20050008572, 2005.

[26] Park J-H, Zhang L, Derfus AM, Sailor MJ, Von Maltzahn GA, Harris T, *et al.* Nanoworms for *in vivo* tumor targeting. US20100254914, 2010.

[27] Gao X. Peptide-bound gold metal nano-clusters as cancer cell killing agents. US9090660, 2015.

[28] Ganss R, Anna Johansson A. Treatment of tumours using peptide-protein conjugates. WO2016041014, 2016.

[29] Sieckman G, Volkert W, Forte L, Hoffman T, Gali H. Therapeutic and diagnostic targeting of cancers cells with tumor homing peptides. US20030232013, 2003.

[30] Arap W, Pasqualini R. Human and mouse targeting peptides identified by phage display. WO2002020769, 2002.

[31] Ruoslahti E, Teesalu T, Sugahara K, Roth L. Truncated LyP-1 peptide and methods and compositions using truncated LyP -1 peptides. US20150259380, 2015.

[32] Van Kuik-Romeijn P, Platenburg GJ. Molecules for targeting compounds to various selected organs, tissues or tumor cells. US8609065, 2013.

[33] Dennis M. Serum albumin binding peptides for tumor targeting. US20050287153, 2005.

[34] Wu HC, Lin CT, Chang DK. Lung cancer targeted peptides and applications thereof. US20080193375, 2008.

[35] Li S, Cutrera J, Xia X. Carcinoma homing peptide (CHP), its analogs, and methods of using. US20120208770, 2012.

[36] Cho CH, Li ZJ. Homing peptide for tumor vasculature. US8247378, 2012.

[37] Robbins SM, Rahn J, Senger DL. Brain tumor targeting peptides and methods. US8530429, 2013.

[38] Arap W, Kolonin MG, Mintz PJ, Pasqualini R, Amado J, Zurita AJ. Compositions and methods of use of targeting peptides for diagnosis and therapy of human cancer. US8507445, 2013.

[39] Ackroyd JE. LY75 as cancer therapeutic and diagnostic target. WO2014072700, 2014.

[40] Hunt DF, Shabanowitz J, Abelin JG, Cobbold M, Penny SA. Target peptides for colorectal cancer therapy and diagnostics. US20150328297, 2014.

[41] Hunt DF, Shabanowitz J, Malaker SA, *et al.* Target peptides for immunotherapy and diagnostics. WO2014036562, 2014.

[42] Hunt DF, Shabanowitz J, Jennifer G, Abelin JG, William H, Hildebrand WH. Target peptides for ovarian cancer therapy and diagnostics. EP2931312, 2015.

[43] Wu CH. Cancer targeting peptides for enhancing anti-cancer drug delivery and therapeutic efficiencies. EP2896403, 2015.

[44] Pietras RJ. Peptide antiestrogen compositions and methods for treating breast cancer. US6306832, 2001.

[45] Bredesen DE, Ellerby M, Ellerby L. Hunter killer peptides and methods of use. WO2005094383, 2005.

[46] Yeaman MR, Yount NY, Brass EP. Peptides and methods for inducing cell death. US8492333, 2013.

[47] Debinski W, Pandya H, Gibo D. Multilevel specific targeting of cancer cells with IL13. US8362207, 2013.

[48] Ruoslahti E, Porkka K, Christian S. HMGN2 peptides and related molecules that selectively home to tumor blood vessels and tumor cells. US8598112, 2013.

[49] Hazlehurst LA, Dalton WS, Emmons M, Gebhard AW. HYD1 peptides for relapsed cancer. US20140080762, 2014.

[50] Okada H. Interleukin-13 receptor alpha2 peptide brain cancer vaccine. JP2013536240, 2014.

[51] Pincus MR, Michl J, Yazdi ES. Membrane resident peptide in anti-cancer peptides causes tumor cell necrosis rather than apoptosis of cancer cells. US8822419, 2014.

[52] Pan CX, Zhang H, Lam KS, Aina OH. Bladder cancer specific ligand peptides. US8946379, 2015.

[53] Simberg D, Duza T, Park JH, *et al.* Biomimetic amplification of nanoparticle homing to tumors. Proc Natl Acad Sci USA 2007; 104(3): 932-6. [http://dx.doi.org/10.1073/pnas.0610298104] [PMID: 17215365]

[54] Elmquist A, Lindgren M, Bartfai T, Langel U . VE-cadherin-derived cell-penetrating peptide, pVEC, with carrier functions. Exp Cell Res 2001; 269(2): 237-44. [http://dx.doi.org/10.1006/excr.2001.5316] [PMID: 11570816]

[55] Shadidi M, Sioud M. Identification of novel carrier peptides for the specific delivery of therapeutics into cancer cells. FASEB J 2003; 17(2): 256-8. [PMID: 12490548]

[56] Regberg J, Srimanee A, Langel U. Applications of cell-penetrating peptides for tumor targeting and future cancer therapies. Pharmaceuticals (Basel) 2012; 5(9): 991-1007. [http://dx.doi.org/10.3390/ph5090991] [PMID: 24280701]

[57] Torchilin VP. Tat peptide-mediated intracellular delivery of pharmaceutical nanocarriers. Adv Drug Deliv Rev 2008; 60(4-5): 548-58. [http://dx.doi.org/10.1016/j.addr.2007.10.008] [PMID: 18053612]

[58] Ruoslahti E, Rajotte D. An address system in the vasculature of normal tissues and tumors. Annu Rev Immunol 2000; 18(1): 813-27. [http://dx.doi.org/10.1146/annurev.immunol.18.1.813] [PMID: 10837076]

[59] Graziadio A, Zanda M, Frau S, *et al.* NGR tumor-homing peptides: Structural requirements for effective APN (CD13) targeting. Bioconjug Chem 2016; 27(5): 1332-40. [http://dx.doi.org/10.1021/acs.bioconjchem.6b00136] [PMID: 27077642]

[60] Liu C, Yang Y, Chen L, Lin YL, Li F. A unified mechanism for aminopeptidase N-based tumor cell motility and tumor-homing therapy. J Biol Chem 2014; 289(50): 34520-9. [http://dx.doi.org/10.1074/jbc.M114.566802] [PMID: 25359769]

[61] Svensen N, Walton JG, Bradley M. Peptides for cell-selective drug delivery. Trends Pharmacol Sci 2012; 33(4): 186-92. [http://dx.doi.org/10.1016/j.tips.2012.02.002] [PMID: 22424670]

[62] Ruoslahti E. Tumor penetrating peptides for improved drug delivery. Adv Drug Deliv Rev 2016; S0169-409X(16): 30094-1.
[http://dx.doi.org/10.1016/j.addr.2016.03.008]

[63] Teesalu T, Sugahara KN, Ruoslahti E. Tumor-penetrating peptides. Front Oncol 2013; 3: 216.
[http://dx.doi.org/10.3389/fonc.2013.00216] [PMID: 23986882]

[64] Kadonosono T, Yamano A, Goto T, *et al.* Cell penetrating peptides improve tumor delivery of cargos through neuropilin-1-dependent extravasation. J Control Release 2015; 201: 14-21.
[http://dx.doi.org/10.1016/j.jconrel.2015.01.011] [PMID: 25592386]

[65] Simón-Gracia L, Hunt H, Scodeller P, *et al.* iRGD peptide conjugation potentiates intraperitoneal tumor delivery of paclitaxel with polymersomes. Biomaterials 2016; 104: 247-57.
[http://dx.doi.org/10.1016/j.biomaterials.2016.07.023] [PMID: 27472162]

[66] Park SH, Zheng JH, Nguyen VH, *et al.* RGD Peptide cell-surface display enhances the targeting and therapeutic efficacy of attenuated Salmonella-mediated cancer therapy. Theranostics 2016; 6(10): 1672-82.
[http://dx.doi.org/10.7150/thno.16135] [PMID: 27446500]

[67] Soker S, Takashima S, Miao HQ, Neufeld G, Klagsbrun M. Neuropilin-1 is expressed by endothelial and tumor cells as an isoform-specific receptor for vascular endothelial growth factor. Cell 1998; 92(6): 735-45.
[http://dx.doi.org/10.1016/S0092-8674(00)81402-6] [PMID: 9529250]

[68] Lin YC, Lim YF, Russo E, *et al.* Multidimensional design of anticancer peptides. Angew Chem Int Ed Engl 2015; 54(35): 10370-4.
[http://dx.doi.org/10.1002/anie.201504018] [PMID: 26119906]

[69] Kandela I, Chou J, Chow K. Registered report: Coadministration of a tumor-penetrating peptide enhances the efficacy of cancer drugs. eLife 2015; 4: e06959.

[70] Joyce JA, Laakkonen P, Bernasconi M, Bergers G, Ruoslahti E, Hanahan D. Stage-specific vascular markers revealed by phage display in a mouse model of pancreatic islet tumorigenesis. Cancer Cell 2003; 4(5): 393-403.
[http://dx.doi.org/10.1016/S1535-6108(03)00271-X] [PMID: 14667506]

[71] Li ZJ, Cho CH. Peptides as targeting probes against tumor vasculature for diagnosis and drug delivery. J Transl Med 2012; 10(1) (Suppl. 1): S1.
[http://dx.doi.org/10.1186/1479-5876-10-S1-S1] [PMID: 23046982]

[72] Wang Y, Huang L. Multifunctional theranostic nanoparticles for brain tumors. Mol Ther 2012; 20(1): 10-1.
[http://dx.doi.org/10.1038/mt.2011.274] [PMID: 22215053]

[73] Feng X, Gao X, Kang T, *et al.* Mammary-derived growth inhibitor targeting peptide-modified PEG-PLA nanoparticles for enhanced targeted glioblastoma therapy. Bioconjug Chem 2015; 26(8): 1850-61.
[http://dx.doi.org/10.1021/acs.bioconjchem.5b00379] [PMID: 26222392]

[74] Layek B, Sadhukha T, Prabha S. Glycoengineered mesenchymal stem cells as an enabling platform for two-step targeting of solid tumors. Biomaterials 2016; 88: 97-109.

[http://dx.doi.org/10.1016/j.biomaterials.2016.02.024] [PMID: 26946263]

[75] Okur AC, Erkoc P, Kizilel S. Targeting cancer cells via tumor-homing peptide CREKA functional PEG nanoparticles. Colloids Surf B Biointerfaces 2016; 147: 191-200. [http://dx.doi.org/10.1016/j.colsurfb.2016.08.005] [PMID: 27513587]

[76] Laakkonen P, Vuorinen K. Homing peptides as targeted delivery vehicles. Integr Biol (Camb) 2010; 2(7-8): 326-37. [http://dx.doi.org/10.1039/c0ib00013b] [PMID: 20657951]

[77] Mäkelä AR, Enbäck J, Laakkonen JP, Vihinen-Ranta M, Laakkonen P, Oker-Blom C. Tumor targeting of baculovirus displaying a lymphatic homing peptide. J Gene Med 2008; 10(9): 1019-31. [http://dx.doi.org/10.1002/jgm.1222] [PMID: 18655234]

[78] Ruoslahti E. Peptides as targeting elements and tissue penetration devices for nanoparticles. Adv Mater 2012; 24(28): 3747-56. [http://dx.doi.org/10.1002/adma.201200454] [PMID: 22550056]

[79] Sharma A, Kapoor P, Gautam A, *et al.* Computational approach for designing tumor homing peptides. Sci Rep 2013; 3: 1607. [http://dx.doi.org/10.1038/srep01607] [PMID: 23558316]

[80] Derossi D, Joliot AH, Chassaing G, Prochiantz A. The third helix of the Antennapedia homeodomain translocates through biological membranes. J Biol Chem 1994; 269(14): 10444-50. [PMID: 8144628]

[81] Falanga A, Galdiero M, Galdiero S. Membranotropic cell penetrating peptides: The outstanding journey. Int J Mol Sci 2015; 16(10): 25323-37. [http://dx.doi.org/10.3390/ijms161025323] [PMID: 26512649]

[82] Mäe M, Langel U. Cell-penetrating peptides as vectors for peptide, protein and oligonucleotide delivery. Curr Opin Pharmacol 2006; 6(5): 509-14. [http://dx.doi.org/10.1016/j.coph.2006.04.004] [PMID: 16860608]

[83] Fonseca SB, Pereira MP, Kelley SO. Recent advances in the use of cell-penetrating peptides for medical and biological applications. Adv Drug Deliv Rev 2009; 61(11): 953-64. [http://dx.doi.org/10.1016/j.addr.2009.06.001] [PMID: 19538995]

[84] Vandenbroucke RE, De Smedt SC, Demeester J, Sanders NN. Cellular entry pathway and gene transfer capacity of TAT-modified lipoplexes. Biochim Biophys Acta 2007; 1768(3): 571-9. [http://dx.doi.org/10.1016/j.bbamem.2006.11.006] [PMID: 17188643]

[85] Mayor S, Pagano RE. Pathways of clathrin-independent endocytosis. Nat Rev Mol Cell Biol 2007; 8(8): 603-12. [http://dx.doi.org/10.1038/nrm2216] [PMID: 17609668]

[86] Duchardt F, Fotin-Mleczek M, Schwarz H, Fischer R, Brock R. A comprehensive model for the cellular uptake of cationic cell-penetrating peptides. Traffic 2007; 8(7): 848-66. [http://dx.doi.org/10.1111/j.1600-0854.2007.00572.x] [PMID: 17587406]

[87] Pack DW, Hoffman AS, Pun S, Stayton PS. Design and development of polymers for gene delivery. Nat Rev Drug Discov 2005; 4(7): 581-93. [http://dx.doi.org/10.1038/nrd1775] [PMID: 16052241]

[88] Ouyang D, Zhang H, Parekh HS, Smith SC. The effect of pH on PAMAM dendrimer-siRNA complexation: Endosomal considerations as determined by molecular dynamics simulation. Biophys Chem 2011; 158(2-3): 126-33.
[http://dx.doi.org/10.1016/j.bpc.2011.06.003] [PMID: 21752532]

[89] Li ZL, Ding HM, Ma YQ. Interaction of peptides with cell membranes: Insights from molecular modeling. J Phys Condens Matter 2016; 28(8): 083001.
[http://dx.doi.org/10.1088/0953-8984/28/8/083001] [PMID: 26828575]

[90] Kawamoto S, Takasu M, Miyakawa T, *et al.* Inverted micelle formation of cell-penetrating peptide studied by coarse-grained simulation: Importance of attractive force between cell-penetrating peptides and lipid head group. J Chem Phys 2011; 134(9): 095103.
[http://dx.doi.org/10.1063/1.3555531] [PMID: 21385001]

[91] Hinz A, Galla HJ. Viral membrane penetration: Lytic activity of a nodaviral fusion peptide. Eur Biophys J 2005; 34(4): 285-93.
[http://dx.doi.org/10.1007/s00249-004-0450-z] [PMID: 15834560]

[92] Mudhakir D, Harashima H. Learning from the viral journey: How to enter cells and how to overcome intracellular barriers to reach the nucleus. AAPS J 2009; 11(1): 65-77.
[http://dx.doi.org/10.1208/s12248-009-9080-9] [PMID: 19194803]

[93] Yang L, Harroun TA, Weiss TM, Ding L, Huang HW. Barrel-stave model or toroidal model? A case study on melittin pores. Biophys J 2001; 81(3): 1475-85.
[http://dx.doi.org/10.1016/S0006-3495(01)75802-X] [PMID: 11509361]

[94] Tréhin R, Merkle HP. Chances and pitfalls of cell penetrating peptides for cellular drug delivery. Eur J Pharm Biopharm 2004; 58(2): 209-23.
[http://dx.doi.org/10.1016/j.ejpb.2004.02.018] [PMID: 15296950]

[95] Alberici L, Roth L, Sugahara KN, *et al. De novo* design of a tumor-penetrating peptide. Cancer Res 2013; 73(2): 804-12.
[http://dx.doi.org/10.1158/0008-5472.CAN-12-1668] [PMID: 23151901]

[96] Patyar S, Joshi R, Byrav DS, Prakash A, Medhi B, Das BK. Bacteria in cancer therapy: A novel experimental strategy. J Biomed Sci 2010; 17(1): 21.
[http://dx.doi.org/10.1186/1423-0127-17-21] [PMID: 20331869]

[97] Iida N, Dzutsev A, Stewart CA, *et al.* Commensal bacteria control cancer response to therapy by modulating the tumor microenvironment. Science 2013; 342(6161): 967-70.
[http://dx.doi.org/10.1126/science.1240527] [PMID: 24264989]

[98] Johnson MD, Garrett CK, Bond JE, Coggan KA, Wolfgang MC, Redinbo MR. *Pseudomonas aeruginosa* PilY1 binds integrin in an RGD- and calcium-dependent manner. PLoS One 2011; 6(12): e29629.
[http://dx.doi.org/10.1371/journal.pone.0029629] [PMID: 22242136]

[99] Nguyen VD, Nguyen HH. Molecular screening of azurin-like anticancer bacteriocins from human gut microflora using bioinformatics. Advanced Computational Methods for Knowledge Engineering. Berlin, Germany: Springer 2015; pp. 219-29.
[http://dx.doi.org/10.1007/978-3-319-17996-4_20]

[100] Mäkelä AR, Oker-Blom C. Baculovirus display: A multifunctional technology for gene delivery and eukaryotic library development. Adv Virus Res 2006; 68: 91-112. [http://dx.doi.org/10.1016/S0065-3527(06)68003-2] [PMID: 16997010]

[101] Tani H, Nishijima M, Ushijima H, Miyamura T, Matsuura Y. Characterization of cell-surface determinants important for baculovirus infection. Virology 2001; 279(1): 343-53. [http://dx.doi.org/10.1006/viro.2000.0699] [PMID: 11145915]

[102] Mäkelä AR, Matilainen H, White DJ, Ruoslahti E, Oker-Blom C. Enhanced baculovirus-mediated transduction of human cancer cells by tumor-homing peptides. J Virol 2006; 80(13): 6603-11. [http://dx.doi.org/10.1128/JVI.00528-06] [PMID: 16775347]

[103] Fang J, Nakamura H, Maeda H. The EPR effect: Unique features of tumor blood vessels for drug delivery, factors involved, and limitations and augmentation of the effect. Adv Drug Deliv Rev 2011; 63(3): 136-51. [http://dx.doi.org/10.1016/j.addr.2010.04.009] [PMID: 20441782]

[104] Cao Y, Langer R. Optimizing the delivery of cancer drugs that block angiogenesis. Science translational medicine 2010; 2(15): 15ps3-3. [http://dx.doi.org/10.1126/scitranslmed.3000399]

[105] Pasqualini R, Koivunen E, Kain R, *et al.* Aminopeptidase N is a receptor for tumor-homing peptides and a target for inhibiting angiogenesis. Cancer Res 2000; 60(3): 722-7. [PMID: 10676659]

[106] Lee SH, Jeong D, Han YS, Baek MJ. Pivotal role of vascular endothelial growth factor pathway in tumor angiogenesis. Ann Surg Treat Res 2015; 89(1): 1-8. [http://dx.doi.org/10.4174/astr.2015.89.1.1] [PMID: 26131438]

[107] Gautam A, Singh H, Tyagi A, *et al.* CPPsite: A curated database of cell penetrating peptides. Database (Oxford) 2012; 2012: bas015. [http://dx.doi.org/10.1093/database/bas015] [PMID: 22403286]

[108] Zitzmann S, Ehemann V, Schwab M. Arginine-glycine-aspartic acid (RGD)-peptide binds to both tumor and tumor-endothelial cells *in vivo.* Cancer Res 2002; 62(18): 5139-43. [PMID: 12234975]

[109] Gao H, Xiong Y, Zhang S, Yang Z, Cao S, Jiang X. RGD and interleukin-13 peptide functionalized nanoparticles for enhanced glioblastoma cells and neovasculature dual targeting delivery and elevated tumor penetration. Mol Pharm 2014; 11(3): 1042-52. [http://dx.doi.org/10.1021/mp400751g] [PMID: 24521297]

[110] Corti A, Curnis F. Tumor vasculature targeting through NGR peptide-based drug delivery systems. Curr Pharm Biotechnol 2011; 12(8): 1128-34. [http://dx.doi.org/10.2174/138920111796117373] [PMID: 21470145]

[111] D'Onofrio N, Caraglia M, Grimaldi A, *et al.* Vascular-homing peptides for targeted drug delivery and molecular imaging: meeting the clinical challenges. Biochimica et Biophysica Acta (BBA)-. Rev Can 2014; 1846(1): 1-12.

[112] Enbäck J, Laakkonen P. Tumour-homing peptides: Tools for targeting, imaging and destruction. Biochem Soc Trans 2007; 35(Pt 4): 780-3.

[http://dx.doi.org/10.1042/BST0350780] [PMID: 17635147]

[113] Thundimadathil J. Cancer treatment using peptides: Current therapies and future prospects. J Amino Acids 2012; 2012: 967347.
[http://dx.doi.org/10.1155/2012/967347] [PMID: 23316341]

[114] Liu Y, Mei L, Yu Q, *et al.* Integrin αvβ3 targeting activity study of different retro-inverso sequences of RGD and their potentiality in the designing of tumor targeting peptides. Amino Acids 2015; 47(12): 2533-9.
[http://dx.doi.org/10.1007/s00726-015-2043-9] [PMID: 26173509]

[115] Gao H, Zhang Q, Yang Y, Jiang X, He Q. Tumor homing cell penetrating peptide decorated nanoparticles used for enhancing tumor targeting delivery and therapy. Int J Pharm 2015; 478(1): 240-50.
[http://dx.doi.org/10.1016/j.ijpharm.2014.11.029] [PMID: 25448586]

[116] Di Matteo P, Mangia P, Tiziano E, *et al.* Anti-metastatic activity of the tumor vascular targeting agent NGR-TNF. Clin Exp Metastasis 2015; 32(3): 289-300.
[http://dx.doi.org/10.1007/s10585-015-9704-7] [PMID: 25648442]

[117] Hart RG, Diener HC, Coutts SB, *et al.* Embolic strokes of undetermined source: The case for a new clinical construct. Lancet Neurol 2014; 13(4): 429-38.
[http://dx.doi.org/10.1016/S1474-4422(13)70310-7] [PMID: 24646875]

[118] Li K, Kaaks R, Linseisen J, Rohrmann S. Associations of dietary calcium intake and calcium supplementation with myocardial infarction and stroke risk and overall cardiovascular mortality in the Heidelberg cohort of the European Prospective Investigation into Cancer and Nutrition study (EPIC-Heidelberg). Heart 2012; 98(12): 920-5.
[http://dx.doi.org/10.1136/heartjnl-2011-301345] [PMID: 22626900]

[119] Laakkonen P, Zhang L, Ruoslahti E. Peptide targeting of tumor lymph vessels. Ann N Y Acad Sci 2008; 1131: 37-43.
[http://dx.doi.org/10.1196/annals.1413.003] [PMID: 18519957]

[120] Choi I, Lee S, Hong YK. The new era of the lymphatic system: No longer secondary to the blood vascular system. Cold Spring Harb Perspect Med 2012; 2(4): a006445.
[http://dx.doi.org/10.1101/cshperspect.a006445] [PMID: 22474611]

[121] Le CP, Nowell CJ, Kim-Fuchs C, *et al.* Chronic stress in mice remodels lymph vasculature to promote tumour cell dissemination. Nat Commun 2016; 7: 10634.
[http://dx.doi.org/10.1038/ncomms10634] [PMID: 26925549]

[122] Laakkonen P, Porkka K, Hoffman JA, Ruoslahti E. A tumor-homing peptide with a targeting specificity related to lymphatic vessels. Nat Med 2002; 8(7): 751-5.
[PMID: 12053175]

[123] Ruoslahti E, Duza T, Zhang L. Vascular homing peptides with cell-penetrating properties. Curr Pharm Des 2005; 11(28): 3655-60.
[http://dx.doi.org/10.2174/138161205774580787] [PMID: 16305501]

[124] Laakkonen P, Akerman ME, Biliran H, *et al.* Antitumor activity of a homing peptide that targets tumor lymphatics and tumor cells. Proc Natl Acad Sci USA 2004; 101(25): 9381-6.

[http://dx.doi.org/10.1073/pnas.0403317101] [PMID: 15197262]

[125] Wall SJ, Jiang Y, Muschel RJ, DeClerck YA. Meeting report: Proteases, extracellular matrix, and cancer: An AACR Special Conference in Cancer Research. Cancer Res 2003; 63(15): 4750-5. [PMID: 12907660]

[126] Lu P, Weaver VM, Werb Z. The extracellular matrix: A dynamic niche in cancer progression. J Cell Biol 2012; 196(4): 395-406. [http://dx.doi.org/10.1083/jcb.201102147] [PMID: 22351925]

[127] Hanahan D, Coussens LM. Accessories to the crime: Functions of cells recruited to the tumor microenvironment. Cancer Cell 2012; 21(3): 309-22. [http://dx.doi.org/10.1016/j.ccr.2012.02.022] [PMID: 22439926]

[128] Weilbaecher KN, Guise TA, McCauley LK. Cancer to bone: A fatal attraction. Nat Rev Cancer 2011; 11(6): 411-25. [http://dx.doi.org/10.1038/nrc3055] [PMID: 21593787]

[129] Pola C, Formenti SC, Schneider RJ. Vitronectin-αvβ3 integrin engagement directs hypoxia-resistant mTOR activity and sustained protein synthesis linked to invasion by breast cancer cells. Cancer Res 2013; 73(14): 4571-8. [http://dx.doi.org/10.1158/0008-5472.CAN-13-0218] [PMID: 23722547]

[130] Joyce JA. Therapeutic targeting of the tumor microenvironment. Cancer Cell 2005; 7(6): 513-20. [http://dx.doi.org/10.1016/j.ccr.2005.05.024] [PMID: 15950901]

[131] Schaefer L, Reinhardt DP. Therapeutic tools and targets in cancer treatment. Advanced drug delivery reviews (Special issue) 2016; 97: 1-3.

[132] Lingasamy P, Tobi A, Hunt H, Säälik P, Salumäe M, Teesalu T. Tenascin-C binding peptides for cancer targeting. Cancer Res 2016; 76(14): 2164-4. [http://dx.doi.org/10.1158/1538-7445.AM2016-2164]

[133] Oskarsson T, Acharyya S, Zhang XH, *et al.* Breast cancer cells produce tenascin C as a metastatic niche component to colonize the lungs. Nat Med 2011; 17(7): 867-74. [http://dx.doi.org/10.1038/nm.2379] [PMID: 21706029]

[134] Naldini L. Gene therapy returns to centre stage. Nature 2015; 526(7573): 351-60. [http://dx.doi.org/10.1038/nature15818] [PMID: 26469046]

[135] Ariatti M. Targeted delivery of peptide-tagged DNA lipoplexes to hepatocellular carcinoma cells. Non-Viral Gene Delivery Vectors: Methods and Protocols 2016; 109-36. [http://dx.doi.org/10.1007/978-1-4939-3718-9_7]

[136] Zarovni N, Monaco L, Corti A. Inhibition of tumor growth by intramuscular injection of cDNA encoding tumor necrosis factor alpha coupled to NGR and RGD tumor-homing peptides. Hum Gene Ther 2004; 15(4): 373-82. [http://dx.doi.org/10.1089/104303404322959524] [PMID: 15053862]

[137] Aigner A, Fischer D. Nanoparticle-mediated delivery of small RNA molecules in tumor therapy. Pharmazie 2016; 71(1): 27-34. [PMID: 26867350]

[138] An S, Jiang X, Shi J, *et al.* Single-component self-assembled RNAi nanoparticles functionalized with tumor-targeting iNGR delivering abundant siRNA for efficient glioma therapy. Biomaterials 2015; 53: 330-40.
[http://dx.doi.org/10.1016/j.biomaterials.2015.02.084] [PMID: 25890731]

[139] Numata K, Mieszawska-Czajkowska AJ, Kvenvold LA, Kaplan DL. Silk-based nanocomplexes with tumor-homing peptides for tumor-specific gene delivery. Macromol Biosci 2012; 12(1): 75-82.
[http://dx.doi.org/10.1002/mabi.201100274] [PMID: 22052706]

[140] Schiffelers RM, Ansari A, Xu J, *et al.* Cancer siRNA therapy by tumor selective delivery with ligand-targeted sterically stabilized nanoparticle. Nucleic Acids Res 2004; 32(19): e149-9.
[http://dx.doi.org/10.1093/nar/gnh140] [PMID: 15520458]

[141] Hyvönen M, Enbäck J, Huhtala T, *et al.* Novel target for peptide-based imaging and treatment of brain tumors. Mol Cancer Ther 2014; 13(4): 996-1007.
[http://dx.doi.org/10.1158/1535-7163.MCT-13-0684] [PMID: 24493698]

[142] Ellerby HM, Arap W, Ellerby LM, *et al.* Anti-cancer activity of targeted pro-apoptotic peptides. Nat Med 1999; 5(9): 1032-8.
[http://dx.doi.org/10.1038/12469] [PMID: 10470080]

[143] Agemy L, Kotamraju VR, Friedmann-Morvinski D, Sharma S, Sugahara KN, Ruoslahti E. Proapoptotic peptide-mediated cancer therapy targeted to cell surface p32. Mol Ther 2013; 21(12): 2195-204.
[http://dx.doi.org/10.1038/mt.2013.191] [PMID: 23959073]

[144] Jiang Y, Lv L, Shi H, *et al.* PEGylated Polyamidoamine dendrimer conjugated with tumor homing peptide as a potential targeted delivery system for glioma. Colloids Surf B Biointerfaces 2016; 147: 242-9.
[http://dx.doi.org/10.1016/j.colsurfb.2016.08.002] [PMID: 27518456]

[145] Säälik P, Hunt H, Tobi A, Willmore AM, Toome K, Sharma S, *et al.* P32-targeting TT1 peptide delivers nanoparticles to intracranial glioblastomas. Cancer Res 2016; 76(14): 1343-3.
[http://dx.doi.org/10.1158/1538-7445.AM2016-1343]

[146] Daquinag AC, Tseng C, Zhang Y, *et al.* Targeted proapoptotic peptides depleting adipose stromal cells inhibit tumor growth. Mol Ther 2016; 24(1): 34-40.
[http://dx.doi.org/10.1038/mt.2015.155] [PMID: 26316391]

[147] Cai Y, Xi Y, Cao Z, *et al.* Dual targeting and enhanced cytotoxicity to HER2-overexpressing tumors by immunoapoptotin-armored mesenchymal stem cells. Cancer Lett 2016; 381(1): 104-12.
[http://dx.doi.org/10.1016/j.canlet.2016.07.027] [PMID: 27473824]

[148] Brigger I, Dubernet C, Couvreur P. Nanoparticles in cancer therapy and diagnosis. Adv Drug Deliv Rev 2002; 54(5): 631-51.
[http://dx.doi.org/10.1016/S0169-409X(02)00044-3] [PMID: 12204596]

[149] Peer D, Karp JM, Hong S, Farokhzad OC, Margalit R, Langer R. Nanocarriers as an emerging platform for cancer therapy. Nat Nanotechnol 2007; 2(12): 751-60.
[http://dx.doi.org/10.1038/nnano.2007.387] [PMID: 18654426]

[150] Galbiati E, Gambini L, Civitarese V, *et al.* Blind targeting in action: From phage display to breast

cancer cell targeting with peptide-gold nanoconjugates. Pharmacol Res 2016; 111: 155-62. [http://dx.doi.org/10.1016/j.phrs.2016.06.007] [PMID: 27293049]

[151] Qin M, Zong H, Kopelman R. Click conjugation of peptide to hydrogel nanoparticles for tumor-targeted drug delivery. Biomacromolecules 2014; 15(10): 3728-34. [http://dx.doi.org/10.1021/bm501028c] [PMID: 25162488]

[152] Zhang WQ, Yu KF, Zhong T, *et al.* Does ligand-receptor mediated competitive effect or penetrating effect of iRGD peptide when co-administration with iRGD-modified SSL? J Drug Target 2015; 23(10): 897-909. [http://dx.doi.org/10.3109/1061186X.2015.1034279] [PMID: 26087869]

[153] Curnis F, Gasparri A, Sacchi A, Fiocchi M, Corti A. Anti-tumor activity of TNF-gold nanodrugs tagged with tumor vasculature-homing peptides containing the NGR or isoDGR motives. Cancer Res 2015; 75(15) (Suppl.): 4387-7. [http://dx.doi.org/10.1158/1538-7445.AM2015-4387]

[154] Fang C, Wang K, Stephen ZR, *et al.* Temozolomide nanoparticles for targeted glioblastoma therapy. ACS Appl Mater Interfaces 2015; 7(12): 6674-82. [http://dx.doi.org/10.1021/am5092165] [PMID: 25751368]

[155] Dardevet L, Rani D, Aziz TA, *et al.* Chlorotoxin: A helpful natural scorpion peptide to diagnose glioma and fight tumor invasion. Toxins (Basel) 2015; 7(4): 1079-101. [http://dx.doi.org/10.3390/toxins7041079] [PMID: 25826056]

[156] Veiseh M, Gabikian P, Bahrami SB, *et al.* Tumor paint: A chlorotoxin:Cy5.5 bioconjugate for intraoperative visualization of cancer foci. Cancer Res 2007; 67(14): 6882-8. [http://dx.doi.org/10.1158/0008-5472.CAN-06-3948] [PMID: 17638899]

[157] Ma J, Zhang D, Ying X, *et al.* A novel NGR-conjugated peptide targets DNA damage responses for radiosensitization. Curr Cancer Drug Targets 2015; 15(6): 533-41. [http://dx.doi.org/10.2174/1568009615666150408114817] [PMID: 25850444]

[158] Drecoll E, Gaertner FC, Miederer M, *et al.* Treatment of peritoneal carcinomatosis by targeted delivery of the radio-labeled tumor homing peptide bi-DTPA-[F3]2 into the nucleus of tumor cells. PLoS One 2009; 4(5): e5715. [http://dx.doi.org/10.1371/journal.pone.0005715] [PMID: 19479088]

[159] Baum RP, Kluge AK, Kulkarni HR, *et al.* 2269 [177Lu-DOTA]-D-Phe1-Tyr3-octreotide (177Lu-DOTATOC) for peptide receptor radiotherapy in patients with advanced neuroendocrine tumours: A retrospective Phase II study of efficacy and safety. Eur J Cancer 2015; 51: S422-3. [http://dx.doi.org/10.1016/S0959-8049(16)31185-6]

[160] Ferretti C, Bruni L, Dangles-Marie V, Pecking AP, Bellet D. Molecular circuits shared by placental and cancer cells, and their implications in the proliferative, invasive and migratory capacities of trophoblasts. Hum Reprod Update 2007; 13(2): 121-41. [http://dx.doi.org/10.1093/humupd/dml048] [PMID: 17068222]

[161] Pijnenborg R, Vercruysse L, Hanssens M. The uterine spiral arteries in human pregnancy: Facts and controversies. Placenta 2006; 27(9-10): 939-58. [http://dx.doi.org/10.1016/j.placenta.2005.12.006] [PMID: 16490251]

[162] Berardi R, Morgese F, Onofri A, *et al.* Role of maspin in cancer. Clin Transl Med 2013; 2(1): 8. [http://dx.doi.org/10.1186/2001-1326-2-8] [PMID: 23497644]

[163] Zha RH, Sur S, Boekhoven J, Shi HY, Zhang M, Stupp SI. Supramolecular assembly of multifunctional maspin-mimetic nanostructures as a potent peptide-based angiogenesis inhibitor. Acta Biomater 2015; 12: 1-10. [http://dx.doi.org/10.1016/j.actbio.2014.11.001] [PMID: 25462852]

[164] Yin R, Guo L, Zhang J, *et al.* RGD and polyhistidine tumor homing peptides potentiates the action of human Maspin as an antineoplastic candidate. Appl Microbiol Biotechnol 2016; 100(14): 6209-18. [http://dx.doi.org/10.1007/s00253-016-7345-7] [PMID: 26846625]

[165] Kapoor P, Singh H, Gautam A, Chaudhary K, Kumar R, Raghava GP. TumorHoPe: A database of tumor homing peptides. PLoS One 2012; 7(4): e35187. [http://dx.doi.org/10.1371/journal.pone.0035187] [PMID: 22523575]

[166] Singh S, Chaudhary K, Dhanda SK, *et al.* SATPdb: A database of structurally annotated therapeutic peptides. Nucleic Acids Res 2016; 44(D1): D1119-26. [http://dx.doi.org/10.1093/nar/gkv1114] [PMID: 26527728]

[167] Yang X, Zhang F, Luo J, *et al.* A new non-muscle-invasive bladder tumor-homing peptide identified by phage display *in vivo.* Oncol Rep 2016; 36(1): 79-89. [http://dx.doi.org/10.3727/096504015X14478843952942] [PMID: 27221614]

[168] Hyvönen M, Laakkonen P. Identification and characterization of homing peptides using *in vivo* peptide phage display. Cell-Penetrating Peptides: Methods and Protocols 2015; 205-22. [http://dx.doi.org/10.1007/978-1-4939-2806-4_14]

[169] Krumpe LR, Mori T. Potential of phage-displayed peptide library technology to identify functional targeting peptides. Expert Opin Drug Discov 2007; 2(4): 525. [http://dx.doi.org/10.1517/17460441.2.4.525] [PMID: 20150977]

[170] Lee KJ, Lee JH, Chung HK, *et al.* Application of peptide displaying phage as a novel diagnostic probe for human lung adenocarcinoma. Amino Acids 2016; 48(4): 1079-86. [http://dx.doi.org/10.1007/s00726-015-2153-4] [PMID: 26759016]

[171] Fogal V, Zhang L, Krajewski S, Ruoslahti E. Mitochondrial/cell-surface protein p32/gC1qR as a molecular target in tumor cells and tumor stroma. Cancer Res 2008; 68(17): 7210-8. [http://dx.doi.org/10.1158/0008-5472.CAN-07-6752] [PMID: 18757437]

[172] Huang P, Wu Q, Rich J, Liu J. CBIO-20 Glioblastoma specific proteins identified through combined *in vitro* and *in vivo* phage display biopanning. Neuro-oncol 2015; 17(5): v59-9.

[173] Yang FF. Identification of cancer specific ligands from one-bead one compound combinatorial libraries to develop theranostics agents against oral squamous cell carcinoma. Doctoral dissertation, University of California, San Francisco 2016.

[174] Qian Z, Upadhyaya P, Pei D. Synthesis and screening of one-bead-one-compound cyclic peptide libraries. Methods Mol Biol 2015; 1248: 39-53. [http://dx.doi.org/10.1007/978-1-4939-2020-4_3] [PMID: 25616324]

[175] Gautam A, Kapoor P, Chaudhary K, Kumar R, Raghava GP. Tumor homing peptides as molecular probes for cancer therapeutics, diagnostics and theranostics. Curr Med Chem 2014; 21(21): 2367-91.

[http://dx.doi.org/10.2174/0929867321666140217122100] [PMID: 24533809]

[176] Krag DN, Shukla GS, Shen GP, *et al.* Selection of tumor-binding ligands in cancer patients with phage display libraries. Cancer Res 2006; 66(15): 7724-33.
[http://dx.doi.org/10.1158/0008-5472.CAN-05-4441] [PMID: 16885375]

[177] Pang HB, Braun GB, She ZG, *et al.* A free cysteine prolongs the half-life of a homing peptide and improves its tumor-penetrating activity. J Control Release 2014; 175: 48-53.
[http://dx.doi.org/10.1016/j.jconrel.2013.12.006] [PMID: 24345789]

[178] Braun GB, Sugahara KN, Yu OM, *et al.* Urokinase-controlled tumor penetrating peptide. J Control Release 2016; 232: 188-95.
[http://dx.doi.org/10.1016/j.jconrel.2016.04.027] [PMID: 27106816]

[179] Paasonen L, Sharma S, Braun GB, *et al.* New p32/gC1qR ligands for targeted tumor drug delivery. ChemBioChem 2016; 17(7): 570-5.
[http://dx.doi.org/10.1002/cbic.201500564] [PMID: 26895508]

[180] Sugahara KN, Scodeller P, Braun GB, *et al.* A tumor-penetrating peptide enhances circulation-independent targeting of peritoneal carcinomatosis. J Control Release 2015; 212: 59-69.
[http://dx.doi.org/10.1016/j.jconrel.2015.06.009] [PMID: 26071630]

[181] Ndinguri MW, Solipuram R, Gambrell RP, Aggarwal S, Hammer RP. Peptide targeting of platinum anti-cancer drugs. Bioconjug Chem 2009; 20(10): 1869-78.
[http://dx.doi.org/10.1021/bc900065r] [PMID: 19775102]

[182] Zou M, Zhang L, Xie Y, Xu W. NGR-based strategies for targeting delivery of chemotherapeutics to tumor vasculature. Anticancer Agents Med Chem 2012; 12(3): 239-46.
[http://dx.doi.org/10.2174/187152012800228751] [PMID: 22263803]

[183] Guo Z, He B, Yuan L, *et al.* Dual targeting for metastatic breast cancer and tumor neovasculature by EphA2-mediated nanocarriers. Int J Pharm 2015; 493(1-2): 380-9.
[http://dx.doi.org/10.1016/j.ijpharm.2015.05.051] [PMID: 26004003]

[184] Aguilera TA. Activatable cell penetrating peptides and their use in clinical contrast agent and therapeutic development. Ph.D. Thesis, University of California. Available from: https://escholarship.org/uc/item/9871p905 2009.

[185] Safarzadeh E, Sandoghchian Shotorbani S, Baradaran B. Herbal medicine as inducers of apoptosis in cancer treatment. Adv Pharm Bull 2014; 4(1) (Suppl. 1): 421-7.
[PMID: 25364657]

[186] Choi JY, Hong WG, Cho JH, *et al.* Podophyllotoxin acetate triggers anticancer effects against non-small cell lung cancer cells by promoting cell death via cell cycle arrest, ER stress and autophagy. Int J Oncol 2015; 47(4): 1257-65.
[PMID: 26314270]

[187] Liang DS, Su HT, Liu YJ, Wang AT, Qi XR. Tumor-specific penetrating peptides-functionalized hyaluronic acid-d-α-tocopheryl succinate based nanoparticles for multi-task delivery to invasive cancers. Biomaterials 2015; 71: 11-23.
[http://dx.doi.org/10.1016/j.biomaterials.2015.08.035] [PMID: 26310359]

[188] Kotamraju VR, Sharma S, Kolhar P, Agemy L, Pavlovich J, Ruoslahti E. Increasing tumor

accessibility with conjugatable disulfide-bridged tumor-penetrating peptides for cancer diagnosis and treatment. Breast Cancer (Auckl) 2016; 9(2) (Suppl. 2): 79-87.
[http://dx.doi.org/10.4137/BCBCR.S29426] [PMID: 27385913]

[189] Qifan W, Fen N, Ying X, Xinwei F, Jun D, Ge Z. iRGD-targeted delivery of a pro-apoptotic peptide activated by cathepsin B inhibits tumor growth and metastasis in mice. Tumour Biol 2016; 37(8): 10643-52.
[http://dx.doi.org/10.1007/s13277-016-4961-x] [PMID: 26867766]

[190] Hamilton AM, Aidoudi-Ahmed S, Sharma S, *et al.* Nanoparticles coated with the tumor-penetrating peptide iRGD reduce experimental breast cancer metastasis in the brain. J Mol Med 2015; 93(9): 991-1001.
[http://dx.doi.org/10.1007/s00109-015-1279-x] [PMID: 25869026]

[191] Lao X, Li B, Liu M, *et al.* A modified thymosin alpha 1 inhibits the growth of breast cancer both *in vitro* and *in vivo*: suppressment of cell proliferation, inducible cell apoptosis and enhancement of targeted anticancer effects. Apoptosis 2015; 20(10): 1307-20.
[http://dx.doi.org/10.1007/s10495-015-1151-z] [PMID: 26283169]

[192] Su T, Yang H, Fan Q, *et al.* Enhancing the circulating half-life and the antitumor effects of a tumor-selective cytotoxic peptide by exploiting endogenous serum albumin as a drug carrier. Int J Pharm 2016; 499(1-2): 195-204.
[http://dx.doi.org/10.1016/j.ijpharm.2015.12.069] [PMID: 26752086]

[193] Ding J, Yao J, Xue J, *et al.* Tumor-homing cell-penetrating peptide linked to colloidal mesoporous silica encapsulated (-)-epigallocatechin-3-gallate as drug delivery system for breast cancer therapy *in vivo.* ACS Appl Mater Interfaces 2015; 7(32): 18145-55.
[http://dx.doi.org/10.1021/acsami.5b05618] [PMID: 26225796]

[194] Arap W, Pasqualini R, Ruoslahti E. Cancer treatment by targeted drug delivery to tumor vasculature in a mouse model. Science 1998; 279(5349): 377-80.
[http://dx.doi.org/10.1126/science.279.5349.377] [PMID: 9430587]

[195] Schiffelers RM, Koning GA, ten Hagen TL, *et al.* Anti-tumor efficacy of tumor vasculature-targeted liposomal doxorubicin. J Control Release 2003; 91(1-2): 115-22.
[http://dx.doi.org/10.1016/S0168-3659(03)00240-2] [PMID: 12932643]

[196] Kolonin MG, Saha PK, Chan L, Pasqualini R, Arap W. Reversal of obesity by targeted ablation of adipose tissue. Nat Med 2004; 10(6): 625-32.
[http://dx.doi.org/10.1038/nm1048] [PMID: 15133506]

[197] Trail PA, King HD, Dubowchik GM. Monoclonal antibody drug immunoconjugates for targeted treatment of cancer. Cancer Immunol Immunother 2003; 52(5): 328-37.
[PMID: 12700948]

[198] Boohaker RJ, Lee MW, Vishnubhotla P, Perez JM, Khaled AR. The use of therapeutic peptides to target and to kill cancer cells. Curr Med Chem 2012; 19(22): 3794-804.
[http://dx.doi.org/10.2174/092986712801661004] [PMID: 22725698]

[199] Gregorc V, Zucali PA, Santoro A, *et al.* Phase II study of asparagine-glycine-arginine-human tumor necrosis factor α, a selective vascular targeting agent, in previously treated patients with malignant pleural mesothelioma. J Clin Oncol 2010; 28(15): 2604-11.

[http://dx.doi.org/10.1200/JCO.2009.27.3649] [PMID: 20406925]

[200] Mas-Moruno C, Rechenmacher F, Kessler H. Cilengitide: The first anti-angiogenic small molecule drug candidate design, synthesis and clinical evaluation. Anticancer Agents Med Chem 2010; 10(10): 753-68.
[http://dx.doi.org/10.2174/187152010794728639] [PMID: 21269250]

CHAPTER 3

Cell-Based Anticancer Drug Delivery Systems

Darinka Gjorgieva Ackova[1], **Katarina Smilkov**[1] and **Darko Bosnakovski**[1,2,3,*]

[1] *Department of Pharmacy, Faculty of Medical Sciences, University Goce Delcev - Stip, R. Macedonia*

[2] *Faculty of Medical Science Università del Piemonte Orientale, Novara, Italy*

[3] *Department of Pediatrics, University of Minnesota, Minneapolis, USA*

Abstract: Most explored approaches to developing cell-based drug delivery systems (DDSs) are encapsulation of the drug into the cells, cell surface modification, genetic modification of cells to secrete desired therapeutic proteins, and generating new biosynthetic systems. Tumor-tropism of mesenchymal stem cells (MSCs), as demonstrated in many studies, can be coupled with appropriate engineering with anticancer genes to enable their employment in anticancer therapy. Furthermore, MSCs can be loaded with nanoparticles (NPs), providing transport across the blood-brain barrier and accumulation of anticancer agent at the tumor site. Another attractive cell type for DDS are dendritic cells (DC), monocytes and macrophages because of their ability to accumulate in large numbers at hypoxic sites of the tumors. To this moment, exosomes are very attractive and investigated cellular entities that are used to be loaded with RNA, proteins, or other small molecules, including anticancer agents. Some of the above-mentioned cells can also be used as membrane sources in the production of anticancer delivery systems. A number of recent research papers and patents in this field are evidence of the growing interest in cell-based DDSs. In this chapter, we summarize recent developments in the field, present a newly established methodology and approaches, give an overview of the recently published inventions (patent databases FPO and Delphion were searched to locate newly published patents: US20150079631, WO2015058148A1, US20160220613, etc.), and discuss further possible developments. Further expansion in this field is expected, although limitations in design and use of DDSs exist and must be overcome before these innovative formulations can reach clinical trials and marketing authorization.

* **Corresponding author Darko Bosnakovski:** Faculty of Medical Sciences, University "Goce Delcev" Stip, Krste Misirkov bb, 2000 Stip, R. Macedonia; Tel: +389 70 516 649; E-mails: darko.bosnakovski@ugd.edu.mk; darko@umn.edu

Atta-ur-Rahman and Khurshid Zaman (Eds.)

Keywords: Anticancer agents, anticancer therapy, cell membrane vesicles, dendritic cells, drug delivery systems, exosomes, genetic engineering, mesenchymal stem cells, nanoparticles, recent patents.

1. INTRODUCTION

The bioavailability of many drugs is often compromised by their poor hydrosolubility, disintegration, metabolic activation/inactivation or excretion. Many of these problems could be resolved through the use of new and modified drug delivery systems (DDSs), which is one of the focuses of current pharmaceutical research [1, 2]. Different DDSs currently in use for pharmaceutical applications (clinical or cosmetic) are artificial and chemically synthesized (liposomes, micelles, nanoparticles, dendrimers…), or based on autologous cells or cell membranes. DDS using similar membrane structures compared to body cells are considered safest with good biocompatibility and low toxicity. In recent years, novel cell membrane-coated particles combining advantages of natural cells and synthetic polymers with various applications, such as drug delivery, have also been developed [3, 4]. Different types of DDSs that are currently in advanced phase of clinical investigation are given in Table **1** [5 - 19]. In addition, as a confirmation of the growing potential of these systems, some cell-based DDS have already been marketed (e.g., sipuleucel-T).

Despite the known advantages, there are also some concerns pointing that these DDSs are not ideal, as possibilities for the development of an antibody-antigen reaction, tumor progression and differentiation or development of toxic response to some of the components exist. Therefore, the selection of suitable cell-type for drug delivery must be accompanied with great attention. As targeting delivery of anticancer agents is still a great challenge, this chapter will focus on three main kinds of DDS for anticancer agents: whole cells - MSCs, immunological cells (DCs) and cell membrane vesicles (particles). This chapter will also present facts about fabrication processes, unique properties and their applications as promising tools to help in the search of effective cancer therapy.

Table 1. Artificial, Whole Cell or Cell Membrane-Based Drug Delivery Systems.

Carrier	Source/Target	Carrier for	Reference
Artificial			
Liposomes	Cationic cardiolipin liposomes/ prostate cancer	Nucleic acid (RAF siRNA)	[5]
Micelles	Styrene-maleic acid-copolymer micelle	Drugs (cisplatin)	[6]
Nanoparticles	Glycoengineered MSCs /ovarian tumor	Drugs (paclitaxel)	[7]
Dendrimers	PAMAM dendritic polymers coupled with folic acid/ human KB cell line	Drugs (methotrexate)	[8]
Whole Cell or Cell Membrane-Based			
Bacteria/Bacterial ghost	Mannheimia haemolytica/human colorectal adenocarcinoma cells (Caco-2) *Vibrio cholerae* ghosts /	Drugs (doxorubicin) Vaccine (outer membrane protein of *Chlamydia trachomatis)*	[9] [10]
Viruses	Adeno-associated virus (AAV)/ liver cancer cells	Nucleic acid (miRNA)	[11]
RBCs/ Erythrocyte ghost	Red blood cell membrane-cloaked nanoparticles Pravastatin chitosan nanogels-loaded erythrocytes/ HepG2 cell lines	Various drugs Various drugs	[3] [12]
Macrophages	Tumor-associated macrophages/ liver metastases	Albumin bound paclitaxel	[13]
Dendritic cells	Regulatory DCs	Nanoparticles encapsulating siRNA	[14]
Mesenchymal stem cells	Gene-manipulated adipose-tissue derived MSCs/colon cancer Gene-manipulated adipose-tissue derived MSCs/colon cancer	Prodrug (5-fluorocytosine) Prodrug (gancyclovir)	[15] [16]
Exosomes	Exosomes Exosomes from MSCs/ human pancreatic cell line CFPAC-1	Drugs (curcumin) Drugs (paclitaxel)	[17] [18]
MSC NGs	Nano ghosts derived from MSCs/ PC3 cell line	Protein (sTRAIL)	[19]

2. AUTOLOGOUS WHOLE CELL-BASED DDSs

2.1. Mesenchymal Stem Cells (MSCs)

2.1.1. Background of MSCs

Mesenchymal stem cells (MSCs) are important cells naturally present in the human organism; they differentiate from mesoderm in the stadium of embryonic development and support osteo- and hematogenesis. Depending on their morphology, MSCs are a heterogeneous population of cells and their description and recognition are based on the combination of established criteria. They can be derived and isolated for manipulations from different tissues (fat, umbilical cord Wharton's jelly, and amniotic fluid) [20, 21]. Many unique properties that MSCs possess, such as hypoimmunogenicity, easy isolation, very easy and fast expansion in *ex vivo* conditions [22, 23], and additionally, their properties for migration and localization at tumor site (tumor-tropism) make them an attractive delivery system for active delivery of anticancer agents [24 - 28]. The tumor-tropism of MSCs is confirmed in many studies including animal studies and studies with different human cancer cell lines [27, 29 - 36].

According to the available information until today, MSCs can be described as cells with both procancer and anticancer attributes; and some researchers description "double-edged sword" is very suitable and describes very closely their tumor interactions [37, 38]. Taking into consideration the fact that stem cells may promote tumor growth and differentiation is a major limitation that these cells have in anticancer therapy applications. Appropriately, gene engineering and mani-pulation with implantation of anticancer genes in MSCs could be a tool of great importance in fight against cancers; and, although the majority of recent investigations are focused on genetically engineered MSCs as DDS [28, 39, 40], non-genetically engineered MSCs have also been studied [24].

2.2. Possibilities for "Loading" of MSCs with Anticancer Agents

2.2.1. Genetically Engineered MSCs as DDS

MSCs are considered as important anticancer DDSs because of their above mentioned attributes of tumor tropism, low immunogenicity and anti-inflammatory properties. MSCs with genetic modification could secrete anticancer therapeutic proteins in tumor tissue [27, 28, 35, 39 - 43], release conditional replicative oncolytic viruses [44, 45] or act as vehicles for targeted chemotherapy with an enzyme prodrug conversion [15, 16, 36, 46] (Fig. (**1**)).

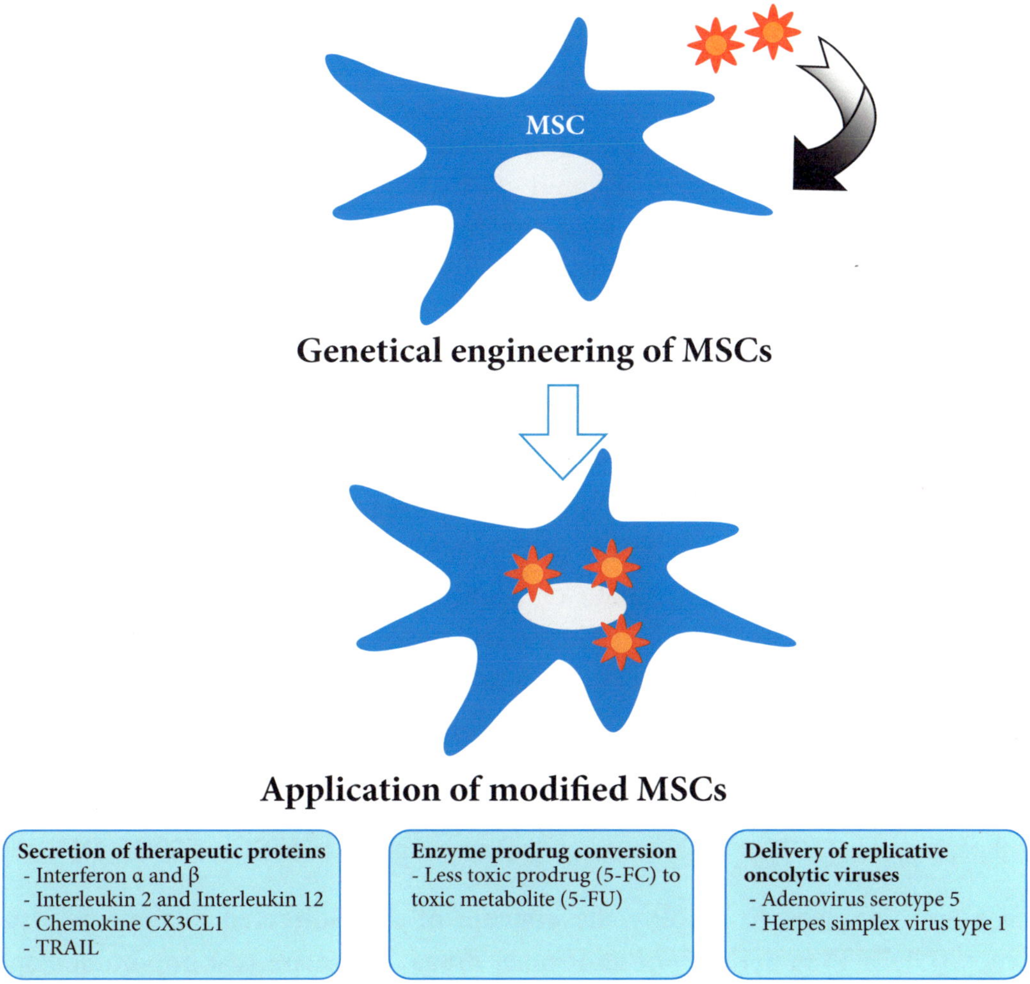

Fig. (1). MSCs genetically engineered as anticancer DDS.

The production of therapeutic proteins can be localized and directed in specific areas because genetically modified MSCs preferentially localize in the target tumor micro environment. Anticancer proteins include, but are not limited to, cytokines, enzymes, signaling molecules, and anti-angiogenic polypeptides. For example, a therapeutic agent may be IFNα or IFNβ, because the application of MSCs engineered to express INFβ in animal tumor models results in decreased tumor mass (regional secretion of IFNβ) and increased animal survival (minimizes systemic toxicity because of decreased systemic levels of IFNβ) [34]. Also, MSCs secreting IL-12 or IL-2 stimulate inflammatory cell infiltration in tumor tissue and do not cause systemic toxicity [41, 47, 48].

Manipulations in the apoptotic pathway which involve Tumor Necrosis Factor-Related Apoptosis Inducing Ligand (TRAIL) and TRAIL-receptors are specifically interesting options in gene engineering of MSCs indicating successful targeting of tumor cells and, furthermore, compatibility with other therapeutic approaches [49 - 51].

Due to low levels of and/or inactive TRAIL-receptors, MSCs and cells of most healthy tissues are resistant to apoptosis induced by TRAIL. The ability to selectively target tumor cells makes this approach an attractive option for the therapy of malignant brain tumors and lung cancers, where significant decreases of lung metastases have been observed [25, 26]. Tumor cells, by still unresolved mechanisms, can also show innate or acquired (at some stages) resistance to apoptosis mediated by TRAIL. Therefore, some therapeutic agents operated collectively can be used in a manner such as to increase responsiveness to TRAIL delivery. There are studies evaluating the inhibitor of lipoxygenase MK886 [52], proteasome inhibitor bortezomib [53], inhibitor of apoptosis protein linked with X-chromosome (XIAP) [54], inhibitor of PI3K/mTOR [55], and different bisphosphonates [56] for their useas cooperative agents to MSCs-TRAIL DDSs.

MSCs are also used to employ the concept of gene-directed enzyme prodrug therapy (GDEPT) in delivery of anticancer drugs. There are two important steps: 1) the transfer of a gene provides genetic information for the enzyme which activates the prodrug, and 2) administration of a prodrug (inactive), which is locally activated into cytotoxic metabolites by the enzyme [57].

Combinations of enzyme and prodrug that have been successfully tested in animal models with malignant tumors in preclinical studies are the fusion of herpes simplex virus thymidine kinase (HSV-TK)/gancyclovir (GCV) [58 - 60], cytosine deaminase (CD)/5-fluorocytosine (5-FC) [46, 61, 62], carboxylesterase (CE)/ irinotecan (CPT-11) [63], and cytochrome P450 (CYP)/cyclophosphamide (CPA) or ifosfamide (IFO) [64, 65].

The application of these different kinds of genetically engineered MSC-based DDSs can be performed by using several methods for application: systemic (intravenous and intra-arterial), directional (intratumoral, intraperitoneal and intracerebral), and semi-directional (intratracheal administration) [35, 40, 44, 47, 66, 67].

By using anticancer genetically-engineered MSCs, tumors can be specifically targeted and affected through multiple mechanisms as presented in Table **2**.

Table 2. Mechanism for Specific Targeting and Affection to Tumors by Anticancer Gene-Engineered MSCs.

Mechanism	Characteristics	Effects
Migration and incorporation of MSCs at tumor site	1) Not affiliated to tumor type 2) Not affiliated to the MSCs delivery route	1) Agents are delivered by MSCs locally and constantly 2) Systemic side effects are minimized
Cancer-specific agents can be delivered or expressed by MSCs	Different anticancer genes can be engineered	Anticancer effects proved on several cancer models
Effects in the tumor microenvironment	Engineered MSCs are a source that constantly produces a specific anticancer agent	Efficiently induce tumor growth inhibition or apoptosis
Modification of the vector construction intended to and suitable for antigen expression in specific organs	MSCs secrete anticancer therapeutic proteins only when are in contact with tumors with specific location and consist of the same cell type	Selectively kills only tumor cells with the same protein (antigen) expression

Tumor tropism of MSCs is exploited for tumor targeting with active proteins, but according to our knowledge, recently, very few studies where MSCs are exploited for delivering small molecules exist. A recently published study by Layek *et al.* from 2016 [7] presents one very new approach of glycoengineered MSCs. The authors developed methods to implement azide groups on the surface of MSCs (groups that are not present naturally on MSCs) at the same time taking care not to affect their viability or capacity for tumor tropism. These artificial surface objects (azide functional groups) are introduced only in the tumor cells (not in the healthy tissues) by the application of this kind of modified MSCs. Subsequent administration of alkynes (such as DBCO- or dibenzylcyclooctyne-labeled fluorophores or nanoparticles), to animal models (mouse) previously treated with these surface-modified MSCs resulted in improved tumor accumulation of active agents [68]. This DBCO-based fluorophoresence can be used for imaging cancer cells. Furthermore, the same authors investigated the application of glycoengineered MSCs together with DBCO-nanoparticles loaded with drug paclitaxel and their results showed significant ($p < 0.05$) inhibition of growth of the tumor in an ovarian tumor model with metastasis [7, 69].

The MSCs labeled with visualizable agents can be monitored *in vivo*. One interesting approach that enables the study of MSC tumor tropism involves genetic manipulation of MSCs with introduction of reporter gene (MSCs-R) for luciferase-enhanced green fluorescence protein (fLuc-eGFP) from fireflies [70]. Non-invasive cell tracking can also be provided through the use of superparamagnetic iron oxide nanoparticles (SPIONs) for labeling and subsequent visualization of various cell types with magnetic resonance imaging (MRI) [71, 72] or through labeling with radioactive markers (^{111}In) for PET and SPECT *in vivo* imaging [73].

Genetically-engineered MSCs are a powerful tool in anticancer therapy, but this approach only allows delivery of protein-based drugs at the tumor site. In addition, the process of genetic modification itself could affect the MSCs innate characteristics. These observations encouraged new directions in recent years for the development of DDSs using MSC-systems based on nanoparticles (NPs) [74].

2.2.2. Non-Genetically Engineered MSCs as DDSs

With genetically engineered MSCs only protein drugs can be delivered. Because of this, researchers now investigate new NP-delivery strategies for delivering non-peptidic drugs. Drug-loaded NP can be associated with MSCs, and as MSCs migrates to the target tumor tissue, the drug can be released in the exact desired location. MSC and NP coupling occurs through either cellular internalization or lipid membrane fusion [74]. Because MSCs possess their own advantages (tumor homing properties, low toxicity and low immunogenicity), these combinations have higher delivery efficiency compared to conventional NP delivery systems.

MSC surface modification is another approach used to improve the cell's homing property and subsequent drug delivery.

2.2.2.1. Incorporation of Therapeutic Agents in MSCs with NPs

Currently, there are two methods proposed for drug incorporation in MSCs by using NPs, both presented in Fig. (**2**).

NPs used are usually polymeric or liposomal. Polymeric NPs are typically prepared using polymer poly-(D, L-lactide) (PLA) and its derivatives. Cellular internalization occurs through endocytosis or pinocytosis and is dependent on the structure, dimension, and surface charge of the NP [74, 75]. In one study using MSCs loaded with PLA-NPs with encapsulated coumarin-6, it was shown that MSC viability was not affected even when MSCs were subjected to high doses of NPs (200μg/mL) [76]. When another derivative of PLA is used, poly-(D,L-lactic acid-co-α,β -malic acid) (PLMA), these NPs are constructed of iron oxide and the suitable fluorescent dye. This kind of systems may be used in two manners, as bifunctional contrast agents for MSCs-tracking with magnetic resonance (MR) on one hand, and for fluorescent visualizations on another [77].

In the second approach, liposomal NPs can interact with the MSCs surface, undergo fusion with the membranes, and can transfer the drug loading on the cell (Fig. (**2B**)). As a final outcome, on the cell surface a synthetic object (receptor) could be formed [74, 77 - 79]. Usually, NPs containing polymers are better organized and efficient in drug loading in comparison with liposomal NPs [80]. When MSCs are associated with NPs, they stay stable and their tumor tropism ability is not influenced, including the ability for crossing the blood-brain barrier [18, 81]. This fact gives advantages of use of MSCs loaded with therapeutic agents over conventional anticancer therapeutics.

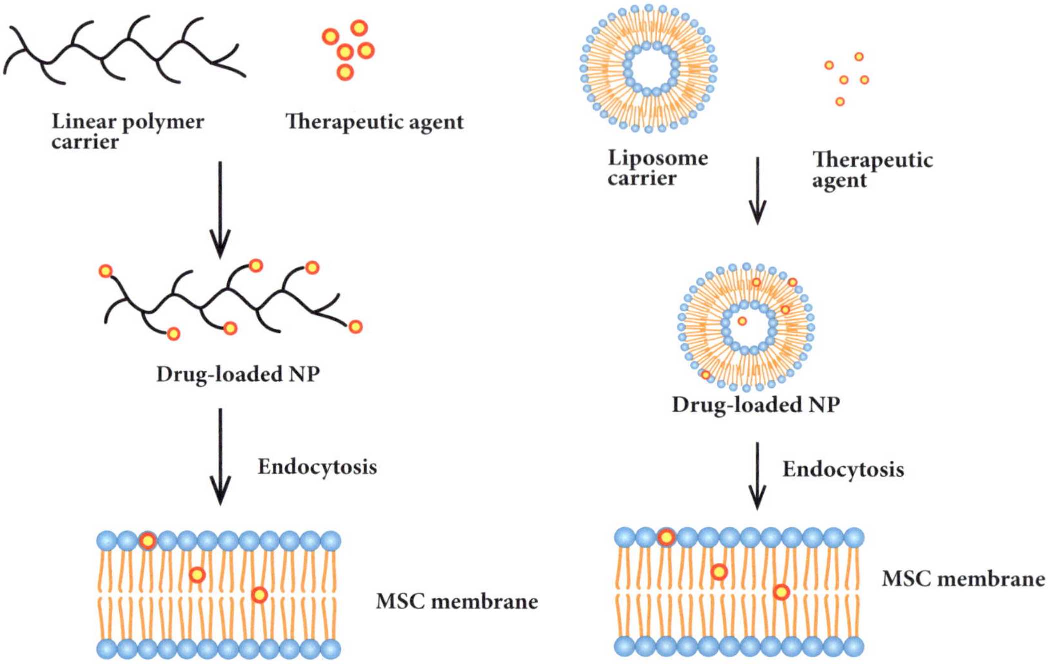

Fig. (2). Mechanisms of coupling MSCs with drug loaded NPs: (**A**) with endocytosis for polymeric NPs and (**B**) fusion of lipid membranes for liposomal NPs.

2.2.2.2. Surface Modification of MSCs

Despite the known advantages of MSCs, application of modifications as genetic manipulations, and previously mentioned coupling of MSCs with NPs loaded with therapeutic agents, delivering of a therapeutically effective dose to the desired site is a challenge.

MSCs surface modification in order to introduce targeting moieties is an attempt to deal with and/or lower the risks associated with multiple MSC-administrations (such as activation of the immunity and systemic toxicity).

The most popular methods for surface modifications are enzymatic modifications [82, 83], chemical modifications via the covalent bioconjugation method [84 - 86], and clinically very attractive - conjugation of antibodies or peptides with MSCs. Conjugation of antibodies is a promising approach in cancer immunotherapy due to the high affinity of antibodies towards the specific and unique tumor antigens overexpressed only on the tumor cells [87 - 89]. In this way, the recognition of antibodies as DDS - non-self for the body can be avoided.

The newest patents concerning MSCs in a role of drug carriers are given in Section 5 of this chapter (Recent patents concerning cell-based DDSs).

2.3. Dendritic Cells (DCs)

Dendritic cells (DCs) are derived from bone marrow and serve as antigen-presenting cells (APCs). Apart from being found everywhere in the body, DCs are highly concentrated in antigen exposed areas, specifically mucosal and epithelial linings. Their function lies in recognizing, capturing and processing exogenous antigens. In fact, DCs tend to migrate from blood into tissues to perform their functions.

Two types of DCs exist:

- Immature DCs, with high phagocytic potential, but low performance as APCs, and
- Mature DCs, cells that have undergone maturation in phenotypic and functional means, thus expressing major histocompatibility complex (MHC) class I and II antigens along with other molecules which add to their function as APCs. Mature DCs have small phagocytic potential, compared to their immature predecessors, but potent T-cell stimulating activity.

Maturation occurs after antigen stimulation, using specific pathogen-related molecular patterns, via toll-like receptors (TLRs), and also by secretion of inflammatory cytokines and prostaglandins in the environment [90]. These different maturation patterns enable the creation of different populations of DCs with various functional capabilities which in turn leaves various populations of DCs open to investigation in immunotherapy.

Recent research had shown that, besides priming the immune response after interacting with T cells, DCs are responsible for preventing autoimmunity in suppressing the regulatory action of T-cells and in inducing antigen-specific unresponsiveness in lymphoid, but also peripheral organs [90 - 92]. Another property of DCs, along with monocytes and macrophages, is their ability to accumulate in large numbers in vascular, hypoxic sites in cancer tumors, therefore making these cells eligible for potential use as drug carriers in breast carcinomas [93, 94]. Their basic role in the immunological system is presented in Fig. (**3**).

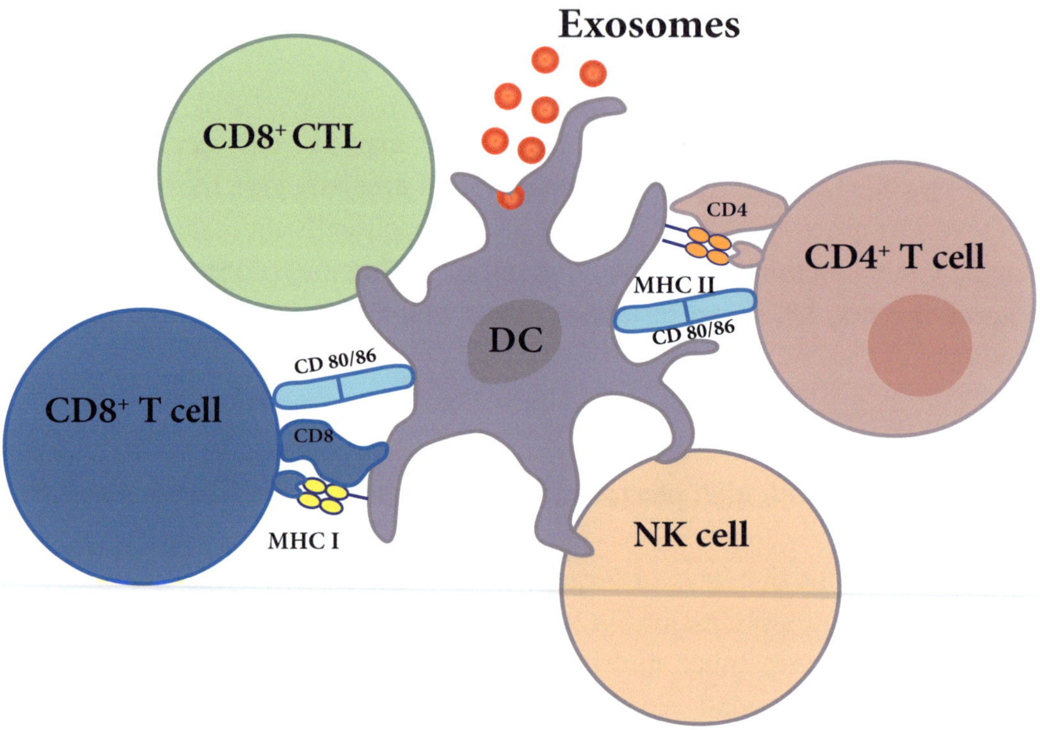

Fig. (3). Basic communication patterns between dendritic cells (DCs) and different types of T cells. DCs migrate to the lymph nodes and act as APC to T cells.

The T-cell receptor recognizes a specific peptide of the MHC molecule in a way that $CD4^+$ T-cells communicate with MHC class II molecules while $CD8^+$ T-cells interact with MHC class I. The interaction of T cells and DCs includes the costimulatory molecules CD80 and CD86, expressed on DCs.

2.3.1. Inclusion of DCs in Anticancer Therapy

Considering the biology of DCs, their capability to accumulate at tumor sites, as well their immunosuppressive action, novel strategies in cancer and immunotherapy can be considered, especially in addition to conventional immunotherapy (Fig. (**4**)):

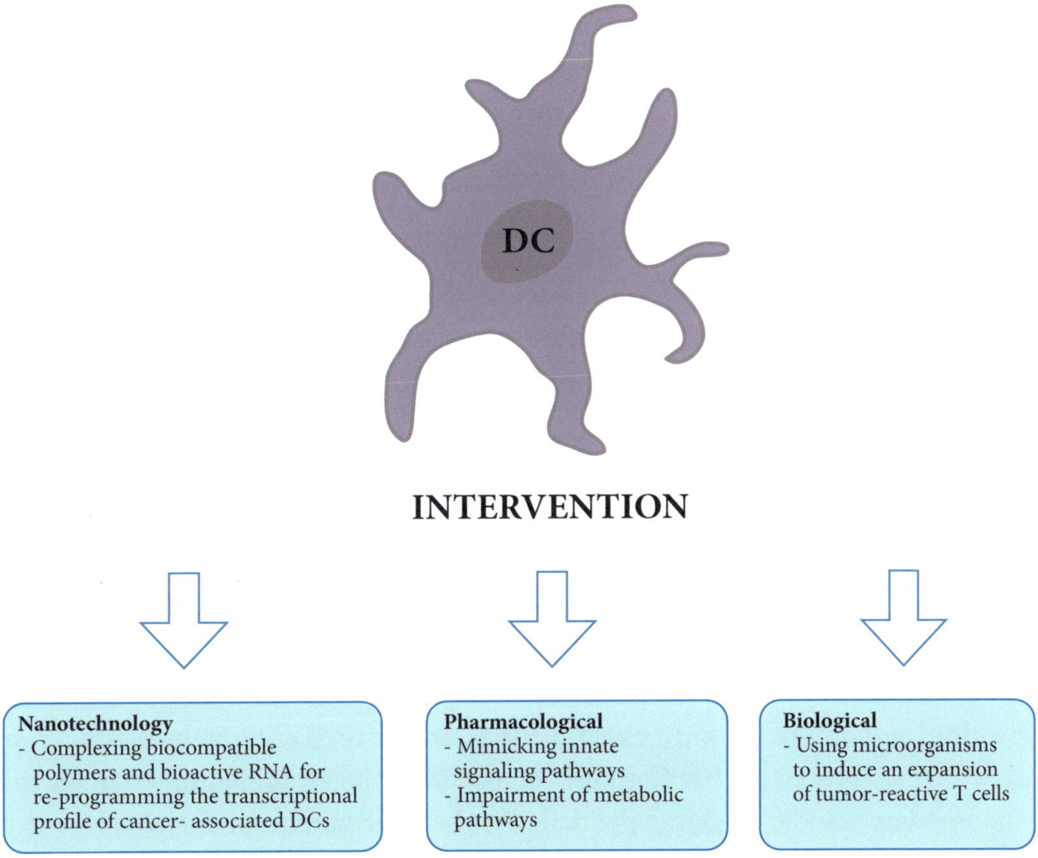

Fig. (4). Interventions made to increase immunostimulatory potential of DCs.

1. Enhancing the immunostimulatory properties of DCs that are associated with tumor cells by using nanomaterials.
2. Applying certain pharmacological and biological interventions.

DCs are in the spotlight of recent investigations for new technologies for vaccine development [95 - 99], moreover, recent patents in this field and clinical trials in progress for different types of cancer (prostate cancer, breast cancer, renal cancer, leukemia) [100, 101] reveal their great potential and use as new drug carriers. The last developments in this field are given in Section 5 of this chapter (Recent patents concerning cell-based DDSs).

3. CELL-DERIVED EXOSOMES FOR DRUG DELIVERY

Exosomes present a family of nanoparticles having a diameter from 30-120nm. Most of the body cell types secrete them, specifically the cells of the immune system, DCs, macrophages, B and T cells, and MSCs, endothelial and epithelial cells [102 - 104]. Thus, they can be located in extracellular fluids: blood, urine, semen, amniotic fluid, ascites fluid, breast milk, saliva, bile and cerebrospinal fluid [105 - 108]. Exosomes and other types of microvesicles are also secreted by a variety of cancer cells [109].

Being discovered 35 years ago as structures helping discard unwanted cell contains, exosomes experienced complete change of perspective. Although described in earlier works, exosomes were first isolated by Johnstone *et al.*, in 1987 [110], as reticulocyte-derived vesicles, suggesting that their formation may be a mechanism for manifestation of specific membrane functions. In addition, it was confirmed that exosomes are used for discarding cell contains that were not processed by lysosomes [111]. Recent research has extended the role of exosomes. Beside the role in intracellular signaling, the roles in B- and T-cell activation, certain immune effector functions and normal antigen presentation by DCs were also proposed. Furthermore, considering the aforementioned, their role in the immune response against the cells that have been malignantly transformed, has also been proposed. Thus, today exosomes are regarded as cellular entities that play specific roles in diseases [112], which have the possibility to be loaded with RNA, proteins, or other small molecules in order to achieve specific effect [113].

The process of exosome formation starts by invagination into endosomal membranes, and subsequent formation of multivesicular bodies [114]. Exosomes are then secreted by fusion of the multivesicular bodies and the cell membrane. Exosomes are increasingly released in cells prone to high proliferation, including MSCs. In experimental conditions, using gene transfection, these cells may be induced to large production of exosomes, without present mediators, or any physiological interventions [115]. In order to select exosomes having the desired characteristics, it is necessary to first select the donor cell type. The produced exosomes must be stable in the body fluids (circulation) within a sufficient period of time, in order to deliver the loaded drug. Also, they have to be produced in cells free of immunological stimulation to prevent inflammatory responses after administration [113]. Limitations of their use as future DDSs that must be taken in consideration are the facts that mammalian cells produce low quantities of exosomes and their complicated purification.

3.1. Exosomes in Anticancer Therapy

Exosomes have several properties that qualify them as potential therapeutics. The possibility of being recognized and taken-up by other cells, their role in intercellular communication associated with tumor progression, metastasis and drug resistance, and again their role in immune response, combined with their *in vivo* and *in vitro* stability and bioavailability, tolerability, regulation of gene expression by miRNA and siRNA transfer to target cells, as well as the fact that they can serve as natural liposomes [116], led to two main directions of their utilization in anticancer therapy:

1. Exosome-augmented immunotherapy, i.e. exploiting the capacity of exosomes to stimulate the immune system using vaccines (exosomes derived from dendritic cells that had been exposed to tumor cells) and
2. Exosomes as anticancer drug carriers, showing the potential of reduced side effects and targeted action, due to their endogenous origin. For example, Sun *et al.* in 2010 [17] incorporated curcumin into exosomes, resulting with its increased solubility, stability, and bioavailability, enhancing/increasing delivery of curcumin to activated monocytes.

In the context of exosomes-augmented immunotherapy, Escudier *et al.*, in 2005 [117] presented the results of their first Phase I clinical trial of the vaccination with autologous exosomes, derived from DCs in patients with metastatic melanoma. Morse *et al.*, in 2005 [118] conducted a trial of dexosome (autologous dendritic cell-derived exosomes) immunotherapy in patients with advanced non-small cell lung cancer, and Dai *et al.*, in 2008 [119] presented the results of Phase I clinical trial of autologous exosomes, derived from ascites fluid, combined with GM-CSF in the treatment of colorectal cancer. The studies continued to emerge, with Hartman *et al.*, 2011 [120] suggesting enhancing the potency of vaccines, using exosome antigen targeting. They suggested an approach of producing adenoviral vectors expressing the extracellular domain of two non-mutated tumor associated antigens, carcinoembryonic antigen and HER2, coupling them to the lactadherin C1C2 domain.

Investigating the expression of specific immunosuppressive molecules in exosomes derived from tumor cells, Zhang *et al.* in 2010 revealed that exosomes which are derived from renal cancer cells attached to IL-12 expressed antigens associated to renal cell carcinoma. These exosomes presented tumor rejection antigens and also possessed enhanced immunogenic and antitumor properties. In their work, they used GPI anchored IL-12 and presented a vaccine that demonstrated increased *in vitro* cytotoxic effects, thus opening the pathway in vaccine treatment based on exosomes in case of renal cell carcinoma [121].

On the other hand, exosomes can serve as versatile drug carriers. Recent studies dealt with different types of load, from different types of RNA [122 - 124] to doxorubicin-loaded, dendritic cell-derived exosomes in treatment of αv integrin-positive breast cancer cells *in vitro* and in tumor tissue in BALB/c nude mice [125]. Again, other cargos have been considered also, such as superparamagnetic iron oxide in B16-exosomes [126], and curcumin- loaded EL-4-derived exosomes [17].

Still, successful delivery of therapeutic cargos to exosomes needs inclusion of a compatible method. In this sense, traditional methods of cell transfection have been exploited, including several novel methods of transfection and/or activation of donor cells. These methods, as well as routes of administration, have thoroughly been reviewed by Johnsen *et al.*, in 2014 [113].

4. CELL MEMBRANE-BASED DDSs

Some of the above mentioned cells can be used as membrane sources, interesting new starting materials for the production of anticancer delivery systems. The most exploited in the recent investigations have been the novel cell membrane-coated particles, consisted of synthetic polymers [3, 4, 127, 128], the Red Blood Cells (RBC)-derived microvesicles [129-131], the mesenchymal stem cell nanoghosts (MSC-NG) [19] and cell membrane-derived microparticles from tumor cells

[132].

These membrane-derived particles can serve for packaging and delivering of therapeutic agents directly to the tumor with enhanced stability and efficiency, and minimized systemic toxicity. For example, Furman *et al.*, in their work from 2013, obtained NGs with extrusion method, which retained > 50% of MSC surface markers, and were loaded with sTRAIL [19]. These sTRAIL-MSC-NGs caused apoptosis of 89% of tumor cells and 70% reduction of tumor growth after single administration. Forming of MSC-NGs where nucleic matter is removed is one promising option to overcome some adverse effects and genetic risks when using MSCs containing therapeutic agents.

5. RECENT PATENTS CONCERNING CELL-BASED DDSs

Recent patents in this field evidenced that cell-based systems could be the new promising drug delivery systems for anticancer agents in very near future. There are number of patents concerning different cells or cell particles as possible DDSs [133]. For example, RBCs loaded with proteins able to form complex with different drugs were investigated a few years ago, and there are already some formulations that granted the designation as "Orphan drug" [134]. Also, between cells/cell particles employed in researches for suitable DDSs, exosomes are probably the leader according to the number of investigations published or in process, at this moment. In one recent report, exosomes (these particles contain at least 70% of proteins in an MSC conditioned medium) derived from MSCs are described as part of pharmaceutical composition together with suitable excipient, diluents or carrier intended for treatment of a disease (cancer) [135]. The same inventor updated his invention with the patent published 2016 [136]. Natural exosomes with Fc receptors that can be produced by any cell that can deliver exosomes - engineered T cells, macrophages, stem cells, mesenchymal stromal cells or combinations, are subject of interest in the patent published by Seeger *et al.*, in 2015 [137]. Interesting in this research is the possibility to form pharmaceutical composition with exosomes where therapeutic agents such as small molecules drugs, nucleic acids, peptides, proteins or antibodies can be included. The authors present ability to target cancer cell with exosome comprise antibodies additionally conjugated with the therapeutic anticancer agent. The treatment of disease such as cancer by delivering anticancer agents to the cancer cells by cell microvesicles is described in quite a new research study by Breakefield *et al.*, from 2015 [138]. Modified stem cells that comprise microparticle or nanoparticle containing an active agent are the subject of interest and discussed as cell-theranostic in the patent published in 2013 [139]. In addition, nanoparticles containing different drugs can be encapsulated with the cell membrane, which presents interesting new DDSs [140].

There is a great interest in the delivery of therapeutic anticancer proteins with cell-carriers. For example, in the invention published in 2014 (The General Hospital Corporation) there is a description of novel compositions comprising multimodal TRAIL agents and cells engineered to express such multimodal TRAIL agents [141]. These multimodal therapeutic agents can be very useful in combinatorial therapies with surgical interventions, radiotherapy, or chemotherapy.

In a patent published in 2014, interactions of MSCs with dendritic cells, two types of helper T-cells, and NK cells were described in a view of the possibility for their usage as anticancer therapy [142]. Dendritic cells are those that are in the center of research where formulation of cancer vaccine is the final goal [143, 144].

Table **3** summarizes the selected, recently published inventions (2013-2016) related to the usage of cells or cell particles as DDSs [135 - 144, 145 - 159].

Table 3. Patents Concerning Cell-Based Anticancer Drug Delivery Systems.

Patent/Year	Inventor(s)	Reference	Description of the Invention
US20130071326 (2013)	Martinez, J.O., Tasciotti, E., Kolonin, M., Ferrari, M.	[139]	Modified stem cells that comprise microparticle or nanoparticle containing active agent
US8455188 (2013)	Taylor, D.D., Gercel-Taylor, C.	[145]	Methods of producing/using modified exosomes in cancer therapy
US8524679 (2013)	Pachuk, C.	[146]	Methods of delivering nucleic acids to mammalian cells via intercellular transfer
US20130052272 (2013)	Cohen, S.	[147]	Cell extracts for treatment and prevention of cancer

(Table 3) contd.....

Patent/Year	Inventor(s)	Reference	Description of the Invention
WO2013052167 (2013)	Zhang, L., Fang, R.H., Hu, C-M., Copp, J.	[140]	Nanoparticles encapsulated with cell membrane
US8697439 (2014)	Mangeot, P., Lotteau, V.	[148]	*In vitro* method for delivering proteins into target cells by using microvesicles
US2014016776 (2014)	Aggarwal, S., Pittenger, M.F., Varney, T.	[142]	Mesenchymal stem cells and their uses
US20140056909 (2014)	Markovic, S.N.	[149]	Cancer treatment
US20140086907 (2014)	The General Hospital Corporation	[141]	Multimodal TRAIL molecules and uses in cellular therapies
US20150374702 (2015)	Kuh, H.J., Kim, J.H.	[150]	Delivery of anticancer agents
US20150175667 (2015)	Wang, P., Yang, L., Baltimore, D.	[143]	Delivery of polynucleotide encoding a gene of interest (usually an antigen) to a DC, where compositions can be used to treat cancer
US20150374714 (2015)	Dhar, S., Marrache, S., Harn, D.A., Tundup, S.	[144]	Activation of DCs to produce INF-γ by NPs containing a photosensitizer with application in enhancing immunogenicity of cancer cells
US20150086515 (2015)	Cheng, Z., Chen, K., Chen, X.	[151]	MSCs as target-delivery vehicle
US2015/0190430 (2015)	Lim, S.K.	[135]	Exosomes derived from MSCs as part of pharmaceutical formulation
US9085778 (2015)	Lötvall, J., Valadi, H.	[152]	Methods of introducing nucleic acids to cells via exosomes
US20150079631 (2015)	Breakefield, X.O., Bolukbasi, M.F., Mizrak, A., Saydam, O.	[138]	Delivering of therapeutic agents by administering microvesicles
WO2015058148 (2015)	Seeger, R.C., Fabbri, M., Jong, A., Wayne, A.S.	[137]	Therapy with exosomes in pharmaceutical composition where antibodies can also be included
WO2015120150 (2015)	Trujillo, K.	[153]	Exosomes as an anticancer therapeutic
WO2015189395 (2015)	Garrido-Fleury, C., Gobbo, J., Seigneuric, R., Marcion, G.	[154]	Compositions for diagnosing, monitoring and treatment of cancer
WO2016022947 (2016)	Quinones-Hinojosa, A., Green, J.	[155]	Modification of MSCs with nanoparticles for treating brain cancer
US20160220613 (2016)	Lim, S.K.	[136]	Exosomes derived from MSCs as part of pharmaceutical formulation
WO2016120853 (2016)	Shrivastava, S.	[156]	Compositions and methods for monitoring, diagnosis, prognosis, detection, and treatment of cancer

(Table 3) contd.....

Patent/Year	Inventor(s)	Reference	Description of the Invention
US20160287665 (2016)	Austyn, J., Preston, S., Nuttall, P., Paesen, G.	[157]	Pharmaceutical compositions comprising the DC modulatory molecule and/or active fragments and antibodies, intended for use in treating diseases including cancers
US20160008397 (2016)	Krams, S.M., Lau, A.H.	[158]	Modified DCs and methods of using them in cellular therapy for treating different immune conditions including cancer
US20160058886 (2016)	de Fonseca, N.A.C., Gomes Da Silva, L.C., Caldeira De Moura, V.L.D.N., De MagalhaesSimoes, S.P., De Almeida Moreira, J.N.S.	[159]	Therapy and diagnostics using NPs that provide targeted delivery of agents to cancer cells and stem cells

6. CURRENT & FUTURE DEVELOPMENTS

The increased understanding of disease processes and mechanisms, along with the inexorable progress in biotechnology, pharmacology and related disciplines, have led the search for new and/or improved treatment methods. In this context, cancer research is probably the leader, joining the scientific efforts of many researchers worldwide.

The pursue for ideal DDS is parallel with the pursue for new therapeutic agents. Still, the need of favorable pharmacokinetics and bioavailability, thus achieving low toxicity, specificity and selectivity, remains a great challenge to be addressed. Cells used as carriers can be isolated from the same patient, which is a great advantage of cell-based DDS and along with the low toxicity and low immunogenicity, this can be a step forward in personalized medicine and individualization of therapy. Another very promising feature of these cell-based systems is the possibility for their use not only for therapy, but also for diagnostic purposes when they are labeled with a suitable agent [69, 71, 72, 77].

In this chapter, we tried to summarize the available to-date approaches and methodologies used in designing cell-based DDS. The versatility of these systems extends beyond cancer treatment so it is expected that some of these strategies will be very important and of clinical significance in the period that follows.

According to the desired therapeutic effect, different approaches to the design of DDS can be selected: encapsulating the drug into the cells/attached to cell surface; engineering the cells to secrete desired therapeutic protein; generating new bio-synthetic systems, etc.

In future, further development of gene-based and RNAi - based therapeutic modalities is expected. The selection of suitable DDS that meets the needs of successful delivery of these agents is expected to be based on cells and cell-membranes, since these natural materials can provide safety, selectivity and efficacy in delivering the cell load. Beside transportation of loaded drugs inside the body, this cell-based DDSs can be used as a new strategy of drug producing cell modules where therapeutic agents will be produced on site and/or released in the blood circulation.

Currently, the rise in clinical trials involving cell therapies is evident, as there are 277 registered ones for various cell types in public clinical trials database (http://www.clinicaltrials.gov (accessed 29.08.2016)). It is expected that in the future, cell-based DDS will be more exploited as delivery systems for known chemotherapeutics, providing reduced systemic side-effects and enhanced site-specificity. Certainly, limitations in the design and usage of DDS do exist and must be overcome before these advanced systems become a standard pharmaceutical formulation and a part of everyday clinical practice. On the one hand, there are the challenges in providing consistent, optimized, large-scale production of these systems, and on the other, the need for regulatory issues evolution regarding these newly designed DDSs for ensuring safe and efficient clinical application of these products.

CONFLICT OF INTEREST

The authors confirm that they have no conflict of interest to declare for this publication.

ACKNOWLEDGEMENTS

The authors want to acknowledge the great assistance of Mr. Slave Dimitrov for the technical support in preparing the figures presented in this text chapter.

REFERENCES

[1] Chertok B, Webber MJ, Succi MD, Langer R. Drug delivery interfaces in the 21st century: From science fiction ideas to viable technologies. Mol Pharm 2013; 10(10): 3531-43. [http://dx.doi.org/10.1021/mp4003283] [PMID: 23915375]

[2] Fliervoet LA, Mastrobattista E. Drug delivery with living cells. Adv Drug Deliv Rev 2016; 106(Pt A): 63-72. [http://dx.doi.org/10.1016/j.addr.2016.04.021] [PMID: 27129442]

[3] Luk BT, Hu C-M, Fang RH, *et al.* Interfacial interactions between natural RBC membranes and synthetic polymeric nanoparticles. Nanoscale 2014; 6(5): 2730-7. [http://dx.doi.org/10.1039/C3NR06371B] [PMID: 24463706]

[4] Fang RH, Hu C-M, Luk BT, *et al.* Cancer cell membrane-coated nanoparticles for anticancer vaccination and drug delivery. Nano Lett 2014; 14(4): 2181-8. [http://dx.doi.org/10.1021/nl500618u] [PMID: 24673373]

[5] Pal A, Ahmad A, Khan S, *et al.* Systemic delivery of RafsiRNA using cationic cardiolipin liposomes silences Raf-1 expression and inhibits tumor growth in xenograft model of human prostate cancer. Int J Oncol 2005; 26(4): 1087-91. [PMID: 15754006]

[6] Saisyo A, Nakamura H, Fang J, *et al.* pH-sensitive polymeric cisplatin-ion complex with styrene-maleic acid copolymer exhibits tumor-selective drug delivery and antitumor activity as a result of the enhanced permeability and retention effect. Colloids Surf B Biointerfaces 2016; 138: 128-37. [http://dx.doi.org/10.1016/j.colsurfb.2015.11.032] [PMID: 26674841]

[7] Layek B, Sadhukha T, Prabha S. Glycoengineered mesenchymal stem cells as an enabling platform for two-step targeting of solid tumors. Biomaterials 2016; 88: 97-109. [http://dx.doi.org/10.1016/j.biomaterials.2016.02.024] [PMID: 26946263]

[8] Kukowska-Latallo JF, Candido KA, Cao Z, *et al.* Nanoparticle targeting of anticancer drug improves therapeutic response in animal model of human epithelial cancer. Cancer Res 2005; 65(12): 5317-24. [http://dx.doi.org/10.1158/0008-5472.CAN-04-3921] [PMID: 15958579]

[9] Paukner S, Kohl G, Lubitz W. Bacterial ghosts as novel advanced drug delivery systems: Antiproliferative activity of loaded doxorubicin in human Caco-2 cells. J Control Release 2004; 94(1): 63-74. [http://dx.doi.org/10.1016/j.jconrel.2003.09.010] [PMID: 14684272]

[10] Eko FO, Lubitz W, McMillan L, *et al.* Recombinant *Vibrio cholerae* ghosts as a delivery vehicle for vaccinating against *Chlamydia trachomatis*. Vaccine 2003; 21(15): 1694-703. [http://dx.doi.org/10.1016/S0264-410X(02)00677-1] [PMID: 12639492]

[11] Kota J, Chivukula RR, ODonnell KA, *et al.* Therapeutic microRNA delivery suppresses tumorigenesis in a murine liver cancer model. Cell 2009; 137(6): 1005-17. [http://dx.doi.org/10.1016/j.cell.2009.04.021] [PMID: 19524505]

[12] Harisa GI, Badran MM, AlQahtani SA, Alanazi FK, Attia SM. Pravastatin chitosan nanogels-loaded erythrocytes as a new delivery strategy for targeting liver cancer. Saudi Pharm J 2016; 24(1): 74-81. [http://dx.doi.org/10.1016/j.jsps.2015.03.024] [PMID: 26903771]

[13] Leonard F, Louis CT, Yesantharao P, Tanei T, Alexander JF, Xuewu L, *et al.* Enhancing therapeutic efficacy of albumin bound paclitaxel in breast cancer liver metastasis by homing to tumor associated macrophages: *In vitro*, *in vivo* and *in silico* studies. In: Proceedings of the 107th Annual Meeting of the American Association for Cancer Research. Cancer Res 2016; 76(14 S): Abstract nr 1324.

[14] Cubillos-Ruiz JR, Engle X, Scarlett UK, *et al.* Polyethylenimine-based siRNA nanocomplexes reprogram tumor-associated dendritic cells via TLR5 to elicit therapeutic antitumor immunity. J Clin Invest 2009; 119(8): 2231-44.
[PMID: 19620771]

[15] Kucerova L, Altanerova V, Matuskova M, Tyciakova S, Altaner C. Adipose tissue-derived human mesenchymal stem cells mediated prodrug cancer gene therapy. Cancer Res 2007; 67(13): 6304-13.
[http://dx.doi.org/10.1158/0008-5472.CAN-06-4024] [PMID: 17616689]

[16] Matuskova M, Hlubinova K, Pastorakova A, *et al.* HSV-tk expressing mesenchymal stem cells exert bystander effect on human glioblastoma cells. Cancer Lett 2010; 290(1): 58-67.
[http://dx.doi.org/10.1016/j.canlet.2009.08.028] [PMID: 19765892]

[17] Sun D, Zhuang X, Xiang X, *et al.* A novel nanoparticle drug delivery system: The anti-inflammatory activity of curcumin is enhanced when encapsulated in exosomes. Mol Ther 2010; 18(9): 1606-14.
[http://dx.doi.org/10.1038/mt.2010.105] [PMID: 20571541]

[18] Pascucci L, Coccè V, Bonomi A, *et al.* Paclitaxel is incorporated by mesenchymal stromal cells and released in exosomes that inhibit *in vitro* tumor growth: A new approach for drug delivery. J Control Release 2014; 192: 262-70.
[http://dx.doi.org/10.1016/j.jconrel.2014.07.042] [PMID: 25084218]

[19] Toledano Furman NE, Lupu-Haber Y, Bronshtein T, *et al.* Reconstructed stem cell nanoghosts: A natural tumor targeting platform. Nano Lett 2013; 13(7): 3248-55.
[http://dx.doi.org/10.1021/nl401376w] [PMID: 23786263]

[20] Shi C. Recent progress toward understanding the physiological function of bone marrow mesenchymal stem cells. Immunology 2012; 136(2): 133-8.
[http://dx.doi.org/10.1111/j.1365-2567.2012.03567.x] [PMID: 22321024]

[21] Dominici M, Le Blanc K, Mueller I, *et al.* Minimal criteria for defining multipotent mesenchymal stromal cells. The International Society for Cellular Therapy Position Statement. Cytotherapy 2006; 8(4): 315-7.
[http://dx.doi.org/10.1080/14653240600855905] [PMID: 16923606]

[22] Dai T, Yang E, Sun Y, *et al.* Preparation and drug release mechanism of CTS-TAX-NP-MSCs drug delivery system. Int J Pharm 2013; 456(1): 186-94.
[http://dx.doi.org/10.1016/j.ijpharm.2013.07.070] [PMID: 23933442]

[23] Porada CD, Almeida-Porada G. Mesenchymal stem cells as therapeutics and vehicles for gene and drug delivery. Adv Drug Deliv Rev 2010; 62(12): 1156-66.
[http://dx.doi.org/10.1016/j.addr.2010.08.010] [PMID: 20828588]

[24] Wang Q, Cheng H, Peng H, Zhou H, Li PY, Langer R. Non-genetic engineering of cells for drug delivery and cell-based therapy. Adv Drug Deliv Rev 2015; 91: 125-40.
[http://dx.doi.org/10.1016/j.addr.2014.12.003] [PMID: 25543006]

[25] Shah K. Mesenchymal stem cells engineered for cancer therapy. Adv Drug Deliv Rev 2012; 64(8): 739-48.
[http://dx.doi.org/10.1016/j.addr.2011.06.010] [PMID: 21740940]

[26] Loebinger MR, Eddaoudi A, Davies D, Janes SM. Mesenchymal stem cell delivery of TRAIL can eliminate metastatic cancer. Cancer Res 2009; 69(10): 4134-42.
[http://dx.doi.org/10.1158/0008-5472.CAN-08-4698] [PMID: 19435900]

[27] Sasportas LS, Kasmieh R, Wakimoto H, *et al.* Assessment of therapeutic efficacy and fate of engineered human mesenchymal stem cells for cancer therapy. Proc Natl Acad Sci USA 2009; 106(12): 4822-7.
[http://dx.doi.org/10.1073/pnas.0806647106] [PMID: 19264968]

[28] Studeny M, Marini FC, Dembinski JL, *et al.* Mesenchymal stem cells: Potential precursors for tumor stroma and targeted-delivery vehicles for anticancer agents. J Natl Cancer Inst 2004; 96(21): 1593-603.
[http://dx.doi.org/10.1093/jnci/djh299] [PMID: 15523088]

[29] Loebinger MR, Kyrtatos PG, Turmaine M, *et al.* Magnetic resonance imaging of mesenchymal stem cells homing to pulmonary metastases using biocompatible magnetic nanoparticles. Cancer Res 2009; 69(23): 8862-7. b
[http://dx.doi.org/10.1158/0008-5472.CAN-09-1912] [PMID: 19920196]

[30] Sonabend AM, Ulasov IV, Tyler MA, Rivera AA, Mathis JM, Lesniak MS. Mesenchymal stem cells effectively deliver an oncolytic adenovirus to intracranial glioma. Stem Cells 2008; 26(3): 831-41.
[http://dx.doi.org/10.1634/stemcells.2007-0758] [PMID: 18192232]

[31] Khakoo AY, Pati S, Anderson SA, *et al.* Human mesenchymal stem cells exert potent antitumorigenic effects in a model of Kaposis sarcoma. J Exp Med 2006; 203(5): 1235-47.
[http://dx.doi.org/10.1084/jem.20051921] [PMID: 16636132]

[32] Patel SA, Meyer JR, Greco SJ, Corcoran KE, Bryan M, Rameshwar P. Mesenchymal stem cells protect breast cancer cells through regulatory T cells: Role of mesenchymal stem cell-derived TGF-beta. J Immunol 2010; 184(10): 5885-94.
[http://dx.doi.org/10.4049/jimmunol.0903143] [PMID: 20382885]

[33] Menon LG, Picinich S, Koneru R, *et al.* Differential gene expression associated with migration of mesenchymal stem cells to conditioned medium from tumor cells or bone marrow cells. Stem Cells 2007; 25(2): 520-8.
[http://dx.doi.org/10.1634/stemcells.2006-0257] [PMID: 17053212]

[34] Kidd S, Caldwell L, Dietrich M, *et al.* Mesenchymal stromal cells alone or expressing interferon-beta suppress pancreatic tumors *in vivo*, an effect countered by anti-inflammatory treatment. Cytotherapy 2010; 12(5): 615-25.
[http://dx.doi.org/10.3109/14653241003631815] [PMID: 20230221]

[35] Studeny M, Marini FC, Champlin RE, Zompetta C, Fidler IJ, Andreeff M. Bone marrow-derived mesenchymal stem cells as vehicles for interferon-beta delivery into tumors. Cancer Res 2002; 62(13): 3603-8.
[PMID: 12097260]

[36] Zischek C, Niess H, Ischenko I, *et al.* Targeting tumor stroma using engineered mesenchymal stem cells reduces the growth of pancreatic carcinoma. Ann Surg 2009; 250(5): 747-53. [http://dx.doi.org/10.1097/SLA.0b013e3181bd62d0] [PMID: 19826249]

[37] Sun X-Y, Nong J, Qin K, Warnock GL, Dai L-J. Mesenchymal stem cell-mediated cancer therapy: A dual-targeted strategy of personalized medicine. World J Stem Cells 2011; 3(11): 96-103. [http://dx.doi.org/10.4252/wjsc.v3.i11.96] [PMID: 22180830]

[38] Mishra PJ, Mishra PJ, Glod JW, Banerjee D. Mesenchymal stem cells: Flip side of the coin. Cancer Res 2009; 69(4): 1255-8. [http://dx.doi.org/10.1158/0008-5472.CAN-08-3562] [PMID: 19208837]

[39] Ren C, Kumar S, Chanda D, Chen J, Mountz JD, Ponnazhagan S. Therapeutic potential of mesenchymal stem cells producing interferon-α in a mouse melanoma lung metastasis model. Stem Cells 2008; 26(9): 2332-8. [http://dx.doi.org/10.1634/stemcells.2008-0084] [PMID: 18617688]

[40] Nakamizo A, Marini F, Amano T, *et al.* Human bone marrow-derived mesenchymal stem cells in the treatment of gliomas. Cancer Res 2005; 65(8): 3307-18. [PMID: 15833864]

[41] Chen XC, Wang R, Zhao X, *et al.* Prophylaxis against carcinogenesis in three kinds of unestablished tumor models via IL12-gene-engineered MSCs. Carcinogenesis 2006; 27(12): 2434-41. [http://dx.doi.org/10.1093/carcin/bgl069] [PMID: 16854952]

[42] Kim SM, Lim JY, Park SI, *et al.* Gene therapy using TRAIL-secreting human umbilical cord blood-derived mesenchymal stem cells against intracranial glioma. Cancer Res 2008; 68(23): 9614-23. [http://dx.doi.org/10.1158/0008-5472.CAN-08-0451] [PMID: 19047138]

[43] Yu R, Deedigan L, Albarenque SM, Mohr A, Zwacka RM. Delivery of sTRAIL variants by MSCs in combination with cytotoxic drug treatment leads to p53-independent enhanced antitumor effects. Cell Death Dis 2013; 4: e503. [http://dx.doi.org/10.1038/cddis.2013.19] [PMID: 23429289]

[44] Komarova S, Kawakami Y, Stoff-Khalili MA, Curiel DT, Pereboeva L. Mesenchymal progenitor cells as cellular vehicles for delivery of oncolytic adenoviruses. Mol Cancer Ther 2006; 5(3): 755-66. [http://dx.doi.org/10.1158/1535-7163.MCT-05-0334] [PMID: 16546991]

[45] Dembinski JL, Spaeth EL, Fueyo J, *et al.* Reduction of nontarget infection and systemic toxicity by targeted delivery of conditionally replicating viruses transported in mesenchymal stem cells. Cancer Gene Ther 2010; 17(4): 289-97. [http://dx.doi.org/10.1038/cgt.2009.67] [PMID: 19876078]

[46] Kucerova L, Matuskova M, Pastorakova A, *et al.* Cytosine deaminase expressing human mesenchymal stem cells mediated tumour regression in melanoma bearing mice. J Gene Med 2008; 10(10): 1071-82. [http://dx.doi.org/10.1002/jgm.1239] [PMID: 18671316]

[47] Nakamura K, Ito Y, Kawano Y, *et al.* Antitumor effect of genetically engineered mesenchymal stem cells in a rat glioma model. Gene Ther 2004; 11(14): 1155-64. [http://dx.doi.org/10.1038/sj.gt.3302276] [PMID: 15141157]

[48] Stagg J, Lejeune L, Paquin A, Galipeau J. Marrow stromal cells for interleukin-2 delivery in cancer

immunotherapy. Hum Gene Ther 2004; 15(6): 597-608.
[http://dx.doi.org/10.1089/104303404323142042] [PMID: 15212718]

[49] Mohr A, Lyons M, Deedigan L, *et al.* Mesenchymal stem cells expressing TRAIL lead to tumour growth inhibition in an experimental lung cancer model. J Cell Mol Med 2008; 12(6B): 2628-43. [http://dx.doi.org/10.1111/j.1582-4934.2008.00317.x] [PMID: 18373740]

[50] Picarda G, Trichet V, Téletchéa S, Heymann D, Rédini F. TRAIL receptor signaling and therapeutic option in bone tumors: The trap of the bone microenvironment. Am J Cancer Res 2012; 2(1): 45-64. [PMID: 22206045]

[51] Burns JS, Safwat A, Grisendi G, Kassem M, Dominici M. Sarcomas as a mise en abyme of mesenchymal stem cells: Exploiting interrelationships for cell mediated anticancer therapy. Cancer Lett 2012; 325(1): 1-10.
[http://dx.doi.org/10.1016/j.canlet.2012.05.027] [PMID: 22659735]

[52] Kim SM, Woo JS, Jeong CH, Ryu CH, Lim JY, Jeun SS. Effective combination therapy for malignant glioma with TRAIL-secreting mesenchymal stem cells and lipoxygenase inhibitor MK886. Cancer Res 2012; 72(18): 4807-17.
[http://dx.doi.org/10.1158/0008-5472.CAN-12-0123] [PMID: 22962275]

[53] Nagy K, Székely-Szüts K, Izeradjene K, *et al.* Proteasome inhibitors sensitize colon carcinoma cells to TRAIL-induced apoptosis via enhanced release of SMAC/DIABLO from the mitochondria. Pathol Oncol Res 2006; 12(3): 133-42.
[http://dx.doi.org/10.1007/BF02893359] [PMID: 16998592]

[54] Mohr A, Albarenque SM, Deedigan L, *et al.* Targeting of XIAP combined with systemic mesenchymal stem cell-mediated delivery of sTRAIL ligand inhibits metastatic growth of pancreatic carcinoma cells. Stem Cells 2010; 28(11): 2109-20.
[http://dx.doi.org/10.1002/stem.533] [PMID: 20882532]

[55] Bagci-Onder T, Wakimoto H, Anderegg M, Cameron C, Shah K. A dual PI3K/mTOR inhibitor, PI-103, cooperates with stem cell-delivered TRAIL in experimental glioma models. Cancer Res 2011; 71(1): 154-63.
[http://dx.doi.org/10.1158/0008-5472.CAN-10-1601] [PMID: 21084267]

[56] Moon MH, Jeong JK, Seo JS, *et al.* Bisphosphonate enhances TRAIL sensitivity to human osteosarcoma cells via death receptor 5 upregulation. Exp Mol Med 2011; 43(3): 138-45. [http://dx.doi.org/10.3858/emm.2011.43.3.016] [PMID: 21297379]

[57] Amara I, Touati W, Beaune P, de Waziers I. Mesenchymal stem cells as cellular vehicles for prodrug gene therapy against tumors. Biochimie 2014; 105: 4-11.
[http://dx.doi.org/10.1016/j.biochi.2014.06.016] [PMID: 24977933]

[58] Fillat C, Carrió M, Cascante A, Sangro B. Suicide gene therapy mediated by the herpes simplex virus thymidine kinase gene/Ganciclovir system: Fifteen years of application. Curr Gene Ther 2003; 3(1): 13-26.
[http://dx.doi.org/10.2174/1566523033347426] [PMID: 12553532]

[59] Menotti L, Cerretani A, Hengel H, Campadelli-Fiume G. Construction of a fully retargeted herpes simplex virus 1 recombinant capable of entering cells solely via human epidermal growth factor receptor 2. J Virol 2008; 82(20): 10153-61.

[http://dx.doi.org/10.1128/JVI.01133-08] [PMID: 18684832]

[60] Xu F, Li S, Li XL, *et al.* Phase I and biodistribution study of recombinant adenovirus vector-mediated herpes simplex virus thymidine kinase gene and ganciclovir administration in patients with head and neck cancer and other malignant tumors. Cancer Gene Ther 2009; 16(9): 723-30. [http://dx.doi.org/10.1038/cgt.2009.19] [PMID: 19363470]

[61] King I, Bermudes D, Lin S, *et al.* Tumor-targeted *Salmonella* expressing cytosine deaminase as an anticancer agent. Hum Gene Ther 2002; 13(10): 1225-33. [http://dx.doi.org/10.1089/104303402320139005] [PMID: 12133275]

[62] Crystal RG, Hirschowitz E, Lieberman M, *et al.* Phase I study of direct administration of a replication deficient adenovirus vector containing the *E. coli* cytosine deaminase gene to metastatic colon carcinoma of the liver in association with the oral administration of the pro-drug 5-fluorocytosine. Hum Gene Ther 1997; 8(8): 985-1001. [http://dx.doi.org/10.1089/hum.1997.8.8-985] [PMID: 9195221]

[63] Wierdl M, Morton CL, Weeks JK, Danks MK, Harris LC, Potter PM. Sensitization of human tumor cells to CPT-11 via adenoviral-mediated delivery of a rabbit liver carboxylesterase. Cancer Res 2001; 61(13): 5078-82. [PMID: 11431344]

[64] Touati W, Tran T, Seguin J, *et al.* A suicide gene therapy combining the improvement of cyclophosphamide tumor cytotoxicity and the development of an anti-tumor immune response. Curr Gene Ther 2014; 14(3): 236-46. [http://dx.doi.org/10.2174/1566523214666140424152734] [PMID: 24766134]

[65] Nguyen TA, Tychopoulos M, Bichat F, *et al.* Improvement of cyclophosphamide activation by CYP2B6 mutants: From *in silico* to *ex vivo.* Mol Pharmacol 2008; 73(4): 1122-33. [http://dx.doi.org/10.1124/mol.107.042861] [PMID: 18212249]

[66] Zhang ZX, Guan LX, Zhang K, Zhang Q, Dai LJ. A combined procedure to deliver autologous mesenchymal stromal cells to patients with traumatic brain injury. Cytotherapy 2008; 10(2): 134-9. [http://dx.doi.org/10.1080/14653240701883061] [PMID: 18368592]

[67] Xin H, Sun R, Kanehira M, *et al.* Intratracheal delivery of CX3CL1-expressing mesenchymal stem cells to multiple lung tumors. Mol Med 2009; 15(9-10): 321-7. [http://dx.doi.org/10.2119/molmed.2009.00059] [PMID: 19603106]

[68] Lee S, Koo H, Na JH, *et al.* Chemical tumor-targeting of nanoparticles based on metabolic glycoengineering and click chemistry. ACS Nano 2014; 8(3): 2048-63. [http://dx.doi.org/10.1021/nn406584y] [PMID: 24499346]

[69] Andreas K, Georgieva R, Ladwig M, *et al.* Highly efficient magnetic stem cell labeling with citrate-coated superparamagnetic iron oxide nanoparticles for MRI tracking. Biomaterials 2012; 33(18): 4515-25. [http://dx.doi.org/10.1016/j.biomaterials.2012.02.064] [PMID: 22445482]

[70] Wang H, Cao F, De A, *et al.* Trafficking mesenchymal stem cell engraftment and differentiation in tumor-bearing mice by bioluminescence imaging. Stem Cells 2009; 27(7): 1548-58. [http://dx.doi.org/10.1002/stem.81] [PMID: 19544460]

[71] Jasmin AL, Torres AL, Nunes HM, *et al.* Optimized labeling of bone marrow mesenchymal cells with superparamagnetic iron oxide nanoparticles and *in vivo* visualization by magnetic resonance imaging. J Nanobiotechnology 2011; 9: 4.
[http://dx.doi.org/10.1186/1477-3155-9-4] [PMID: 21542946]

[72] Li L, Jiang W, Luo K, *et al.* Superparamagnetic iron oxide nanoparticles as MRI contrast agents for non-invasive stem cell labeling and tracking. Theranostics 2013; 3(8): 595-615.
[http://dx.doi.org/10.7150/thno.5366] [PMID: 23946825]

[73] Villa C, Erratico S, Razini P, *et al.* Stem cell tracking by nanotechnologies. Int J Mol Sci 2010; 11(3): 1070-81.
[http://dx.doi.org/10.3390/ijms11031070] [PMID: 20480000]

[74] Park JS, Suryaprakash S, Lao Y-H, Leong KW. Engineering mesenchymal stem cells for regenerative medicine and drug delivery. Methods 2015; 84: 3-16.
[http://dx.doi.org/10.1016/j.ymeth.2015.03.002] [PMID: 25770356]

[75] Gratton SE, Ropp PA, Pohlhaus PD, *et al.* The effect of particle design on cellular internalization pathways. Proc Natl Acad Sci USA 2008; 105(33): 11613-8.
[http://dx.doi.org/10.1073/pnas.0801763105] [PMID: 18697944]

[76] Roger M, Clavreul A, Venier-Julienne MC, *et al.* Mesenchymal stem cells as cellular vehicles for delivery of nanoparticles to brain tumors. Biomaterials 2010; 31(32): 8393-401.
[http://dx.doi.org/10.1016/j.biomaterials.2010.07.048] [PMID: 20688391]

[77] Wang L, Neoh KG, Kang ET, Shuter B, Wang SC. Biodegradable magnetic-fluorescent magnetite/poly(dl-lactic acid-co-alpha,beta-malic acid) composite nanoparticles for stem cell labeling. Biomaterials 2010; 31(13): 3502-11.
[http://dx.doi.org/10.1016/j.biomaterials.2010.01.081] [PMID: 20144844]

[78] Sarkar D, Vemula PK, Zhao W, Gupta A, Karnik R, Karp JM. Engineered mesenchymal stem cells with self-assembled vesicles for systemic cell targeting. Biomaterials 2010; 31(19): 5266-74.
[http://dx.doi.org/10.1016/j.biomaterials.2010.03.006] [PMID: 20381141]

[79] Landázuri N, Tong S, Suo J, *et al.* Magnetic targeting of human mesenchymal stem cells with internalized superparamagnetic iron oxide nanoparticles. Small 2013; 9(23): 4017-26.
[http://dx.doi.org/10.1002/smll.201300570] [PMID: 23766267]

[80] Riegler J, Liew A, Hynes SO, *et al.* Superparamagnetic iron oxide nanoparticle targeting of MSCs in vascular injury. Biomaterials 2013; 34(8): 1987-94.
[http://dx.doi.org/10.1016/j.biomaterials.2012.11.040] [PMID: 23237516]

[81] Huang X, Zhang F, Wang H, *et al.* Mesenchymal stem cell-based cell engineering with multifunctional mesoporous silica nanoparticles for tumor delivery. Biomaterials 2013; 34(7): 1772-80.
[http://dx.doi.org/10.1016/j.biomaterials.2012.11.032] [PMID: 23228423]

[82] Sackstein R, Merzaban JS, Cain DW, *et al. Ex vivo* glycan engineering of CD44 programs human multipotent mesenchymal stromal cell trafficking to bone. Nat Med 2008; 14(2): 181-7.
[http://dx.doi.org/10.1038/nm1703] [PMID: 18193058]

[83] Xia L, McDaniel JM, Yago T, Doeden A, McEver RP. Surface fucosylation of human cord blood cells augments binding to P-selectin and E-selectin and enhances engraftment in bone marrow. Blood 2004;

104(10): 3091-6.
[http://dx.doi.org/10.1182/blood-2004-02-0650] [PMID: 15280192]

[84] Sarkar D, Spencer JA, Phillips JA, *et al.* Engineered cell homing. Blood 2011; 118(25): e184-91.
[http://dx.doi.org/10.1182/blood-2010-10-311464] [PMID: 22034631]

[85] Cheng H, Byrska-Bishop M, Zhang CT, *et al.* Stem cell membrane engineering for cell rolling using peptide conjugation and tuning of cell-selectin interaction kinetics. Biomaterials 2012; 33(20): 5004-12.
[http://dx.doi.org/10.1016/j.biomaterials.2012.03.065] [PMID: 22494889]

[86] DSouza S, Murata H, Jose MV, *et al.* Engineering of cell membranes with a bisphosphonate-containing polymer using ATRP synthesis for bone targeting. Biomaterials 2014; 35(35): 9447-58.
[http://dx.doi.org/10.1016/j.biomaterials.2014.07.041] [PMID: 25150889]

[87] Dennis JE, Cohen N, Goldberg VM, Caplan AI. Targeted delivery of progenitor cells for cartilage repair. J Orthop Res 2004; 22(4): 735-41.
[http://dx.doi.org/10.1016/j.orthres.2003.12.002] [PMID: 15183428]

[88] Chen A, Zheng G, Tykocinski ML. Hierarchical costimulator thresholds for distinct immune responses: Application of a novel two-step Fc fusion protein transfer method. J Immunol 2000; 164(2): 705-11.
[http://dx.doi.org/10.4049/jimmunol.164.2.705] [PMID: 10623813]

[89] Li J, Law HK, Lau YL, Chan GC. Differential damage and recovery of human mesenchymal stem cells after exposure to chemotherapeutic agents. Br J Haematol 2004; 127(3): 326-34.
[http://dx.doi.org/10.1111/j.1365-2141.2004.05200.x] [PMID: 15491295]

[90] Nencioni A, Grünebach F, Schmidt SM, *et al.* The use of dendritic cells in cancer immunotherapy. Crit Rev Oncol Hematol 2008; 65(3): 191-9.
[http://dx.doi.org/10.1016/j.critrevonc.2007.10.002] [PMID: 18055210]

[91] Morelli AE, Thomson AW. Tolerogenic dendritic cells and the quest for transplant tolerance. Nat Rev Immunol 2007; 7(8): 610-21.
[http://dx.doi.org/10.1038/nri2132] [PMID: 17627284]

[92] Sakaguchi S, Sakaguchi N, Asano M, Itoh M, Toda M. Immunologic self-tolerance maintained by activated T cells expressing IL-2 receptor alpha-chains (CD25). Breakdown of a single mechanism of self-tolerance causes various autoimmune diseases. J Immunol 1995; 155(3): 1151-64.
[PMID: 7636184]

[93] Leek RD, Lewis CE, Whitehouse R, Greenall M, Clarke J, Harris AL. Association of macrophage infiltration with angiogenesis and prognosis in invasive breast carcinoma. Cancer Res 1996; 56(20): 4625-9.
[PMID: 8840975]

[94] Lewis JS, Landers RJ, Underwood JC, Harris AL, Lewis CE. Expression of vascular endothelial growth factor by macrophages is up-regulated in poorly vascularized areas of breast carcinomas. J Pathol 2000; 192(2): 150-8.
[http://dx.doi.org/10.1002/1096-9896(2000)9999:9999<::AID-PATH687>3.0.CO;2-G] [PMID: 11004690]

[95] Conejo-Garcia JR, Rutkowski MR, Cubillos-Ruiz JR. State-of-the-art of regulatory dendritic cells in cancer. Pharmacol Therapeut 2016. http://dx.doi.org/10.1016/j.pharmthera.2016.04.003. [http://dx.doi.org/10.1016/j.pharmthera.2016.04.003]

[96] Paczesny S, Ueno H, Fay J, Banchereau J, Palucka AK. Dendritic cells as vectors for immunotherapy of cancer. Semin Cancer Biol 2003; 13(6): 439-47. [http://dx.doi.org/10.1016/j.semcancer.2003.09.008] [PMID: 15001163]

[97] Nouri-Shirazi M, Banchereau J, Fay J, Palucka K. Dendritic cell based tumor vaccines. Immunol Lett 2000; 74(1): 5-10. [http://dx.doi.org/10.1016/S0165-2478(00)00243-1] [PMID: 10996622]

[98] Banchereau J, Palucka AK. Dendritic cells as therapeutic vaccines against cancer. Nat Rev Immunol 2005; 5(4): 296-306. [http://dx.doi.org/10.1038/nri1592] [PMID: 15803149]

[99] Ballestrero A, Boy D, Moran E, Cirmena G, Brossart P, Nencioni A. Immunotherapy with dendritic cells for cancer. Adv Drug Deliv Rev 2008; 60(2): 173-83. [http://dx.doi.org/10.1016/j.addr.2007.08.026] [PMID: 17977615]

[100] Davis ID, Jefford M, Parente P, Cebon J. Rational approaches to human cancer immunotherapy. J Leukoc Biol 2003; 73(1): 3-29. [http://dx.doi.org/10.1189/jlb.0502261] [PMID: 12525559]

[101] Wang D, Zhang B, Gao H, *et al.* Clinical research of genetically modified dendritic cells in combination with cytokine-induced killer cell treatment in advanced renal cancer. BMC Cancer 2014; 14: 251. [http://dx.doi.org/10.1186/1471-2407-14-251] [PMID: 24720900]

[102] Thèry C, Amigorena S, Raposo G, Clayton A. Isolation and characterization of exosomes from cell culture supernatants and biological fluids. Curr Protoc Cell Biol 2006; 30: 3.22:3.22.1-3.22.29.

[103] Lai RC, Yeo RW, Tan KH, Lim SK. Exosomes for drug delivery - a novel application for the mesenchymal stem cell. Biotechnol Adv 2013; 31(5): 543-51. [http://dx.doi.org/10.1016/j.biotechadv.2012.08.008] [PMID: 22959595]

[104] Lai RC, Yeo RW, Lim SK. Mesenchymal stem cell exosomes. Semin Cell Dev Biol 2015; 40: 82-8. [http://dx.doi.org/10.1016/j.semcdb.2015.03.001] [PMID: 25765629]

[105] Record M, Subra C, Silvente-Poirot S, Poirot M. Exosomes as intercellular signalosomes and pharmacological effectors. Biochem Pharmacol 2011; 81(10): 1171-82. [http://dx.doi.org/10.1016/j.bcp.2011.02.011] [PMID: 21371441]

[106] Vlassov AV, Magdaleno S, Setterquist R, Conrad R. Exosomes: Current knowledgeof their composition, biological functions, and diagnostic and therapeutic potentials. Biochim Biophys Acta 2012; 1820: 940-8.

[107] Jia S, Zocco D, Samuels ML, *et al.* Emerging technologies in extracellular vesicle-based molecular diagnostics. Expert Rev Mol Diagn 2014; 14(3): 307-21. [http://dx.doi.org/10.1586/14737159.2014.893828] [PMID: 24575799]

[108] Ferguson SW, Nguyen J. Exosomes as therapeutics: The implications of molecular composition and exosomal heterogeneity. J Control Release 2016; 228: 179-90.

[http://dx.doi.org/10.1016/j.jconrel.2016.02.037] [PMID: 26941033]

[109] Benito-Martin A, Di Giannatale A, Ceder S, Peinado H. The new deal: A potential role for secreted vesicles in innate immunity and tumor progression. Front Immunol 2015; 6: 66. [http://dx.doi.org/10.3389/fimmu.2015.00066] [PMID: 25759690]

[110] Johnstone RM, Adam M, Hammond JR, Orr L, Turbide C. Vesicle formation during reticulocyte maturation. Association of plasma membrane activities with released vesicles (exosomes). J Biol Chem 1987; 262(19): 9412-20. [PMID: 3597417]

[111] Johnstone RM, Mathew A, Mason AB, Teng K. Exosome formation during maturation of mammalian and avian reticulocytes: Evidence that exosome release is a major route for externalization of obsolete membrane proteins. J Cell Physiol 1991; 147(1): 27-36. [http://dx.doi.org/10.1002/jcp.1041470105] [PMID: 2037622]

[112] Robinson SM, Fan L, White SA, Charnley RM, Mann J. The role of exosomes in the pathogenesis of pancreatic ductal adenocarcinoma. Int J Biochem Cell Biol 2016; 75: 131-9. [http://dx.doi.org/10.1016/j.biocel.2016.03.009] [PMID: 27017975]

[113] Johnsen KB, Gudbergsson JM, Skov MN, Pilgaard L, Moos T, Duroux M. Acomprehensive overview of exosomes as drug delivery vehicles - Endogenous nanocarriers for targeted cancer therapy. Biochim Biophys Acta 2014; 1846: 75-87.

[114] Raposo G, Nijman HW, Stoorvogel W, *et al.* B Lymphocytes secrete antigen-presenting vesicles. J Exp Med 1996; 183(3): 1161-72. [http://dx.doi.org/10.1084/jem.183.3.1161] [PMID: 8642258]

[115] Yeo RW, Lai RC, Zhang B, *et al.* Mesenchymal stem cell: An efficient mass producer of exosomes for drug delivery. Adv Drug Deliv Rev 2013; 65(3): 336-41. [http://dx.doi.org/10.1016/j.addr.2012.07.001] [PMID: 22780955]

[116] De Toro J, Herschlik L, Waldner C, Mongini C. Emerging roles of exosomes in normal and pathological conditions: New insights for diagnosis and therapeutic applications. Front Immunol 2015; 6: 203. [http://dx.doi.org/10.3389/fimmu.2015.00203] [PMID: 25999947]

[117] Escudier B, Dorval T, Chaput N, *et al.* Vaccination of metastatic melanoma patients with autologous dendritic cell (DC) derived-exosomes: Results of thefirst phase I clinical trial. J Transl Med 2005; 3(1): 10. [http://dx.doi.org/10.1186/1479-5876-3-10] [PMID: 15740633]

[118] Morse MA, Garst J, Osada T, *et al.* A Phase I study of dexosome immunotherapy in patients with advanced non-small cell lung cancer. J Transl Med 2005; 3(1): 9. [http://dx.doi.org/10.1186/1479-5876-3-9] [PMID: 15723705]

[119] Dai S, Wei D, Wu Z, *et al.* Phase I clinical trial of autologous ascites-derived exosomes combined with GM-CSF for colorectal cancer. Mol Ther 2008; 16(4): 782-90. [http://dx.doi.org/10.1038/mt.2008.1] [PMID: 18362931]

[120] Hartman ZC, Wei J, Glass OK, *et al.* Increasing vaccine potency through exosome antigen targeting. Vaccine 2011; 29(50): 9361-7.

[http://dx.doi.org/10.1016/j.vaccine.2011.09.133] [PMID: 22001882]

[121] Zhang Y, Luo CL, He BC, Zhang JM, Cheng G, Wu XH. Exosomes derived from IL-12-anchored renal cancer cells increase induction of specific antitumor response *in vitro*: A novel vaccine for renal cell carcinoma. Int J Oncol 2010; 36(1): 133-40.
[PMID: 19956842]

[122] Alvarez-Erviti L, Seow Y, Yin H, Betts C, Lakhal S, Wood MJ. Delivery of siRNA to the mouse brain by systemic injection of targeted exosomes. Nat Biotechnol 2011; 29(4): 341-5.
[http://dx.doi.org/10.1038/nbt.1807] [PMID: 21423189]

[123] Pan Q, Ramakrishnaiah V, Henry S, *et al.* Hepatic cell-to-cell transmission of small silencing RNA can extend the therapeutic reach of RNA interference (RNAi). Gut 2012; 61(9): 1330-9.
[http://dx.doi.org/10.1136/gutjnl-2011-300449] [PMID: 22198713]

[124] Shtam TA, Kovalev RA, Varfolomeeva EY, Makarov EM, Kil YV, Filatov MV. Exosomes are natural carriers of exogenous siRNA to human cells *in vitro*. Cell Commun Signal 2013; 11: 88.
[http://dx.doi.org/10.1186/1478-811X-11-88] [PMID: 24245560]

[125] Tian Y, Li S, Song J, *et al.* A doxorubicin delivery platform using engineered natural membrane vesicle exosomes for targeted tumor therapy. Biomaterials 2014; 35(7): 2383-90.
[http://dx.doi.org/10.1016/j.biomaterials.2013.11.083] [PMID: 24345736]

[126] Hood JL, Scott MJ, Wickline SA. Maximizing exosome colloidal stability following electroporation. Anal Biochem 2014; 448: 41-9.
[http://dx.doi.org/10.1016/j.ab.2013.12.001] [PMID: 24333249]

[127] Aryal S, Hu C-M, Fang RH, *et al.* Erythrocyte membrane-cloaked polymeric nanoparticles for controlled drug loading and release. Nanomedicine (Lond) 2013; 8(8): 1271-80.
[http://dx.doi.org/10.2217/nnm.12.153] [PMID: 23409747]

[128] Hu C-M, Fang RH, Luk BT, Zhang L. Nanoparticle-detained toxins for safe and effective vaccination. Nat Nanotechnol 2013; 8(12): 933-8.
[http://dx.doi.org/10.1038/nnano.2013.254] [PMID: 24292514]

[129] Bahmani B, Bacon D, Anvari B. Erythrocyte-derived photo-theranostic agents: Hybrid nano-vesicles containing indocyanine green for near infrared imaging and therapeutic applications. Sci Rep 2013; 3: 2180.
[http://dx.doi.org/10.1038/srep02180] [PMID: 23846447]

[130] Gupta N, Patel B, Ahsan F. Nano-engineered erythrocyte ghosts as inhalational carriers for delivery of fasudil: Preparation and characterization. Pharm Res 2014; 31(6): 1553-65.
[http://dx.doi.org/10.1007/s11095-013-1261-7] [PMID: 24449438]

[131] Chang M, Hsiao J-K, Yao M, *et al.* Homologous RBC-derived vesicles as ultrasmall carriers of iron oxide for magnetic resonance imaging of stem cells. Nanotechnology 2010; 21(23): 235103.
[http://dx.doi.org/10.1088/0957-4484/21/23/235103] [PMID: 20479509]

[132] Tang K, Zhang Y, Zhang H, *et al.* Delivery of chemotherapeutic drugs in tumour cell-derived microparticles. Nat Commun 2012; 3: 1282.
[http://dx.doi.org/10.1038/ncomms2282] [PMID: 23250412]

[133] Ackova DG, Kanjevac T, Rimondini L, Bosnakovski D. Perspectives in engineered mesenchymal

stem/stromal cells based anti- cancer drug delivery systems. Recent Patents Anticancer Drug Discov 2016; 11(1): 98-111.
[http://dx.doi.org/10.2174/1574892811666151111142721] [PMID: 26554397]

[134] Magnani M, Rossi L, Biagiotti S, Bianchi M. Drug delivery system. US20120141540, 2012.

[135] Lim SK. Mesenchymal stem cell particles. US20150190430, 2015.

[136] Lim SK. Method. US20160220613, 2016.

[137] Seeger RC, Fabbri M, Jong A, Wayne AS. Antibody dependent exosome therapy. WO2015058148, 2015.

[138] Breakefield XO, Bolukbasi MF, Mizrak A, Saydam O. Microvesicle-mediated delivery of therapeutic molecules. US20150079631, 2015.

[139] Martinez JO, Tasciotti E, Kolonin M, Ferrari M. Universal cell-directed theranostics. US20130071326, 2013.

[140] Zhang L, Fang RH, Hu C-M, Copp J. Membrane encapsulated nanoparticles and method of use. WO2013052167, 2013.

[141] The general hospital corporation. Multimodal TRAIL molecules and uses in cellular therapies. US20140086907, 2014.

[142] Aggarwal S, Pittenger MF, Varney T. Mesenchymal stem cellsand uses thereof. US2014016776, 2014.

[143] Wang P, Yang L, Baltimore D. Targeted gene delivery for dendritic cell vaccination. US20150175667, 2015.

[144] Dhar S, Marrache S, Harn DA, Tundup S. Generation of functional dendritic cellc. US20150374714, 2015.

[145] Taylor DD, Gercel-Taylor C. Modification of exosomal components to use as a vaccine. US8455188, 2013.

[146] Pachuk C. Generation of functional dendritic cellc. US20150374714, 2015.

[147] Cohen S. Pharmaceutical compositions and methods for the treatment and prevention of cancer. US20130052272, 2013.

[148] Mangeot P, Lotteau V. Direct protein delivery with engineered microvesicles. US8697439, 2014.

[149] Markovic SN. Treating cancer. US20140056909, 2014.

[150] Kuh HJ, Kim JH. Anticancer adjuvant containing pentoxifylline. US20150374702, 2015.

[151] Cheng Z, Chen K, Chen X. Imaging-aided gene therapy using mesenchymal stem cells as target-delivery vehicle. WO20150086515, 2015.

[152] Lötvall J, Valadi H. Exosome transfer of nucleic acids to cells. US9085778, 2015.

[153] Trujillo K. Exosomes as a therapeutic for cancer. WO2015120150, 2015.

[154] Garrido-Fleury C, Gobbo J, Seigneuric R, Marcion G. Methods and compositions for diagnosing, monitoring and treating cancer. WO2015189395, 2015.

[155] Quinones-Hinojosa A, Green J. Nanoparticle modification of human adipose-derived mesenchymal

stem cells for treating brain cancer and other neurological diseases. WO2016022947, 2016.

[156] Shrivastava S. Compositions and methods for monitoring, diagnosis, prognosis, detection, and treatment of cancer. WO2016120853, 2016.

[157] Austyn J, Preston S, Nuttall P, Paesen G. Dendritic cell modulatory molecule. US20160287665, 2016.

[158] Krams SM, Lau AH. Immunomodulation by controlling expression levels of microRNAs in dendritic cells. US2016008397, 2016.

[159] de Fonseca NAC, Gomes Da Silva LC, Caldeira De Moura VLDN, De Magalhaes Simoes SP, De Almeida Moreira JNS. Platform for targeted delivery to stem cells and tumor cells and uses thereof. US20160058886, 2016.

CHAPTER 4

Studies on Patents and the Associated Anti-cancer Drug Development in China

Jinhua Shen[1,*,#], **Guohua Zhu**[2,*,#], **Lichun Sun**[3,4,*,#], **Gengping Zhang**[1], **Leyang Qin**[1], **Feng Yang**[1], **Ruru Gao**[5] and **Xinhong Fan**[2]

[1] *Tongji University Library, Shanghai 200092, P.R. China*

[2] *Tongji Law School, Shanghai 200092, P.R. China*

[3] *Hunan Province Cooperative Innovation Center for Molecular Target New Drug Study, Institute of Pharmacy & Pharmacology, University of South China, Hengyang, 421001, P.R. China*

[4] *Department of Medicine, Tulane University Health Sciences Center, New Orleans, LA 70002, USA*

[5] *Department of Chemistry, Tongji University, Shanghai 200092, P.R. China*

Abstract: This chapter consists of five sections. The first part analyzes the macro policies of Chinese anti-cancer drugs, sorts the existing policies and regulations in China and clarifies the main departments of Chinese domestic drug regulation.

The second part is the analysis of Chinese domestic anti-cancer drug patents. Based on the domestic Chinese invention patents as the data source, this section analyzes Chinese domestic anti-cancer drug patents, major competitive countries and regions, developmental characteristics of patented technology, and the main applicants. It can be found that Chinese local patent applications have increased yearly since China began to protect drug patents in 1992. Up to the retrieval date, there is a total of 57,280 pieces of invention patents in China. Patent applications of China, the United States,

* **Corresponding author Lichun Sun:** Department of Medicine, Tulane University Health Sciences Center, New Orleans, LA 70002, USA, Phone: 504-988-1179, Email: peptide612@gmail.com, lsun@tulane.edu.

* **Corresponding author Jinhua Shen:** Tongji University Library, Shanghai 200092, P.R. China, Phone: 86-21-6598-2823, Email: jhshen@lib.tongji.edu.cn.

* **Corresponding author Guohua Zhu:** Tongji Law School, Shanghai 200092, P.R. China, Phone: 86-21-6598-553, Email: Chonghu666@163.com.

# Equal contribution

Atta-ur-Rahman and Khurshid Zaman (Eds.)

Japan, Germany and Britain occupy the top 5 positions. Among them China has the most patent applications. However, high-level patents are few The patent applications of the United States rank second, but the patent quality is considerably ahead, with rapid development in the Chinese patent markets. In addition to the focus and hotspots of patent applications of China, the United States, Japan, Germany and Britain also are analyzed in this part. Bode Gene Dev. Co., Ltd. Shanghai, Roche Holding Ltd., Merck & Co., Ltd., Pfizer Inc., Novartis AG are the top 5 patentees in terms of patent applications, with differences in development in the Chinese market, technical focus and hotspots.

The third part is the analysis of patent applications in foreign countries by Chinese applicants. Up to the retrieval date, Chinese applicants have a total of 4,036 invention patents in foreign countries. Since China's accession to the WTO, the amount of patent applications through the WIPO and EPO has increased rapidly. The United States is the most popular country for Chinese inventors. From the view of technical fields, patent applications in the field of A61K 31/00 (pharmaceutical preparations containing organic components) are the highest, up to 645 pieces. The top 10 of the International Patent Classification (IPC) accounts for 45% of the total applications. From the view of applicants, Roche Holding Ltd. is the most powerful company, occupying the leading position through their technical strength and number of patents. The patent applications of Medipharma SA are far ahead, but are relatively weak in strength. There is a large gap between these two companies and the other companies both in strength and the number of patents.

The fourth part is a case study. According to the statistics of GLOBOCAN, new liver cancer cases in China accounted for about 50% of cases (up to 782,000) in 2012. Based on the analysis of Chinese local anti-cancer drugs, the attention of Chinese inventors concerning liver cancer has increased in recent years. From the perspective of Chinese domestic patents, China's patent applications account for 74.6% of total applications, however important patents and core patents account for only 2%. The number of top 10 IPC patent applications is 2,430, accounting for 43% of the total. From the perspective of applicants, the applications of Fudan University and the Chinese Academy of Sciences are the highest, at 80 pieces each. The technical strength of the Chinese Academy of Sciences is the highest, while GlaxoSmithKline plc. is relatively weak. From the perspective of Chinese applicants in foreign countries, Chinese inventors contributed 738 pieces of patents for liver cancer drugs from 1985 to 2015. The United States, Japan, South Korea, Canada and Australia are the main countries where Chinese inventors apply for patents. The five countries account for 67.8% of the total patent applications. The patent applications of the top 10 IPCs is up to 371, accounting for 50.3% of the total. Among them, A61K 31/00 (pharmaceutical preparations containing effective organic components) is the key IPC. Hangzhou Bensheng Pharmaceutical

Co., Ltd. has applied for 34 pieces of patents, located at the right end of the horizontal axis, indicating the patentee's powerful technology.

Keywords: Anti-cancer drugs, bubble analysis, Chinese applicants, competitor analysis, competitive countries, China market, design, IPC distribution, liver cancer, patent analysis, policies analysis, patent application analysis, patent application, patent for invention, patent strength, technical fields, text clustering, utility model.

INTRODUCTION

The incidence of cancers in China is not optimistic. However, it takes time, higher costs and higher risks for scientists from industry and academia to pursue anti-cancer drug R&D. Mining information from patent data can provide decisive support for inventors, investigators and competitors in the field. The present work aims to study the development of Chinese anti-cancer drugs. On the basis of macro policies of anti-cancer drugs in China, we systematically analyzed the competitive status of anti-cancer drugs in the Chinese domestic markets, explored patent distributions and trends of inventors in the field of anti-cancer drugs, and did a deep analysis using liver-associated cancer drugs as a specific case.

The patent is a kind of scientific and technical document which records the contents of the invention and contains technical, legal and economic information. Many inventions were published in patents which could not be found in other scientific literature. The British Derwent Information Ltd. believes 70%-90% of patents are not published in other publications, however, the European Patent Office (EPO) believes that this ratio is 80%.

China is changing from labor-intensive to knowledge-intensive endeavors, and the importance of intellectual property rights is increasing. In 2008, the State Council of the PRC promulgated the "National Program for Intellectual Property" in which the creation, application, protection and management of intellectual property rights have been promoted to the national strategic level. In 2016, the first year of China's 13th Five-Year Plan, it was put forward to implement the strategy of innovation-driven development, put the developmental basis on innovation with scientific and technological innovation at its core, and develop talent as support, promote the combination between technological innovation and mass entrepreneurship and innovation and build more leading developments which rely on innovation driven and a first mover advantage [1].

The excellent results of China's policy for guidance and market development can be seen from the amount of patent applications. From the perspective of the amount of invention patents, Chinese invention patents in 2011 were more than 520,000 and ranked first in the world for the first time [2]. The amount in 2015 was more than 1 million and was first in the world for five consecutive years [3]. From the perspective that China submits the applications of international patents through the Patent Cooperation Treaty (PCT), the Chinese patent applications in 2015 were 29,846 pieces, accounting for 13.69% of global applications [4]. The growth rate was 16.8% and ranked third in the world for three consecutive years. These data verify the vast Chinese market, as well as the inventor's awareness of intellectual property rights and the ability of technological innovation.

According to "World Cancer Report 2014" announced by WHO, China's new cancer cases in 2012, for the first time, topped the worldwide total. Chinese new cases and deaths from liver cancer, esophageal cancer, gastric cancer and lung cancer are ranked first in the world. An estimated 782,500 new liver cancer cases and 745,500 deaths occurred worldwide during 2012, with China alone accounting for about 50% of the total number of cases and/or deaths [5].

The high incidence of cancer in China has led the Chinese market to counter the growing demand for anti-cancer drugs. The industrialization of the cancer drug industry has gradually emerged, while the domestic patent applications are rapidly increasing. With the enhancement of awareness about intellectual property protection, Chinese inventors have been developing a global cancer drug market.

There are four chapters in this paper. The first chapter mainly elaborates the laws and regulations that must be obeyed during the registration, approval, production and listing of Chinese anti-cancer drugs. The second chapter introduces the general situation of the Chinese patent application for anti-cancer drugs. By text clustering, the section clarifies the scope of applications from the top 5 applicant countries. Also, the section analyzes the application trends, IPC and research focus of the top 5 applicants. From the perspective that China submits their applications for international patents through the Patent Cooperation Treaty (PCT), the third chapter studies the trend of PCT applications and the key technologies. This part also sorts out the main applicants' development venation, research focus and other technical information. The last chapter studies the competitive situation of anti-liver cancer drugs by using liver cancer as an example as this cancer leads to the highest incidence and mortality rate in China.

METHODOLOGY

This article combines the qualitative and quantitative analysis. Qualitative analysis mainly includes macro policies about anti-cancer drugs and patent information. Through the quantitative analysis, both the status of the Chinese domestic anti-cancer drug market and the patent applications in foreign countries by Chinese inventor applicants are described.

All the macro policies are from Chinese government websites, including laws and regulations.

The patent data is from the INNOGRAPHY® platform.

1. The retrieval strategy of anti-cancer drugs is as follows:
   @(abstract, claims, title) (Drug or compound or agent or medicine or inhibitor or resistance) and (cancer* or tumor* or tumour* or neoplas* or carcinogen* or carcinoma* or sarcoma*)
2. The retrieval strategy of anti-liver cancer drugs is as follows:
   @ (abstract, claims, title) (Drug or compound or agent or medicine or inhibitor or resistance) and ("liver cancer" or "hepatic carcinoma" or hepatoma or "hepatic cancer")

Patent applications represent the current status of the technology in the field of anti-cancer drugs. Therefore, the thesis mainly analyzes the patent applications in this field.

The INNOGRAPHY® PALTFORM is based on big data architecture, and it performs a global patent search using data from more than 100 public sources [6]. The definition of concepts in patent analysis as follows.

1. Patent Strength [7]
   Innography®'s PatentStrength is a proprietary algorithm that predicts patent value and relevance, by deriving the likelihood that a patent will eventually be litigated. Starting with a well-regarded study on patent value correlations, Innography® has refined and improved the predictive capability of the algorithm over years of analysis [2].
   Patent Strength is the index of the INNOGRAPHY® platform based on the research paper "Valuable Patent". In this paper, "the data conclusively demonstrate that valuable patents differ in substantial ways from ordinary patents at the time the applications are filed and during their prosecution". This suggests that valuable patents can be identified beforehand [8]. There are more than 10 indexes to calculate the patent strength, Specially, the INNOGRAPHY® platform uses 1 to 100 scales to measure the patent strength. The larger the number, the more valuable the patent.
2. Core Patent & Important Patent & General patent
   In the INNOGRAPHY® platform, patents usually are divided into three classes according to the patent strength. In one patent set, core patents cover the top 20 scores, which means the number of core patents are higher than the remainder of patents in the same set. General patents cover the lower 30%, and patents with 31% to 79% scores are important patents.
3. Text Clustering
   In the thesis, text clustering is a patent analysis method. Through word frequency statistics of title, abstract, claims and specifications, it visualizes the technology distribution in the patent set.
4. IPC Distribution
   The use of "IP Classifications" in patent documents to make statistics the frequency of each IPC section, class, subclass or group. From the results, allows mastery of the distribution fields of the subject.

Patent literature integrates technology, economic and law information. Our object in this thesis is to try to describe the status of the anti-cancer drug market in China from the patent aspect, including the trend patent application number by time, major competitive countries, research directions and main applicants. Secondly, we explain the worldwide performance of Chinese applicants. Moreover, this paper takes anti-liver cancer drugs as the case for the high incidence of liver cancer in China, to show the competitive landscape in this field.

1. ANALYSIS ON MACRO POLICIES OF CHINESE ANTI-CANCER DRUGS AND PATENT INFORMATION ANALYSIS

1.1. Laws and Regulations Related to Chinese Anti-cancer Drugs

The registration, approval, production and commercialization of anti-cancer drugs need to comply with the relevant laws and regulations in China. The existing rules and regulations are listed in Table **1**. "Medicine Administration Law of the People's Republic of China" is the core administrative law and regulator in the field of medicine. Formal implementation of the second revised edition was in April 2015. The law stipulates that the development, production, medical procedures, and the units or individuals responsible for the supervision and administration must abide by this law. It makes clear how the management of administration of pharmaceutical producing enterprises, administration of pharmaceutical trading enterprise, control over medicines in medical institutions, drug control, control over drug packaging, control over drug price and advertisement, drug supervision and legal liability must be done. At the same time, the law provides for the functions of drug administration within the territory of China:

1. The pharmaceutical supervisory and administrative department of the State Council (China Food and Drug Administration, CFDA) is in charge of national drug supervision and management. The relevant departments under the State Council shall be responsible for the supervision and administration of drugs within the scope of their respective duties.
2. The drug regulatory agencies of the provinces, autonomous regions and municipalities directly under the central government shall be responsible for the supervision and control of pharmaceuticals related to the scope of their functions.
3. The drug supervision and administration department under the State Council shall cooperate with the competent department of the State Council in charge of the economy, and formulate the development plan and industrial policy of the

pharmaceutical industry.

Table 1. Drug Related Policies and Regulations [9 - 28].

Laws and Regulations	Classification	Implementation Date
*"Medicine Administration Law of the People's Republic of China"**	Law	2001.02.28
*"Regulations for the Implementation of Drug Administration Law of the People's Republic of China"**	Administrative Regulations	2002.09.15
"Rules for the Implementation of the Regulations on the Administration of Pharmaceuticals"	Regulation	2000.10.24
"Good Preparation Practice"	Regulation	2001.03.13
"Provisions on the Supervision and Administrative Punishment Procedures of Drugs"	Regulation	2003.07.01
"GCP"	Regulation	2003.09.01
"GLP"	Regulation	2003.09.01
"Measures for the Administration of Drug Import"	Regulation	2004.01.01
"Measures for the Administration of Drug Business License"	Regulation	2004.04.01
"Measures for the Supervision and Administration of Drug Production"	Regulation	2004.05.28
"Administrative Measures for Supervision and Administration of Medical Institutions" (Trial Implementation)	Regulation	2005.06.01
"Administrative Measures for the Registration of Medical Institutions"	Regulation	2005.08.01
"State Food and Drug Administration Drug Special Approval Procedures"	Regulation	2005.11.18
"Measures for the Administration of Imported Medicinal Materials" (Trial Implementation)	Regulation	2006.02.01
"Measures for the Examination of Drug Advertisements"	Regulation	2007.05.01
"Drug Advertisement Examination and Issue Standard"	Regulation	2007.05.01
"Measures for the Supervision and Administration of Drug Circulation"	Regulation	2007.05.01
*"Provisions for Drug Registration"**	Regulation	2007.07.10
"Provisions for Drug Recall"	Regulation	2007.12.10
"Good Practices in the Manufacture and Quality Control of Drugs"	Regulation	2011.03.01

Note: * represents core laws and regulations

1.2. The Development of Chinese Medicine Related Laws and Regulations

With the improvement of living standards in China, people's diets have changed, and the negative effects of cancer on the Chinese people's health has increased. In 2012, China added 3,700,000 cancer patients, and experienced about 2,200,000 deaths, accounting for 21.9% and 26.8% of the global total, respectively. The increase in breast cancer and lung cancer in the recent 30 years accounts for 96% and 465%, respectively [5]. In order to cope with the rapid growth of cancer incidence, the Chinese government has taken some measures.

To encourage the development of anti-cancer drugs, strengthen the role of science and technological innovation, the Chinese Association for Cancer Science and Technology award was established in 2006. As the 156th non-governmental award, the award is the only one in the field of cancer tumors in China. Its purpose is to reward medical workers and units who make outstanding contributions in the progress of medical science and technology.

There was also a need to speed up the approval process of cancer drugs to meet the needs of public medication. The clinical evaluation and approval of Chinese medicine take a long time. According to "Provisions for Drug Registration" the technical review time for clinical trial and production of a new drug is 90 working days and 150 working days, respectively. According to the forty-fifth provision in "Provisions for Drug Registration", new drugs with obvious clinical advantages for the treatment of AIDS, malignant tumors, rare diseases and other diseases apply to "Provisions on the Administration of Special Examination and Approval of New Drug Registration". The approval procedures draw heavily on the FDA priority review and fast channel program. It can shorten the time limit, early communication, and rolling review. In August 2015, the State Council of the PRC published "Comments on the Reform of the Examination and Approval System of Medical Devices for Drugs" which said "speed up the review and approval of innovative drugs, the implementation of special reviews and approval systems for innovative drugs; speed up the approval of innovative drugs for AIDS, cancer, major infectious diseases and other rare diseases; put these drugs into the national major projects and national key R & D program of drugs; transfer to domestic innovative drugs and drugs for children as well as innovative drugs with obvious therapeutic advantages".

The Chinese government has gradually incorporated anti-tumor drugs into the scope of its medical insurance in order to adapt to changes in the insured drug demand. Ministry of human resources and social security published the notice on issuing the catalogue of national basic medical insurance, work-related injury insurance and maternity insurance on November 27, 2009. The directory is the basic medical insurance, work-related injury insurance and maternity insurance fund to pay the insured drug costs and strengthen the policy basis and standard of medical service management of medical insurance. It clearly lists the related contents of anti-tumor drugs. A new Chinese medical directory set a two-year limit for clinical use. Some provinces and cities will actively supplement the reimbursement list of local medical insurance. In 2015, in order to raise the level of protection of serious diseases, improve the accessibility of drugs for insured patients, and promote the use of generic drugs, Jiangsu Provincial Department of human society published a notice about ImatinibMesylate Tablets (Xin dimension) and other special drugs included in the medical insurance fund payment. The notice said "Imatinib", a domestic life-saving medicine for treating leukemia was to be put into the insurance coverage. And Jiangsu became the first region to do so.

1.3. Laws and Regulations Related to Patent Information Analysis in China

In 1985, Patent Law was formally launched. Up to now, it has been revised three times (in 1992, 2000 and 2008). Patent related law and rule in China can be found in Table **2**.

Table 2. Patent Related Law and Rule [29 - 32].

Laws and Regulations	Classification	Implementation Date
"Patent Law"(4th Edition)	Law	April 1, 1985
"Implementing Regulations of the Patent Law of the People's Republic of China"	Rules	April 1, 1985
"Regulations on the Protection of Layout-Designs of Integrated Circuits"	Rules	October 1, 2001
"Regulations on Patent Commissioning"	Rules	March 4, 1991

In recent years, The Chinese government published a series of polices to encourage innovation, and protect intellectual property. Some of the policies are listed in Table **3**. These polices activate the whole intellectual property industry, including patent agency, lawyers, patent analysis, patent transfer and other IP related services. China published "The Outline of the National Intellectual Property Strategy" in 2008, which means IPR protection was upgraded to a national strategy. In 2015, the invention patent applications in China were over 1millon for the first time. With the development of China and with the increasing importance of innovation, patent analysis has room for further growth.

Table 3. Related IP Policies in China.

Policy	Published Data
"The Outline of the National Intellectual Property Strategy"	June, 2008
"Speed up the Cultivation and Guidance for the Development of Intellectual Property Services"	Nov., 2012
"In-depth Implementation of National Intellectual Property Strategy(2014-2020)"	Dec., 2014
"National Innovation Driven Development Strategy"	May, 2016

2. ANALYSIS OF CHINESE DOMESTIC ANTI-CANCER DRUG PATENTS

Cancer is one of the major diseases which seriously threatens human health, and it has been a research topic worldwide. In 2012, new Chinese incidences accounted for about 36% of the lung cancer cases in the world, according to the latest statistics from the World Health Organization. The proportion of Chinese cancer patients accounted for worldwide has far exceeded the proportion of the Chinese population (19%) [1]. China has become one of the main battle fields for cancer. The government and enterprises pay more attention to research and development of cancer drugs. By using the Innography® platform and combining it with the theory of patent intelligence analysis, it completely analyzed the competitive status of anti-cancer drugs in the Chinese domestic market and explored patented distribution and trends of the Chinese inventors in the field of foreign anti-cancer drugs.

Innography® is a retrieval and analysis platform for patented information which was launched by Dialog ProQuest. It contains invention patents and utility model patents from more than 90 countries and regions and includes more than 80 million pieces of global patents from which we can query and have access to patents, legal status and the original patents. In addition, it also contains the Patent litigation data of the United States federal court electronic filing system (PACER), dun & Bradstreet business data and the United States trademark data [2].

2.1. Data Source

The patent data is from the Innography® platform, with the retrieval date updated to October 7, 2015 The retrieval strategy includes (abstract, claims, title) (Drug or compound or agent or medicine or inhibitor or resistance) and (cancer* or tumor* or tumour* or neoplas* or carcinogen* or carcinoma* or sarcoma*). There are 501,918 pieces of patent total. The patent applications represent the current status of the technology in the field of anti-cancer drugs, therefore this paper mainly analyzes the patent applications in this field. We chose "Application China" as the source part, which represents the amount of patent applications in the field of Chinese domestic cancer drugs. The number was 57,392.

The Chinese patent right includes invention, utility model and appearance design. The invention refers to a new technical proposal for a product, a process or an improvement. The utility model is a novel technical scheme which is suitable for the shape, the structure, or the combination of the product. The appearance design is a kind of new design which concerns shape, pattern, color or their combination of products and is suitable for industrial applications [3]. The study aim is to analyze the status of the Chinese anti-cancer drug technology based on invention patents. In view of the above 57,392 patents for screening, the amount of invention patents was 57,280.

2.2. General Situation of Patents

Figure **1** shows the development trend of patent technology in the field of anti-cancer drugs. The amount of patent applications received by the patent institution reflects whether the technology is active, and whether the inventor has the initiative to seek patent protection. Patent applications can also represent annual development of patents more accurately, but it can't reflect the amount of patent applications of the past 2-3 years because general patents need 18 months to more than 3 years from application to public use. While the number of annual public patents can't reflect the amount of annual technical applications accurately, it can generally reflect the technical development in the past 2-3 years.

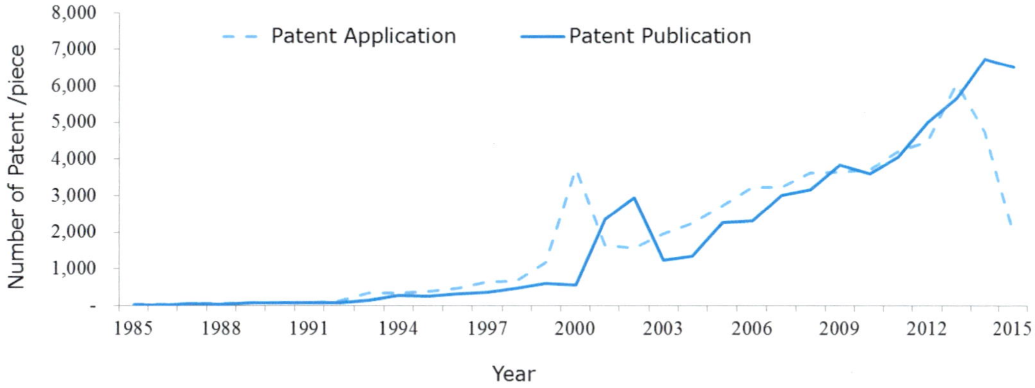

Fig. (1). Developing trends of the anti-cancer drugs patents.

Since the implementation of China's patent law in April 1, 1985, it has been revised three times. The fourth revision was underway in 2015 with the existing law useing the version in 2008 as the standard. In accordance with the provision of Article 25(5) of the patent law implemented in 1985, it states that drugs and substances obtained by chemical methods can't be granted patent rights. The subsection was removed from the patent law in 1992 and was implemented in January 1, 1993. As shown in Fig. (**1**), China's patent applications for anti-cancer drugs began to increase in 1993. The patent applications about anti-cancer drugs increased to 3,741 in 2000. From the view of patentees, Bode Gene Development Co. Ltd. has applied for 2,256 pieces of patents. In recent years, the declining health brought on by the rapid aging of the Chinese population and urbanization caused the morbidity and mortality of Chinese cancer patients to increase gradually. The demand for anti-cancer drugs is growing fast also. At the same time, the amount of patent applications in the field of anti-cancer drugs has maintained a rising trend with the gradual improvements in the Chinese legal system.

2.3. Major Competitive Countries and Regions

1. American patents keep ahead in quality; the patent applications of China are the highest, however, its high-level patents are few.

Generally speaking, the higher the number of patents, the higher the degree and value it is to the patent. The correspondence between the intensity and type of patents is shown in Table **4**.

Table 4. Distribution of Patent Strength.

Patent Strength %	Types	Number of Patents / Pieces	Proportion%
80-100	Core patent	13	0.02
30-80	Important patent	7,395	12.91
0-30	General patent	49,872	87.07

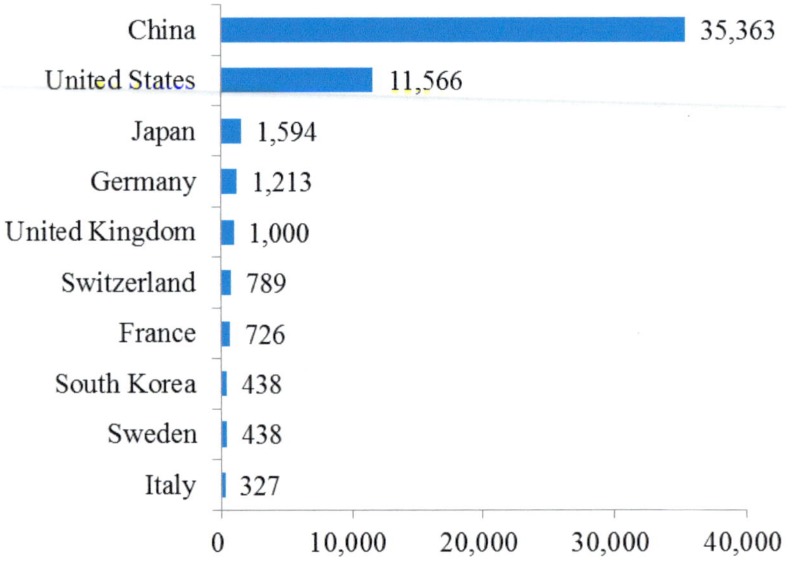

Fig. (2). Distribution of patent applications for major countries (top 10) (unit: piece).

By comparing Fig. (**2**) and Fig. (**3**), it is clearly shown that both China and the United States have a large number of patent applications, but the proportion of core patents in China is small while it is large in the United States and the United

Kingdom with 43% and 30% respectively. Although the patent applications of China occupys first place in the world, it is short of important and core patents, accounting for only 1% of its applications while ranking last in the top 10 countries for patent applications. On the one hand, it reflects that China has great development potential in the field of anti-cancer drugs. However, on the other hand, the Chinese patent documents don't contain the patent citation information needed for Patent Strength analysis, which leads to the inferior position of Chinese patents in the Innography® patent strength evaluation.

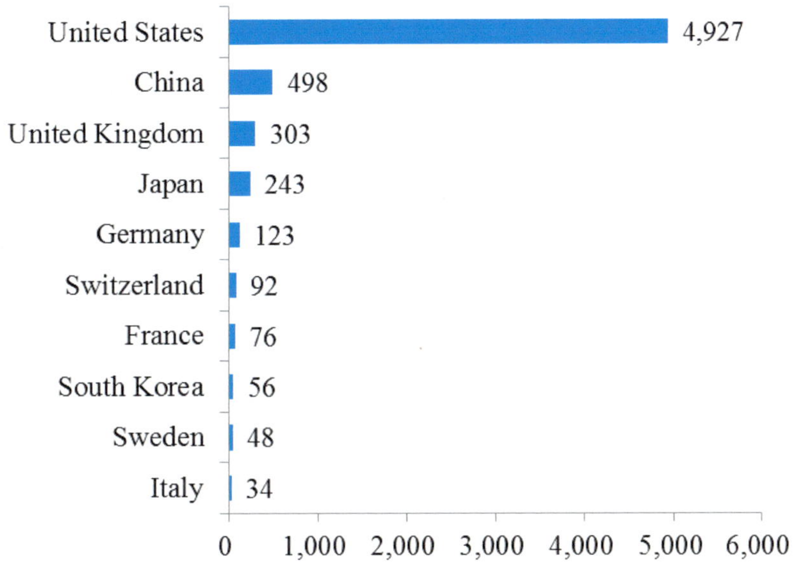

Fig. (3). Distribution of patent applications (intensity >30%) for major countries top 10 (unit: piece).

2. The patent applications of the United States quickly are distributed in the Chinese market

Figure **4** shows the patent application changes of the major countries (top 5). American inventors are very optimistic about the Chinese anti-cancer drug market for the amount of patent applications in China is increasing year by year. China's patent applications began their rapid growth in 1993. During 2003-2007, the annual patent applications of Japan, Germany, and the United Kingdom in China had exceeded 100.

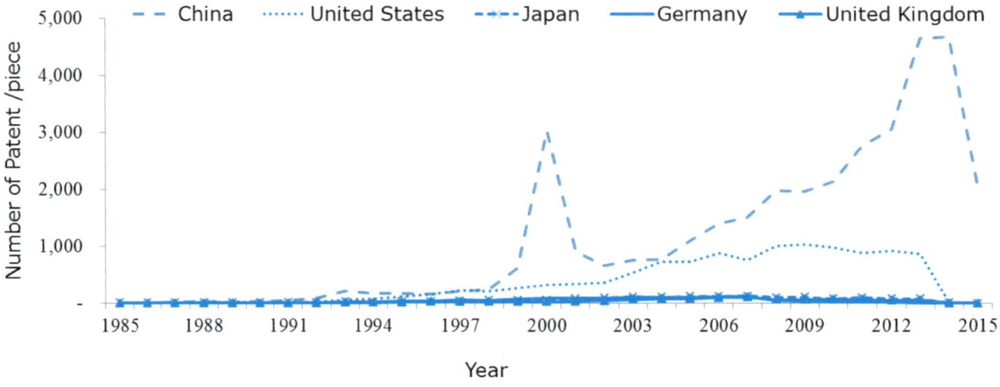

Fig. (4). Patent applications for major countries (Top 5).

Despite the decline in the number of patent applications in Germany and Britain in recent years, they are still interested in the Chinese Market. Figure **5** shows the trend of EPO patent applications in China. It can be found that the patent applications of Germany and the United Kingdom in China have been rapidly reduced since 2008, but at the same time the EP applications in China had increased in 2008, from 42 to 246 pieces. However, as EPO entered the Chinese market as a whole, there is no specific national identity. We are unable to conduct a detailed analysis of the EPO. In view of the 18-month patent open period, data in 2014 and 2015 was not fully open, therefore these data are not included in the analysis.

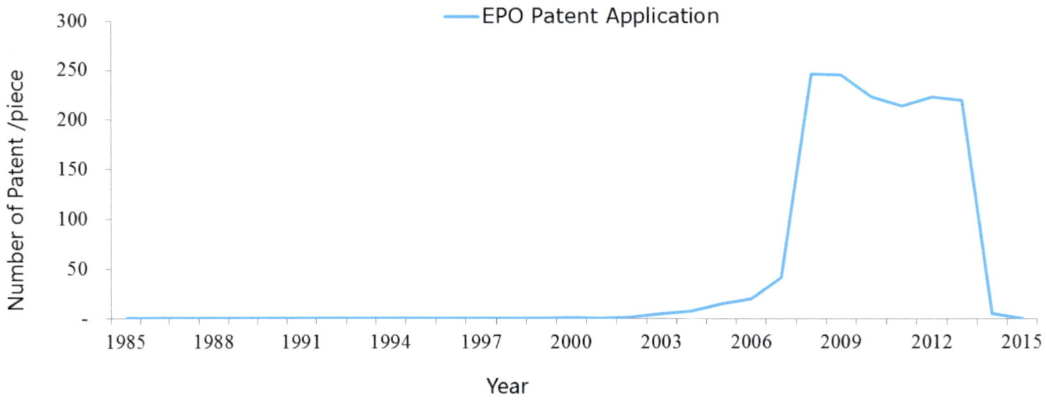

Fig. (5). Trend of EPO patent applications.

2.4. Developmental Characteristics of Patented Technology

Table **5** shows the text clustering of patent titles and abstracts in descending order of frequency. We can know that the main research focus of anti-cancer drugs changed little, mainly including cancer cells, traditional Chinese medicine, pharmaceutical compositions, liver cancer and raw materials. But there is a little change in frequency, for example: patent applications related to raw materials increased. Chinese inventors have begun to pay more attention to lung cancer in recent the years.

Table 5. Text Clustering Statistics for Patent Applications.

Number	IPC Top 10 (1986-2015)	IPC Top 10 (2012 & 2013)
1	Cancer cells	Cancer cells (containing tumor cancers)
2	Traditional Chinese Medicine	Traditional Chinese Medicine
3	DNA recombination	Raw materials
4	Pharmaceutical compositions	Pharmaceutical compositions
5	Raw materials	Liver cancer
6	Liver cancer	Lung cancer

1. Distribution of IPC in the field of anti-cancer drugs

Table **6** is the distribution of the IPC top 10. There are 29,698 pieces of patents, accounting for 51% of the total patent applications, which indicates anti-cancer drugs are involved widely.

Table 6. Distribution of the IPC Top 10.

Number	IPC/ Group	Amount / Pieces
1	A61K 31/00 Pharmaceutical preparations containing effective organic components	6,669
2	A61K 36/00 Pharmaceutical preparations containing algae, moss, fungi, or plants such as a traditional herbal medicine	4,732
3	C12N 15/00 Mutation or genetic engineering; DNA or RNA involved ingenetic engineering, vectors, such as plasmids, or their separation, preparation, or purification; the host	3,408
4	A61P 35/00 Anti-cancer drugs	3,052

(Table 6) contd.....

Number	IPC/ Group	Amount / Pieces
5	A61K 38/00 Pharmaceutical preparations containing peptides	2,861
6	A61K 9/00 Pharmaceutical preparations with special physical shapes	2,511
7	A23L 1/00 Food or feed; their preparation or processing (usually stored in A23L 3/00)	1,766
8	G01N 33/00 Materials are studied or analyzed using special methods not included in the G01N 1/00, G01N 31/00 groups	1,760
9	C12Q 1/00 Methods for the determination or examination of enzymes or microorganisms; compositions thereof; methods for preparing such compositions	1,517
10	C07K 16/00 Immunoglobulin, for example, monoclonal or polyclonal antibodies	1,222

2. Text clustering analysis in the field of anti-cancer drugs

The major IPC code sorting accounted for 26% of total patent applications. Its cluster analysis is shown in Fig. (**6**). The main research focus of anti-cancer drugs includes cancer cells, traditional Chinese medicine, pharmaceutical compositions, DNA recombination, liver cancer and medicaments for treatment.

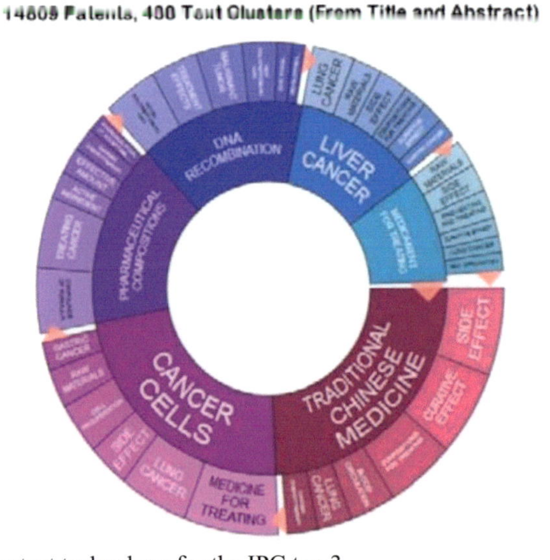

Fig. (6). Distribution of patent technology for the IPC top 3.

The clustering analysis of the ranked 4-10 patents in IPC sorting is shown in Fig. (**7**). The main research focus of anti-cancer drugs includes DNA recombination, cancer cells, raw materials, tumor cells, traditional Chinese medicine and pharmaceutical compositions.

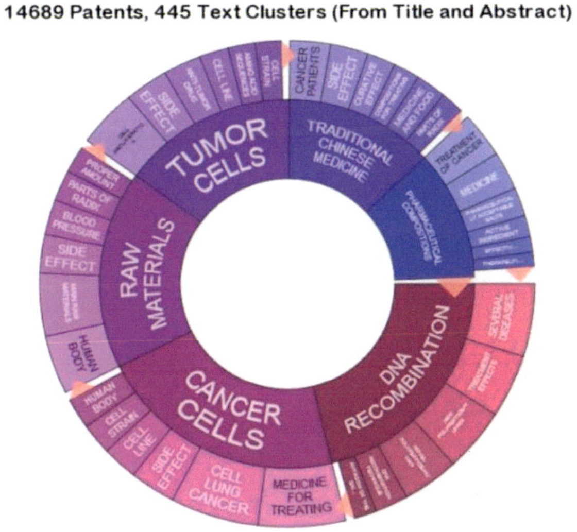

Fig. (7). Distribution of patent technology for the IPC ranked 4-10.

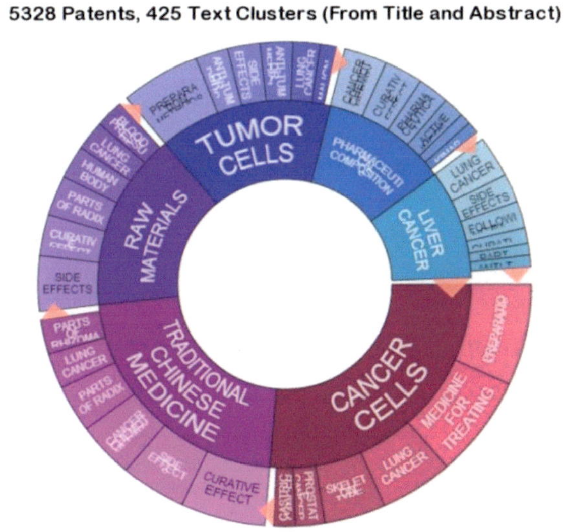

Fig. (8). Distribution of patent technology for IPC top 10 (2012 & 2013).

Figure **8** shows the cluster analysis of the top 10 patent applications in 2012 and 2013 (IP classification). The main research focus of anti-cancer drugs in the last two years includes cancer cells (including tumors), traditional Chinese medicine, raw materials, pharmaceutical compositions, liver cancer and lung cancer.

2.5. General Situation of the Development of Anti-cancer Drugs

2.5.1. Technical Fields the Chinese Inventors Focus on

Table **7** shows the text clustering of patent title and abstracts in descending order of frequency. We can know that the main research focus of anti-cancer drugs has changed little, it mainly includes traditional Chinese medicine, raw materials, cancer cells (including tumor cells), pharmaceutical compositions (including medicament compositions) and liver cancer.

Table 7. Text Clustering Statistics for Patent Applications (China).

Number	IPC Top 10 (1986-2015)	IPC Top 10 (2012 & 2013)
1	Traditional Chinese Medicine	Cancer cells (including tumor cancers)
2	Cancer cells (including tumors)	Traditional Chinese Medicine
3	Raw materials	Raw materials
4	DNA recombination	Liver cancer
5	Medicament compositions	Lung cancer
6	Liver cancer	Pharmaceutical compositions

1. Distribution of the IPC in the field of anti-cancer drugs

Table **8** is the distribution of the IPC top 10. There are 20,322 pieces of patents, accounting for 57% of the total patent applications.

Table 8. Distribution of the IPC Top 10.

Number	IPC / Group	Applications / Piece
1	A61K 36/00 Pharmaceutical preparations containing algae, moss, fungi, or plants such as a traditional herbal medicine	4,582
2	A61K 31/00 Pharmaceutical preparations containing effective organic components	2,830
3	A61P 35/00 Anti-cancer drugs	2,559
4	C12N 15/00 Mutation or genetic engineering; DNA or RNA involved in genetic engineering, vectors, such as plasmids, or their separation, preparation, or purification; the host	2,404
5	A61K 38/00 Pharmaceutical preparations containing peptides	2,057

(Table 8) contd.....

Number	IPC / Group	Applications / Piece
6	A61K 9/00 Pharmaceutical preparations with special physical shapes	1,749
7	A23L 1/00 Food or feed; their preparation or processing (usually stored in A23L 3/00)	1,678
8	A61K 35/00 Medical preparations containing raw materials with unknown structure or its reaction products	894
9	C12Q 1/00 Methods for the determination or examination of enzymes or microorganisms; compositions thereof; methods for preparing such compositions	889
10	G01N 33/00 Materials are studied or analyzed using special methods not included in the G01N 1/00, G01N 31/00 groups	680

2. Text clustering analysis in the field of anti-cancer drugs

The major IPC code sorting accounts for 28% of the total patent applications. Its cluster analysis is shown in Fig. (**9**). The main research focus of anti-cancer drugs includes traditional Chinese medicine, medicament composition, cancer cells, raw materials, side-effect and liver cancer.

9971 Patents, 431 Text Clusters (From Title and Abstract)

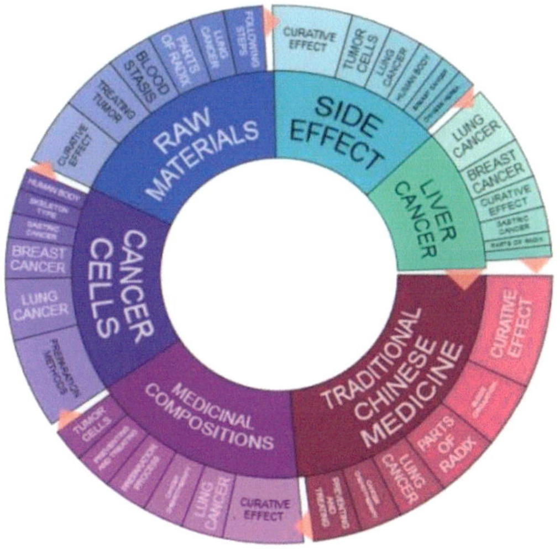

Fig. (9). Distribution of patent technology for the IPC top 3 (China).

The clustering analysis of the ranked 4-10 patents in IPC sorting is shown in Fig. (**10**). The main research focus of anti-cancer drugs includes DNA recombination,

Chinese medicine, raw materials, tumor cells, liver cancer and the health care fields.

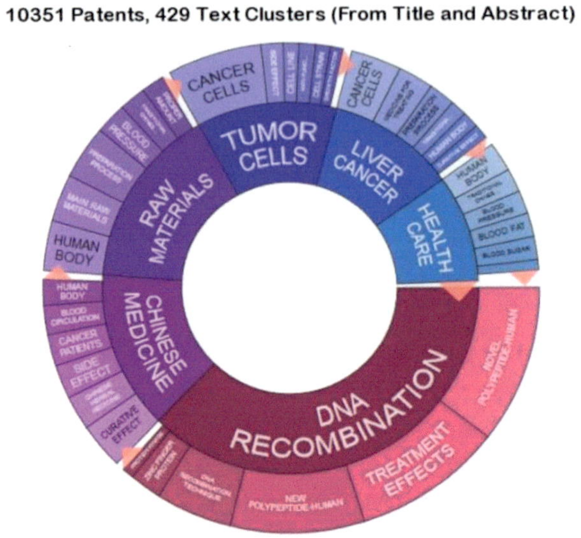

Fig. (10). Distribution of patent technology for the IPC ranked 4-10 (China).

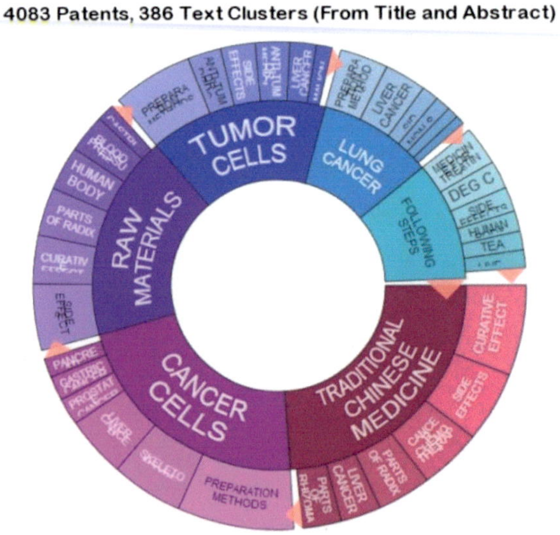

Fig. (11). Distribution of patent technology for the IPC top 10 (China, 2012 & 2013).

Figure **11** shows the cluster analysis of the top 10 patent applications in 2012 and 2013 (IP classification). The main research focus of anti-cancer drugs in the last two years includes cancer cells (including tumors), traditional Chinese medicine, raw materials, liver cancer and lung cancer.

2.5.2. Technical Fields the American Inventors Focus on

Table **9** shows the text clustering of patent titles and abstracts in descending order of frequency. American inventors continue to pay attention to pharmaceutical composition and nucleic acids. In the past 2 years, the patent layout in China has changed. Treating cancer, pharmaceutically acceptable salts and kinase inhibitors have become new research hotspots.

Table 9. Text Clustering Statistics for Patent Applications (US).

Number	IPC Top 10 (1986-2015)	IPC Top 10 (2012 & 2013)
1	Pharmaceutical composition	Treating cancer
2	Compound of formula	Pharmaceutical compositions
3	Effective amount	Pharmaceutically acceptable salt
4	Nucleic acid	Kinase inhibitors
5	Therapeutic agents	Effective amount
6	Breast cancer	Nucleic acid

1. Distribution of the IPC in the field of anti-cancer drugs

Table **10** is the distribution of the IPC top 10. There are 6,042 pieces of patents, accounting for 52% of the total patent applications of American inventors in China. The main IPC field is A61K 31/00 (pharmaceutical distributions containing the effective components).

Table 10. Distribution of the IPC Top 10 (U.S.A).

Number	IPC / Group	Applications / Piece
1	A61K 31/00 Pharmaceutical preparations containing effective organic components	2,048
2	G01N 33/00 Materials are studied or analyzed using special methods not included in the G01N 1/00, G01N 31/00 groups	614
3	C07K 16/00 Immunoglobulin, for example, monoclonal or polyclonal antibodies	564

(Table 10) contd.....

Number	IPC / Group	Applications / Piece
4	A61K 39/00 Pharmaceutical preparations containing antigen or antibody (immune test material into G01N 33/53)	504
5	C12N 15/00 Mutation or genetic engineering; DNA or RNA involved in genetic engineering, vectors, such as plasmids, or their separation, preparation, or purification; the host	463
6	A61K 38/00 Pharmaceutical preparations containing peptides	423
7	A61K 9/00 Pharmaceutical preparations with special physical shapes	387
8	C12Q 1/00 Methods for the determination or examination of enzymes or microorganisms; compositions thereof; methods for preparing such compositions	367
9	C07D 487/00 Heterocyclic compounds containing nitrogen atoms in a fused ring system as a heteroatom only, not included in the C07D 45 1/00, C07D 477/00 groups	359
10	C07D 401/00 Heterocyclic compounds, containing two or more heterocyclic rings, with nitrogen atoms as the only heterocyclic atom. There is at least one hexatomic ring containing only a nitrogen atom.	313

2. Text clustering analysis in the field of anti-cancer drugs

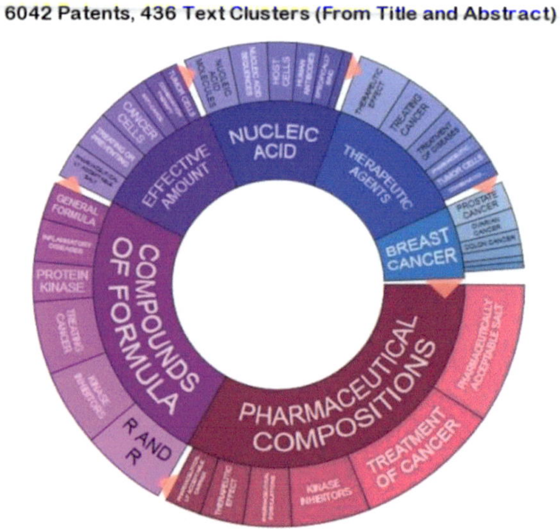

Fig. (12). Distribution of patent technology for the IPC top 10 (U.S.A).

The cluster analysis of the top 10 patents in the IPC sorting is shown in Fig. (**12**). In the Chinese market, the main research focus of the American inventors includes pharmaceutical composition, compound of formula, effective amount, nucleic acid, therapeutic agents and breast cancer.

Figure **13** shows the cluster analysis of the top 10 patent applications in 2012 and 2013 (IP classification). The main research focus of American inventors in the past two years includes treating cancer, pharmaceutical compositions, pharmaceutically acceptable salts, kinase inhibitors, effective amounts and nucleic acid.

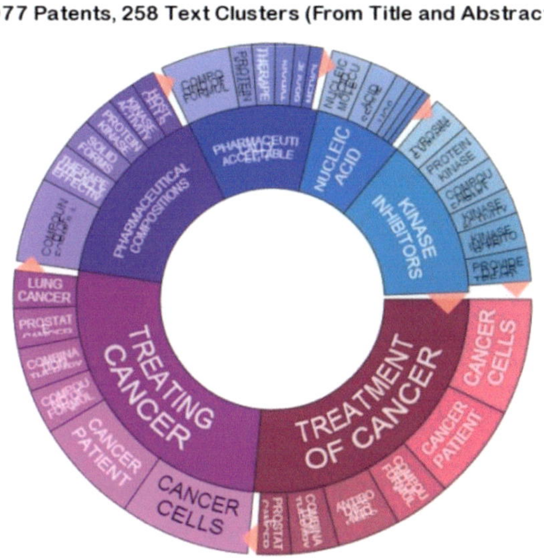

Fig. (13). Distribution of patent technology for the IPC top 10 (U.S.A, 2012 & 2013).

2.5.3. Technical Fields Focused on by Japanese Inventors

Table **11** shows the text clustering of patent titles and abstracts in descending order of frequency. In the Chinese market, the main research focus of Japanese inventors includes ingredients, cancer cells, amino acids, and agents (therapeutic agents, anti-cancer agents and therapeutic agents).

Table 11. Text Clustering Statistics for Patent Applications (Japan).

Number	IPC Top 10 (1986-2015)	IPC Top 10 (2012 & 2013)
1	Active ingredient	Active ingredient
2	Cancer cell	Cancer cell
3	Therapeutic agent	Amino acid

(Table 11) contd.....

Number	IPC Top 10 (1986-2015)	IPC Top 10 (2012 & 2013)
4	Pharmaceutical	Treatment and/or prevention
5	Amino acids	Therapeutic agent
6	Anti-cancer agent	Medicinal agent

1. Distribution of the IPC in the field of anti-cancer drugs

Table **12** is the distribution of the IPC top 10. There are 852 pieces of patents, accounting for 53% of the total patent applications of Japanese inventors in China. The main IPC fields are A61K 31/00 (pharmaceutical distributions containing the effective components), C12N 15/00 (mutation or genetic engineering; DNA or RNA involved in genetic engineering, vectors, such as plasmids, or their separation, preparation, or purification; the host or the separation, preparation or purification; the host) and G01N 33/00 (materials are studied or analyzed using special methods not included in the G01N 1/00, G01N 31/00 groups).

Table 12. Distribution of the IPC Top 10 (Japan).

Number	IPC / Group	Applications / Piece
1	A61K 31/00 Pharmaceutical distributions containing the effective components	284
2	C12N 15/00 Mutation or genetic engineering; DNA or RNA involved in genetic engineering, vectors, such as plasmids, or their separation, preparation, or purification; the host	129
3	G01N 33/00 Materials are studied or analyzed using special methods not included in the G01N1/00, G01N31/00 groups	91
4	C07K 16/00 Immunoglobulin, for example, monoclonal or polyclonal antibodies	60
5	C12Q 1/00 Methods for the determination or examination of enzymes or microorganisms; compositions thereof; methods for preparing such compositions	60
6	A61K 38/00 Pharmaceutical preparations containing peptides	56
7	A61K 9/00 Pharmaceutical preparations with special physical shapes	52
8	A61K 39/00 Pharmaceutical preparations containing antigen or antibody (immune test material into G01N33/53)	49
9	C07D 401/00 Heterocyclic compounds, containing two or more heterocyclic rings, with nitrogen atoms as the only heterocyclic atom. There is at least one hexatomic ring containing only a nitrogen atom	36

(Table 12) contd.....

Number	IPC / Group	Applications / Piece
10	A61K 45/00 Medical preparations containing the effective components, not included in the A61K 31/00 to A61K 41/00 groups	35

2. Text clustering analysis in the field of anti-cancer drugs

The cluster analysis of the top 10 patents using IPC sorting is shown in Fig. (**14**). In the Chinese market, the main research focus of Japanese inventors includes active ingredients, cancer cells, therapeutic agents, pharmaceutical compositions, amino acids and anti-cancer agents.

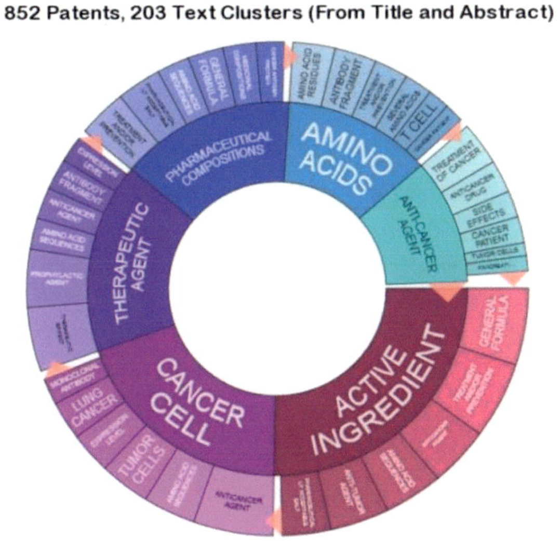

Fig. (14). Distribution of patent technology for the IPC top 10 (Japan).

Figure **15** shows the cluster analysis of the top 10 patent applications in 2012 and 2013 (IP classification). In the Chinese market, the main research focus of Japanese inventors in the past two years includes active ingredients, cancer cells, amino acids, treatments and/or prevention, therapeutic agents and medicinal agents.

2.5.4. Technical Fields the German Inventors Focus on

In recent years, German patent applications in China have decreased year by year, as shown in Fig. (**16**). The amount of patents in 2012 and 2013 were 10 and 1, respectively.

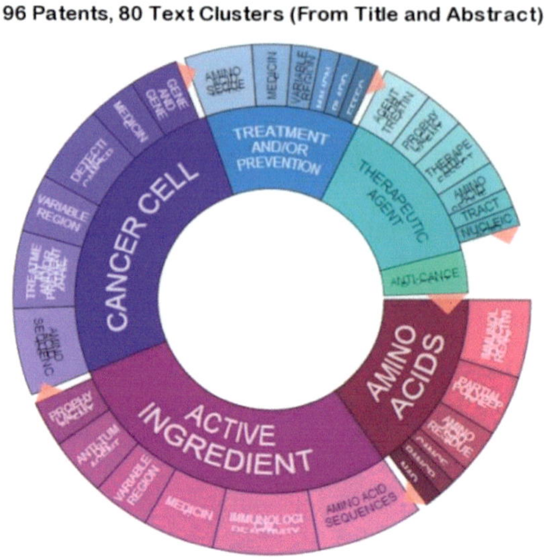

Fig. (15). Distribution of patent technology for the IPC top 10 (Japan, 2012 & 2013).

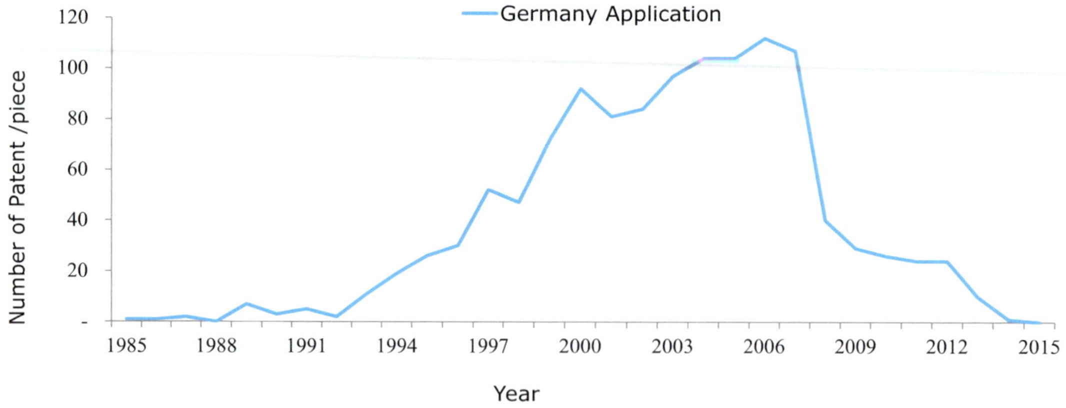

Fig. (16). Developing trends of the anti-cancer drugs patents of German inventors in China.

1. Distribution of IPC in the field of anti-cancer drugs

Table **13** is the distribution of the IPC top 10. There are 590 pieces of patents, accounting for 48% of the total patent applications of German inventors in China. Its concentration of technical patents is slightly lower. The main IPC field is A61K 31/00 (pharmaceutical distributions containing the effective components).

Table 13. Distribution of the IPC Top 10 (Germany).

Number	IPC / Group	Applications / Piece
1	A61K 31/00 Pharmaceutical distributions containing the effective components	266
2	G01N 33/00 Materials are studied or analyzed using special methods not included in the G01N 1/00, G01N 31/00 groups	62
3	A61K 38/00 Pharmaceutical preparations containing peptides	47
4	C07D 401/00 Heterocyclic compounds, containing two or more heterocyclic rings, with nitrogen atoms as the only heterocyclic atom. There is at least one hexatomic ring containing only a nitrogen atom	38
5	A61K 9/00 Pharmaceutical preparations with special physical shapes	37
6	C07D 295/00 Heterocyclic compounds containing multiple methylene imine rings, there are at least one five membered ring, 3 - diazabicyclo [3.2.2]-nonane, piperazinemorpholine or thiomorpholine ring, only hydrogen atoms attached directly to the carbon atoms of the ring	26
7	C07D 487/00 Heterocyclic compounds containing nitrogen atoms in a fused ring system as a heteroatom only, not included in the C07D 451/00, C07D 477/00 groups	26
8	C07D 471/00 Nitrogen atoms are used as the only heterocyclic atoms in a fused ring system. At least one ring is a six membered heterocyclic compound containing a nitrogen atom and not included in the C07D 451/00, C07D 463/00 groups	24
9	A61K 45/00 Medical preparations containing the effective components, not included in the A61K 31/00 to A61K 41/00 groups	24
10	C07K 14/00 Peptides with more than 20 amino acids; gastrin; growth hormone release inhibitory factor; stimulating hormone; its derivatives	20
11	C07K 16/00 Immunoglobulin, for example, monoclonal or polyclonal antibodies	20

2. Text clustering analysis in the field of anti-cancer drugs

The cluster analysis of the top 10 patents from IPC sorting is shown in Fig. (**17**). In the Chinese market, the main research focus of German inventors includes compounds of formulas, general formulas, pharmaceutical compositions, acceptable salts, cell proliferation and tyrosine kinase.

2.5.5. Technical Fields Focused on by British Inventors

As in Germany, in recent years, the amount of patent applications in China or for applications from the United Kingdom in China has decreased year by year due to the establishment of the European Patent Office. As shown in Fig. (**18**), the amount of patents in 2012 and 2013 were 55 and 0, respectively.

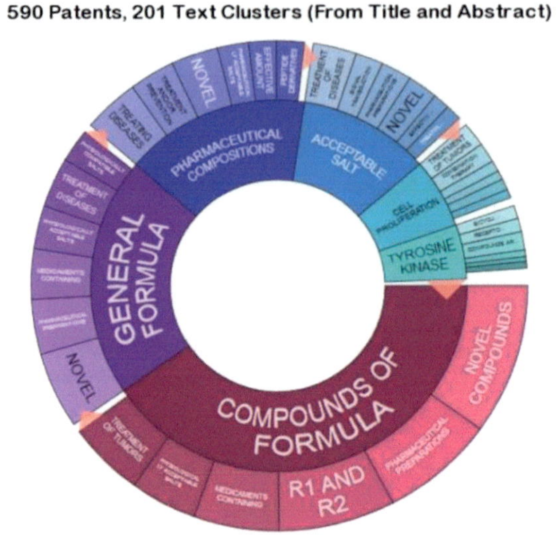

Fig. (17). Distribution of patent technology for the IPC top 10 (Germany).

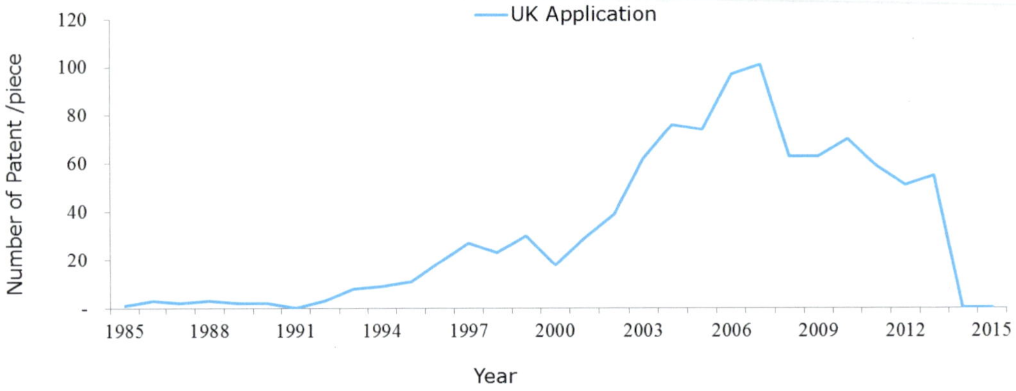

Fig. (18). Developing trend of the anti-cancer drugs patents of British inventors in China.

1. Distribution of IPC in the field of anti-cancer drugs

Table **14** is the distribution of the IPC top 10. There are 339 pieces of patents, accounting for 38% of the total patent applications of British inventors in China. Its concentration of technical patents is slightly lower compared with Germany. The main IPC field is A61K 31/00 (pharmaceutical distributions containing the effective components).

Table 14. Distribution of the IPC Top 10 (Britain).

Number	IPC / Group	Applications / Piece
1	A61K 31/00 Pharmaceutical distributions containing the effective components	173
2	C12N 15/00 Mutation or genetic engineering; DNA or RNA involved in genetic engineering, vectors, such as plasmids, or their separation, preparation, or purification; the host	66
3	A61K 9/00 Pharmaceutical preparations with special physical shapes	50
4	G01N 33/00 Materials are studied or analyzed using special methods not included in the G01N 1/00, G01N 31/00 groups	50
5	C07D 471/00 Nitrogen atoms are used as the only heterocyclic atoms in a fused ring system. At least one ring is a six membered heterocyclic compounds containing a nitrogen atom and not included in the C07D 451/00, C07D 463/00 groups	32
6	A61K 39/00 Pharmaceutical preparations containing antigen or antibody (immune test material into G01N 33/53)	30
7	C12Q 1/00 Method for the determination or examination of enzymes or microorganisms; compositions thereof; methods for preparing such compositions	27
8	A61K 38/00 Pharmaceutical preparations containing peptides	27
9	A61P 35/00 Anti-cancer drugs	25
10	C07D 401/00 Heterocyclic compounds, containing two or more heterocyclic rings, with nitrogen atoms as the only heterocyclic atom. There is at least one hexatomic ring containing only a nitrogen atom	24

2. Text clustering analysis in the field of anti-cancer drugs

The cluster analysis of the top 10 patents from the IPC sorting is shown in Fig. (**19**). In the Chinese market, the main research focus of British inventors includes pharmaceutical compositions, compounds of formulas, pharmaceutical acceptable salts, nucleic acids, medicaments for treatment, and gene expression.

2.6. Analysis of the Main Applicants

This part is based mainly on the Innography® bubble chart analyzing the technical gap in competitors in the field of anti-cancer drugs. The horizontal axis of the bubble chart represents relative technical strength which comprehensively takes the number of patent applications, patent categories and patent citations into consideration. The greater the numerical value of the horizontal axis, the stronger the technology is. The vertical axis of the bubble chart represents the resources of the companies, which comprehensively takes income, geographical position and legal status into consideration. The greater the value of the vertical coordinate, the stronger the strength for the patentee. The bubble area represents the number of patents for the patentee. The larger the bubble, the more patent applications there are.

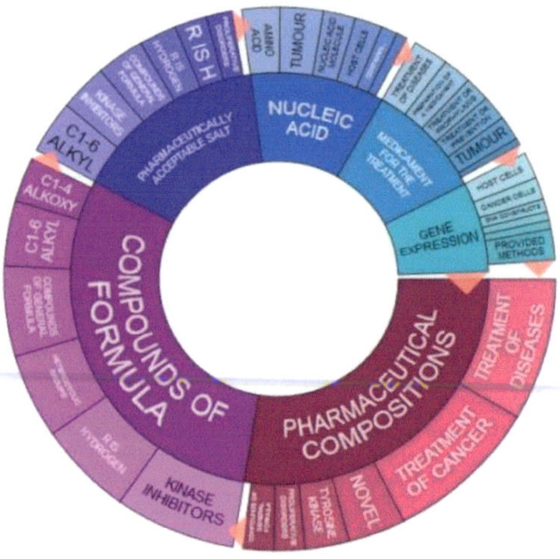

Fig. (19). Distribution of patent technology for the IPC top 10 (Britain).

The bubble chart (patent applications of the top 10) of the patentees in the field of anti-cancer drugs is shown in Fig. (**20**). Because income parameters of some patentees is difficult to calculate, the system automatically sets the parameter to 0, leading to the low value of the vertical axis. For example, the bubble of Bode Gene Dev. Co. Ltd. Shanghai, Fudan University and the Chinese Academy of Sciences finally land on the horizontal axis since to their income parameter is 0.

According to Fig. (**20**), the bubble of Bode Gene Dev. Co. Ltd. Shanghai is the largest, indicating the most patent applications (1,960 pieces); Pfizer Inc., at the far right side of the coordinate, indicates that its relative technological strength is the most comprehensive in the field of anti-cancer drugs in China; and Roche

Holding Ltd., having the most abundant resources. The analysis for patentees (top 5 patent applications) is from three aspects, change in trends of applications, key research fields, active grants and active applications.

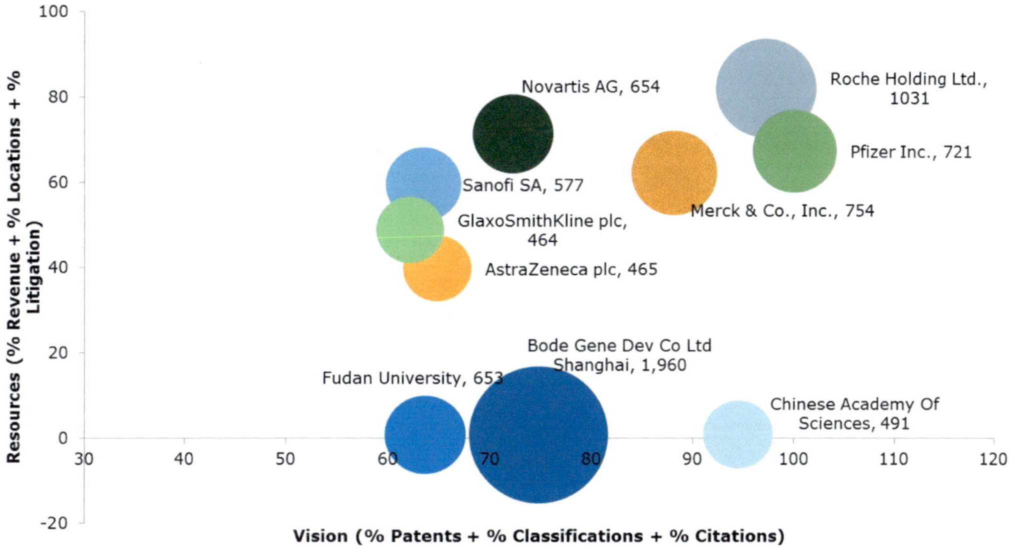

Fig. (20). Bubble analysis of patentees (top 10 patent applications).

2.6.1. Bode Gene Dev. Co., Ltd. Shanghai

1. The time of patent applications particularly is concentrated, the applications in 2000 account for 90% of the total applications.

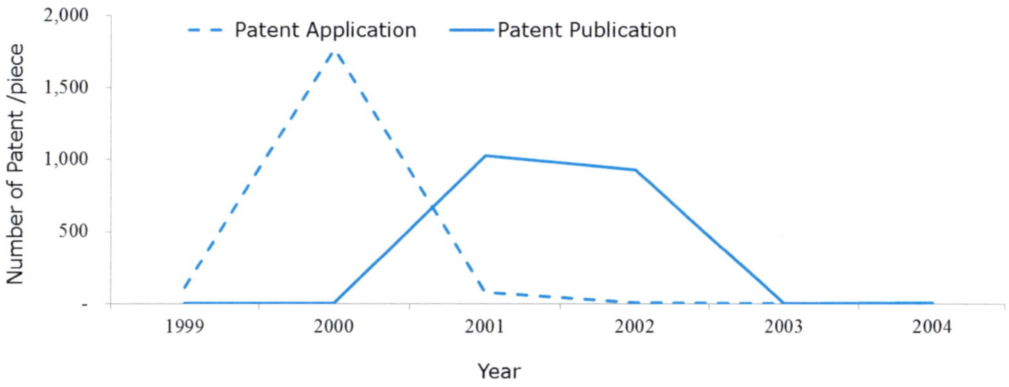

Fig. (21). Development trend of patents.

The development trend for the patents of Bode Gene Dev. Co., Ltd. Shanghai is shown in Fig. (**21**), in which patent applications were concentrated during 1999-2002, especially in 2000, and its patent application amounts reached 1,766.

2. The distribution of the IPC is concentrated, and the IPC top 3 accounts for 87% of the total applications.

Table **15** is the distribution of the IPC top 3. There are 1,700 pieces of patents, accounting for 87% of the total patent applications in China. The concentration of technical patents is high. The main IPC field is C12N 15/00 (mutation or genetic engineering; DNA or RNA involved in genetic engineering, vectors, such as plasmids, or their separation, preparation, or purification; the host).

Table 15. Distribution of the IPC Top 3 (1,960 Pieces).

Number	IPC / Group	Applications / Piece
1	C12N 15/00 Mutation or genetic engineering; DNA or RNA involved in genetic engineering, vectors, such as plasmids, or their separation, preparation, or purification; the host	780
2	C07K 14/00 Peptides with more than 20 amino acids; gastrin; growth hormone release inhibitory factor; stimulating hormone; its derivatives	137
3	A61K 38/00 Pharmaceutical preparations containing peptides	783

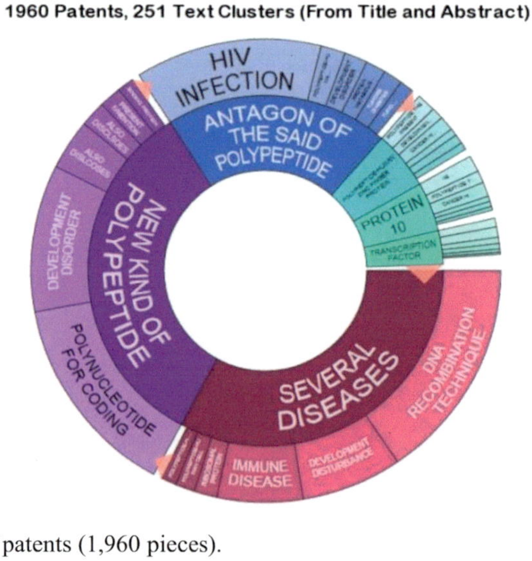

Fig. (22). Text clustering of patents (1,960 pieces).

The text clustering of the anti-cancer drug patents for Bode is shown in Fig. (**22**). The main patent fields in China include three categories, several diseases (key words are DNA recombination technique, development disturbance, immune disease), new kinds of polypeptides (key words are polynucleotide for coding) and antagonists of the said polypeptides (key words are HIV Infection).

3. The sum of active grants and active applications account for 6.3% of the total patent applications.

According to statistics, the sum of active grants and active applications is 125, accounting for 6.3% of total patent applications.

Table **16** shows the distribution of the IPC top 3. There are 113 pieces of patents, accounting for 90% of the effective patents. The main IPC field is A61K 38/00 (pharmaceutical products containing peptides).

Table 16. Distribution of the IPC Top 3 (125 Pieces of Effective Patent).

Number	IPC / Group	Application / Piece
1	A61K 38/00 Pharmaceutical preparations containing peptides	52
2	C12N 15/00 Mutation or genetic engineering; DNA or RNA involved in genetic engineering, vectors, such as plasmids, or their separation, preparation, or purification; the host	41
3	C07K 14/00 Immunoglobulin, for example, monoclonal or polyclonal antibodies	20

The text clustering of the effective 125 patents is shown in Fig. (**23**). The fields involved include development disturbance, polynucleotide for coding IT protein 10, ribosomes, related proteins and polypeptides for treating various diseases.

2.6.2. Roche Holding Ltd.

1. Patent applications began to grow rapidly from 2005 and the amount of patent applications has been relatively stable in recent years.

The development trend of patent technology for Roche Holding Ltd. is shown in Fig. (**24**). At the beginning of the implementation of the patent law in China in

1985, Roche Holding Ltd. had applied for patents for cancer drugs. Patent applications have grown rapidly since 2005. The amount of patent applications has been relatively stable in recent years.

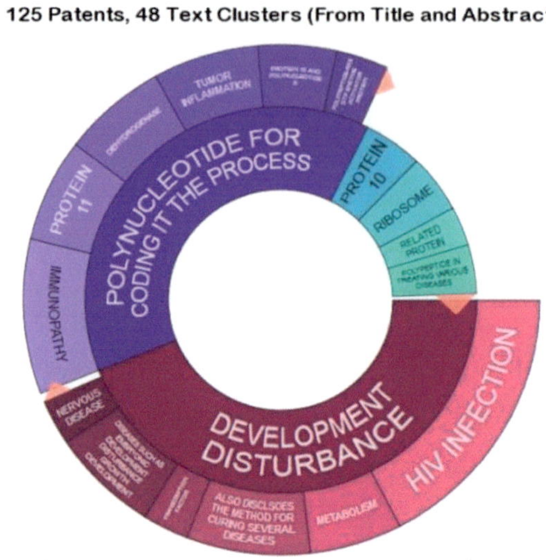

Fig. (23). Text clustering of the 125 effective patents.

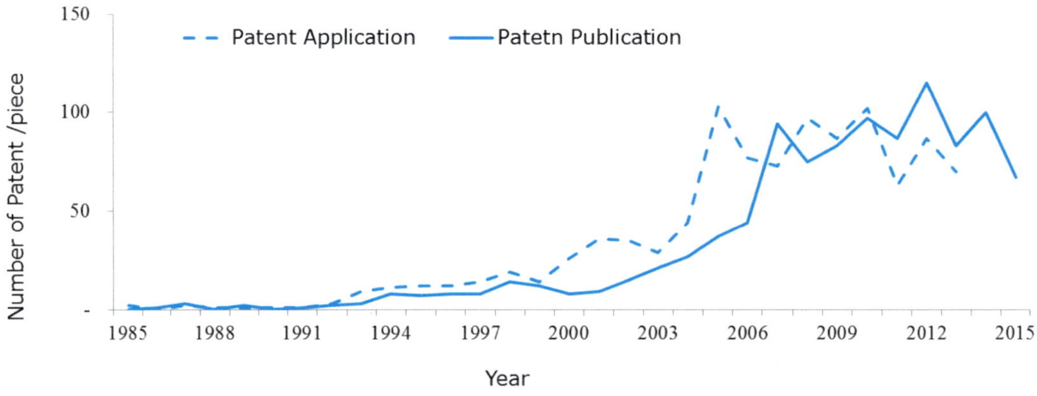

Fig. (24). Development trend of patents.

2. The patents for IPC distributed in the 102 IPC groups and the IPC top 3 account for only 33% of the total applications.

Table **17** is the distribution of the IPC top 3. There are 1,031 pieces of patents, accounting for 33% of the total patent applications in China. Its distribution of patents is wide. The main IPC fields include C07K 16/00 (immunoglobulin, for example, monoclonal or polyclonal antibodies) and A61K 31/00 (pharmaceutical preparations containing effective organic components).

Table 17. Distribution of the IPC Top 3 (1,031 Pieces).

Number	IPC / Group	Application / Piece
1	C07K 16/00 Immunoglobulin, for example, monoclonal or polyclonal antibodies	149
2	A61K 31/00 Pharmaceutical preparations containing organic effective components	132
3	G01N 33/00 Materials are studied or analyzed using special methods not included in the G01N 1/00, G01N 31/00 groups	63

The text clustering of anti-cancer drug patents for patent applicants is shown in Fig. (**25**). The main patent fields in China include pharmaceutically acceptable salts, pharmaceutical compositions, kinase inhibitors, and general formulas.

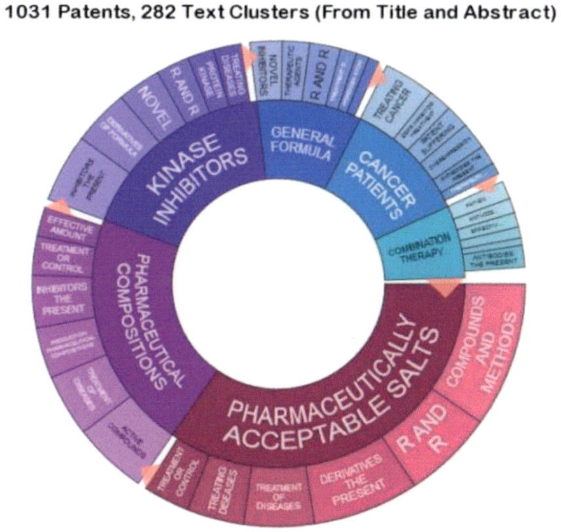

Fig. (25). Text clustering of patents (1,031 pieces).

3. The sum of active grants and active applications account for the 29.7% of total patent applications.

The statistics on the effectiveness of the Chinese patents for anti-cancer drugs say the sum of active grants and active applications is 306, accounting for 29.7% of total patent applications.

Table **18** shows the distribution of the IPC top 3. There are 113 pieces of patents, accounting for 37% of effective patents. The main IPC field is C07K 16/00 (immunoglobulin, for example, monoclonal or polyclonal antibodies).

Table 18. Distribution of the IPC Top 3 (306 Pieces of Effective Patents).

Number	IPC / Group	Application / Piece
1	C07K 16/00 Immunoglobulin, for example, monoclonal or polyclonal antibodies	59
2	A61K 39/00 Pharmaceutical preparations containing antigen or antibody (immune test material into G01N 33/53)	27
3	G01N 33/00 Materials are studied or analyzed using special methods not included in the G01N 1/00, G01N 31/00 groups	27

The text clustering of the effective 306 patents is shown in Fig. (**26**). The fields involved include pharmaceutically acceptable salts, R1 and R2, antibodies and methods, antigen binding and biomarkers.

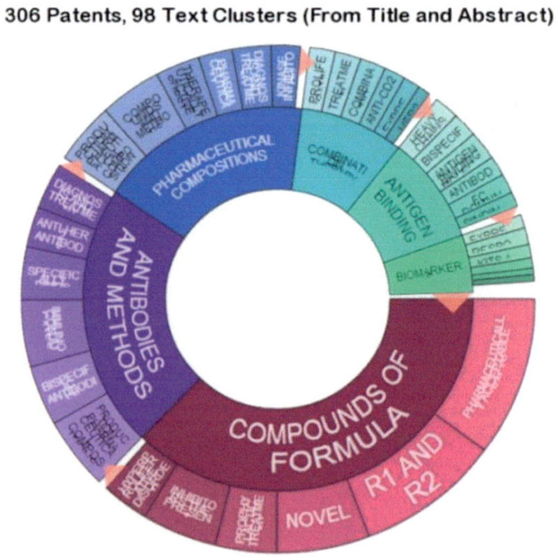

Fig. (26). Text clustering of the 306 effective patents.

2.6.3. Merck & Co., Inc.

1. Since 2000, patent applications began to grow rapidly, but have decreased in recent years, after a peak in 2006.

The development trend of patent technology for Merck & Co., Inc. is shown in Fig. (**27**). Patent applications were concentrated in 2003-2008 and then maintained a downward trend. It has decreased in recent years after a peak in 2006.

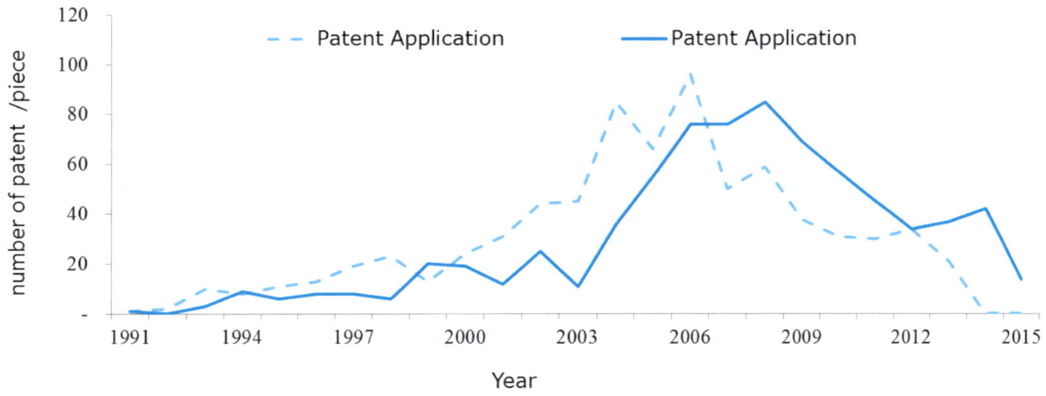

Fig. (27). Development trend of patents.

2. The patents of IPC distributed in the 100 IPC groups, and the IPC top 3 account for 36% of the total applications.

Table 19. Distribution of the IPC Top 3 (754 Pieces).

Number	IPC / Group	Application / Piece
1	A61K 31/00 Pharmaceutical preparations containing effective organic components	177
2	C07D 401/00 Heterocyclic compounds, containing two or more heterocyclic rings, with nitrogen atoms as the only heterocyclic atom. There is at least one hexatomic ring containing only a nitrogen atom	51
3	C07D 487/00 Heterocyclic compounds containing nitrogen atoms in fused a ring system as a heteroatom only, not included in the C07D 451/00, C07D 477/00 groups	49

Merck & Co., Inc.'s 754 patents are distributed within the 100 IPC groups. Table **19** is the distribution of the top 3 IPCs. There are 277 pieces of patents, accounting for 36% of the total patent applications in China. The main IPC field is A61K 31/00 (pharmaceutical preparations containing effective organic components).

The text clustering of the anti-cancer drug patents for patent applicants is shown in Fig. (**28**). The main fields of patents in China include pharmaceutically acceptable salts, pharmaceutical compositions, kinase inhibitors, treating cancer (treatment of tumors) and R1, R2 and R3.

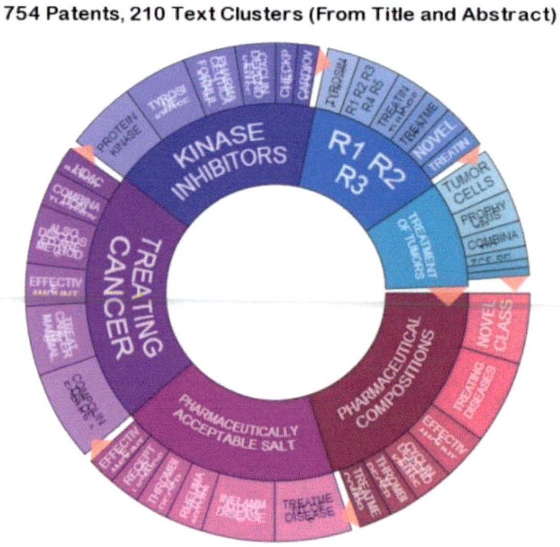

Fig. (28). Text clustering of patents (754 pieces).

3. The sum of active grants and active applications account for 14.2% of the total patent applications.

Statistics on the effectiveness of Chinese patents for anti-cancer drugs say the sum of active grants and active applications is 107, accounting for 14.2% of total patent applications.

There are 107 effective patents of patentees in China, distributed in 47 IPC groups. The distribution of effective patents is wide. Table **20** shows the distribution of the IPC top 3. The total number is 25, accounting for 24% of the effective patents. The main IPC fields include C07D 471/00 (nitrogen atoms are used as the only heterocyclic atoms in a fused ring system. At least one ring is a six membered heterocyclic compound containing a nitrogen atom and not included in the C07D 451/00, C07D 463/00 groups), C07D 487/00 (heterocyclic compounds containing nitrogen atoms in fused ring systems as a heteroatom only, not included in the C07D 451/00, C07D 477/00 groups).

Table 20. Distribution of the IPC Top 3 (107 Pieces of Effective Patent).

Number	IPC / Group	Application / Piece
1	C07D 471/00 Nitrogen atoms are used as the only heterocyclic atoms in a fused ring system. At least one ring is a six membered heterocyclic compound containing a nitrogen atom and not included in the C07D 451/00, C07D 463/00 groups	10
2	C07D 487/00 Heterocyclic compounds containing nitrogen atoms in a fused ring system as a heteroatom only, not included in the C07D 451/00, C07D 477/00 groups	9
3	C07D 401/00 Heterocyclic compounds, containing two or more heterocyclic rings, with nitrogen atoms as the only heterocyclic atom. There is at least one hexatomic ring containing only a nitrogen atom	6

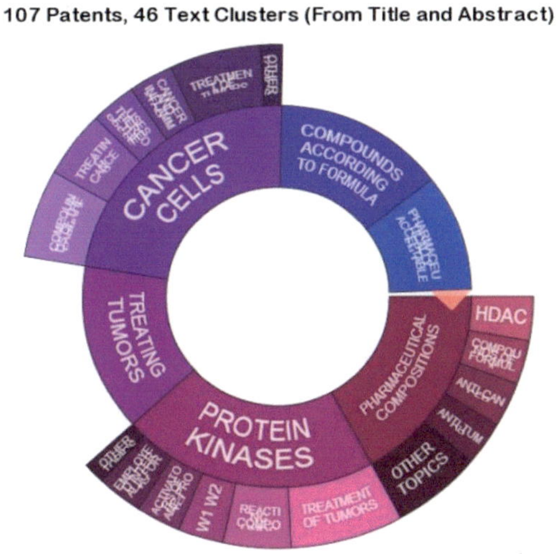

Fig. (29). Text clustering of the 107 effective patents.

The text clustering of the 107 effective patents is shown in Fig. (**29**). The main fields of the patents in China include protein kinases, HDAC, reacting compounds, W1 and W2.

2.6.4. Pfizer Inc.

1. Since 1995, patent applications began to grow rapidly and continues to decline after its peak in 2004. In recent years, the number of patent applications has been low.

The development trend of patent technology for Pfizer Inc. is shown in Fig. (**30**). Pfizer began to apply for patents for anti-cancer drugs as soon as the implementation of the patent law in China came into effect. The patent applications were concentrated in 2000-2005 and have maintained a downward trend since then.

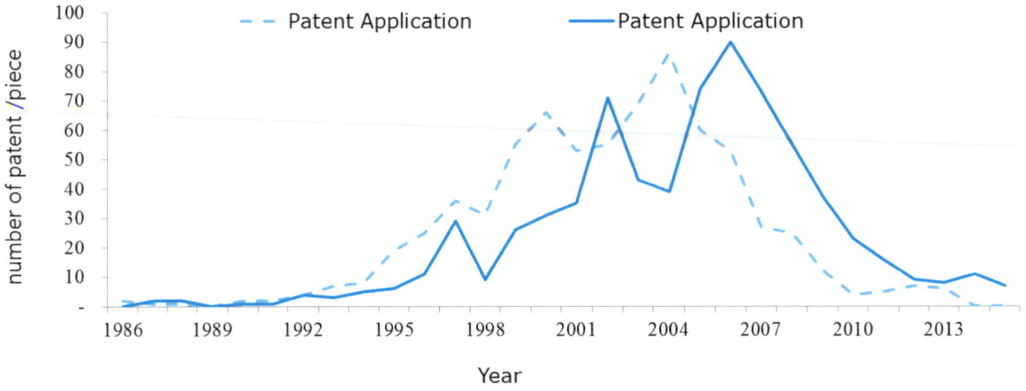

Fig. (30). Development trend of patents.

2. The distribution of the IPC is wide, distributed in 87 IPC groups. The IPC top 3 account for 46% of the total applications.

Merck & Co., Inc.'s 721 patents are distributed in 87 IPC groups. Table **21** is the distribution of the IPC Top 3. There are 330 pieces of patents, accounting for 46% of the total patent applications in China. The main IPC field is A61K 31/00 (pharmaceutical preparations containing effective organic components).

Table 21. Distribution of the IPC Top 3 (721 Pieces).

Number	IPC / Group	Application / Piece
1	A61K 31/00 Pharmaceutical preparations containing effective organic components	271
2	C07D 401/00 Heterocyclic compounds, containing two or more heterocyclic rings, with nitrogen atoms as the only heterocyclic atom. There is at least one hexatomic ring containing only a nitrogen atom	30
3	C07D 487/00 Heterocyclic compounds containing nitrogen atoms in a fused ring system as a heteroatom only, not included in the C07D 451/00, C07D 477/00 groups	29

The text clustering of the anti-cancer drug patents for patent applicants is shown in Fig. (**31**). The main fields of the patents in China include pharmaceutical compositions, pharmaceutically acceptable salts, R and R, protein kinase and effective amounts.

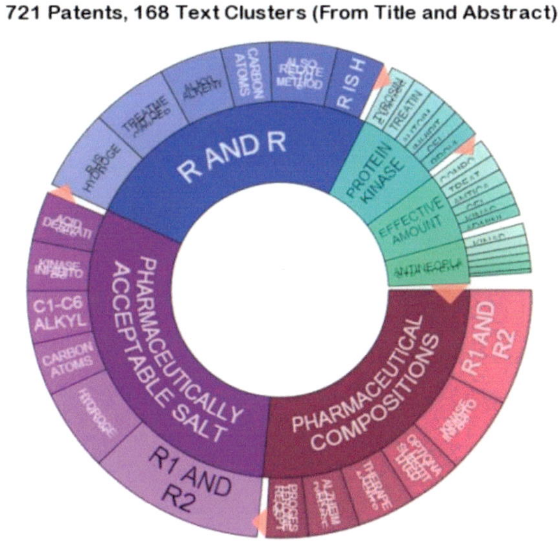

Fig. (31). Text clustering of patents (721 pieces).

3. The sum of active grants and active applications account for 4.2% of the total patent applications.

Statistics on the effectiveness of Chinese patents for anti-cancer drugs say the sum of active grants and active applications is 30, accounting for 4.2% of the total patent applications. Table **22** shows the distribution of the IPC top 3. There are 12 effective patents of the patentees in China, accounting for 40% of the effective patents. The main IPC field is A61K 31/00 (pharmaceutical products containing peptides).

Table 22. Distribution of the IPC Top 3 (30 Pieces of Effective Patent).

Number	IPC / Group	Application / Piece
1	A61K 31/00 Pharmaceutical preparations containing effective organic components	5
2	A61K 39/00 Pharmaceutical preparations containing antigen or antibody (immune test material into G01N 33/53)	4
3	C07D 487/00 Heterocyclic compounds containing nitrogen atoms in a fused ring system as a heteroatom only, not included in the C07D 451/00, C07D 477/00 groups	3

Text clustering of the 30 effective patents is shown in Fig. (**32**). The main fields of the patents in China include pharmaceutical compositions, acceptable salts, R1, R2, R3, R4, CD40 and temsirolimus.

30 Patents, 17 Text Clusters (From Title and Abstract)

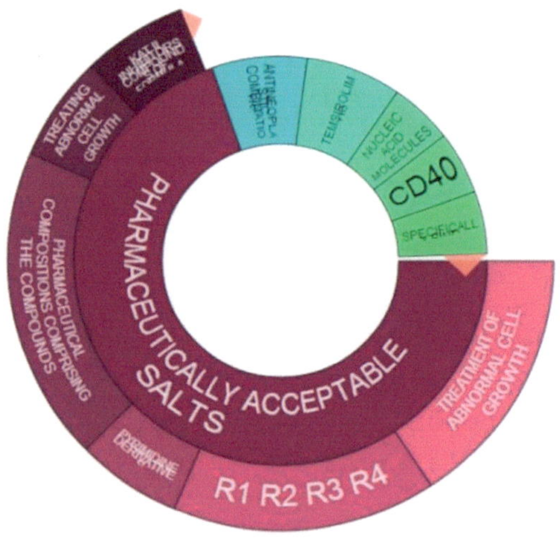

Fig. (32). Clustering analysis for the 30 effective patents.

2.6.5. Novartis AG

1. Since 2002, patent applications began to grow rapidly and has been relatively stable in recent years.

The development trend of patent technology for Novartis AG is shown in Fig. (**33**). Since 2002, the amount of applications began to grow rapidly and has been relatively stable since 2004.

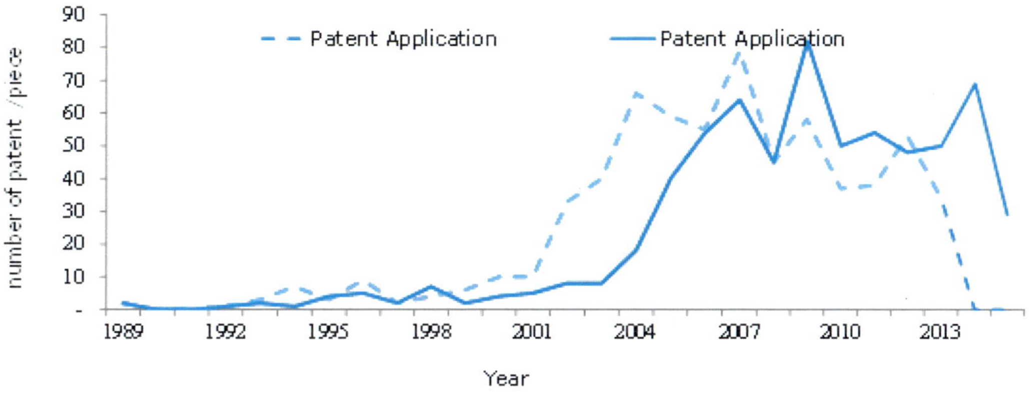

Fig. (33). Development trend of patents.

2. The distribution of IPC is wide, distributed in 77 IPC groups. The IPC top 3 account for 37% of the total applications.

Table 23. Distribution of the IPC Top 3 (654 Pieces).

Number	IPC / Group	Applications / Piece
1	A61K 31/00 Pharmaceutical preparations containing effective organic components	161
2	C07D 401/00 Heterocyclic compounds, containing two or more heterocyclic rings, with nitrogen atoms as the only heterocyclic atom. There is at least one hexatomic ring containing only a nitrogen atom	44
3	A61P 35/00 Anti-cancer drugs	35

Novartis AG's 654 patents are distributed in 77 IPC groups. Table **23** is the distribution of the IPC top 3. There are 240 pieces of patents, accounting for 37% of total patent applications in China. The main IPC field is A61K 31/00 (pharmaceutical preparations containing effective organic components).

The text clustering of the anti-cancer drug patents for patent applicants is shown in Fig. (**34**). The main fields of patents in China include pharmaceutical compositions, pharmaceutically acceptable salts, kinase inhibitors, and proliferative diseases.

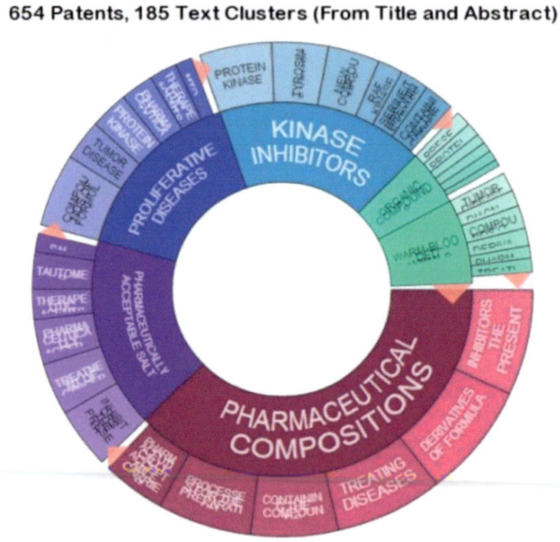

Fig. (34). Text clustering of patents (654 pieces).

3. The sum of active grants and active applications account for 24.3% of total patent applications.

Statistics on the effectiveness of the Chinese patents for anti-cancer drugs say the sum of active grants and active application is 159, accounting for 24.3% of the total patent applications.

There are 159 pieces of effective patents in China, which are distributed in 41 IPC groups. Table **24** shows the distribution of the IPC top 3. The IPC top 3 totals 62, accounting for 39% of the effective patents. The main IPC fields include A61K 31/00 (pharmaceutical products containing peptides), A61P 35/00 (anti-cancer drugs) and C07K 16/00 (immunoglobulin, for example, monoclonal or polyclonal antibodies).

Table 24. Distribution of the IPC Top 3 (119 Effective Patents).

Number	IPC / Group	Application / Piece
1	A61K 31/00 Pharmaceutical preparations containing organic effective components	31
2	A61P 35/00 Anti-cancer drugs	17
3	C07K 16/00 Immunoglobulin, for example, monoclonal or polyclonal antibodies	14

Figure **35** shows the text clustering analysis for the 159 effective patents. The key technology includes kinase inhibitors, proliferative disease, biomarkers and PI3K.

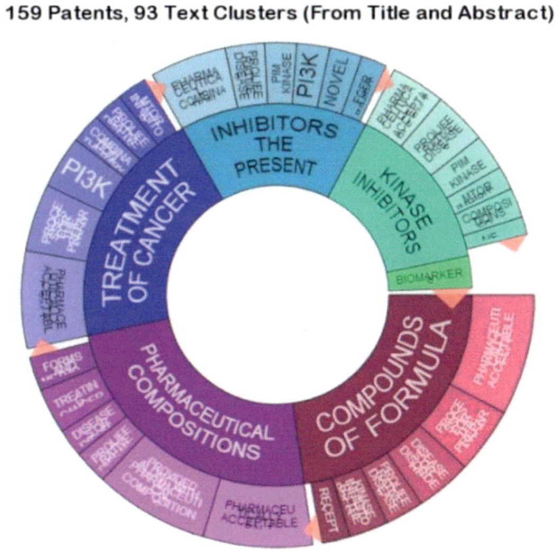

Fig. (35). Text clustering of the 159 effective patents.

3. ANALYSIS OF PATENT APPLICATIONS IN FOREIGN COUNTRIES BY CHINESE APPLICANTS

3.1. Data Sources

The patent data is from an Innography® platform. The retrieval date is updated to September 28, 2015. The retrieval strategy includes @ (abstract, claims, title) (Drug or compound or agent or medicine or inhibitor or resistance) and (cancer* or tumor* or tumour* or neoplas* or carcinogen* or carcinoma* or sarcoma*). The countries were set to other countries other than China; The keywords are "kind_code_a or kind_code_a1 or kind_code_a2 or kind_code_y or kind_code_u"; Inventor's location was set to China. Finally, the patent applications of Chinese inventors in other countries total 4,036 pieces, which are confirmed to be invention patents.

3.2. General Situation of Patents

1. The patent applications of Chinese inventors in foreign countries began early. Since 2001, applications began to grow rapidly and reached a peak in 2012.

Figure **36** is the development trend of China's inventors in foreign countries in the field of anti-cancer drugs, investigated in terms of the number of annual public patents and annual patent applications. The amount of patent applications by Chinese inventors in foreign countries and public patents is roughly the same. China began to apply for foreign patents from the beginning of the implementation of the patent law but the numbers were low at that time. From the beginning of 2001, the applications in foreign countries entered a rapid growth phase, and reached a peak in 2012. Then the number remained relatively stable after a decline. The patent disclosures in 2015 are not sufficient and part of the patent data is not included, and therefore not included in the scope of the trend analysis.

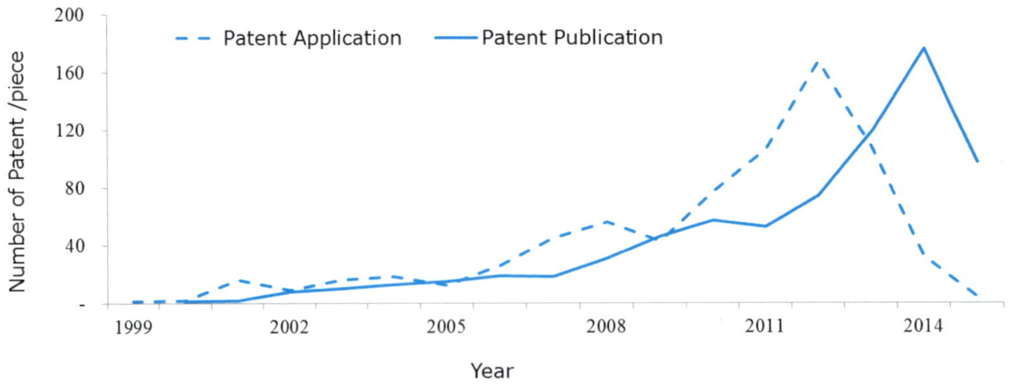

Fig. (36). Development trend of patents (Chinese applications in foreign countries).

2. Chinese applicants focus on the WIPO (World Intellectual Property Office) and EPO to carry out the layout of their patents. The United States is the largest

applying country.

The national distribution of anti-cancer drug patents and the trends of applying countries are shown in Figs. (**37** and **38**). On the whole, the layout of Chinese patents mainly concentrates in the WIPO, EPO, the United States and Japan. The total number is 2,977, accounting for 74% of the total applications in foreign countries. The Chinese inventors welcome patent application through EPO and the WIPO. The amount is 1,081 and 568, accounting for 27% and 14% of the total foreign applications, respectively. The United States is the largest applying country that Chinese patent applicants are concerned about. The amount is 897, accounting for 22% of the total foreign applications. Followed by Japan, the amount being 431, accounting for 11%.

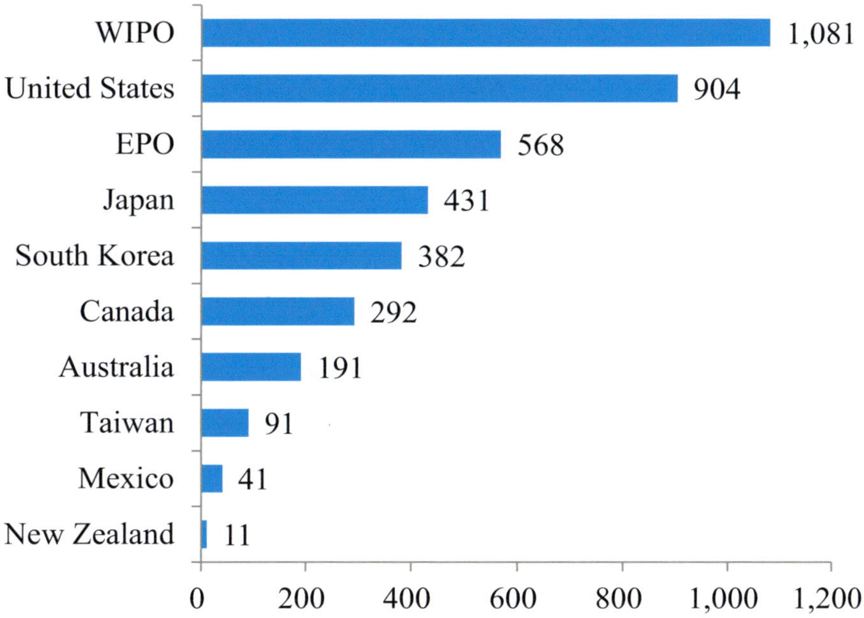

Fig. (37). Distribution of patent applications for main applying countries (top 10) (unit: piece).

3. Lack of important patents and core patents in the layout of foreign countries

The intensity distribution of the Chinese patents in foreign countries for anti-cancer drugs is shown in Table **25**. The patent applications continue to rise. However, there is a lack of core patents and important patents, which indicates

China has great potential for technological development. At the same time, the Chinese patent literature did not add citation information, which led to an inferior position in the evaluation of patent strength according to the unified standard of Innography®.

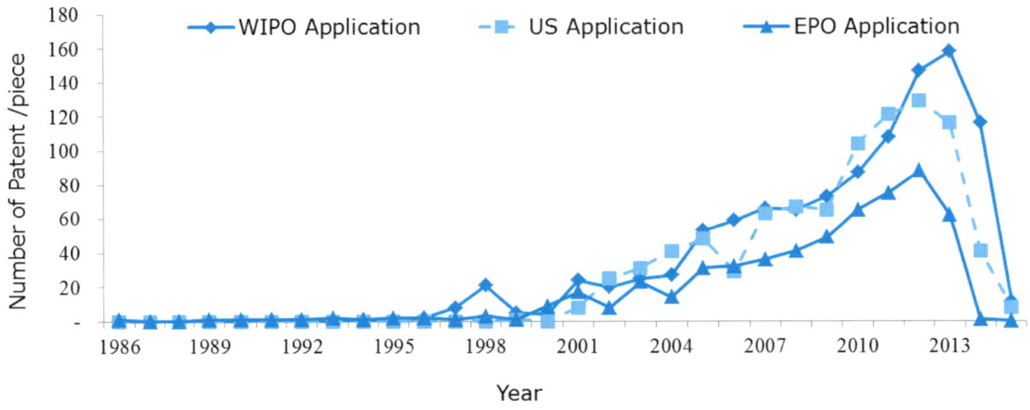

Fig. (38). Development trend of main applying countries (Chinese inventors in foreign applications).

Table 25. Patent Strength for Anti-Cancer Drugs (Chinese Inventors Apply Abroad).

Patent Strength%	Type	Amount/ Pieces	Proportion %
80-100	Core patent	11	0.27
30-80	Important patent	674	16.7
0-30	General patent	3351	83.03

3.3. Developmental Characteristics of Patented Technology

Table **26** shows the text clustering of patent titles and abstracts in descending order of frequency. We can know that the main research focus of anti-cancer drugs has changed little, mainly including cancer cells, traditional Chinese medicine, pharmaceutical compositions, liver cancer and raw materials. But there is a small change in frequency. For example, in recent years Chinese inventors have begun to pay more attention to lung cancer.

1. Distribution of the IPC in the field of anti-cancer drugs

Table **27** is the distribution of the IPC top10. There are 1,814 pieces of patents, accounting for 45% of the total patent applications by Chinese inventors in foreign countries.

Table 26. Text Clustering Statistics of Patent Applications (Chinese Inventors in Foreign Countries).

Number	IPC Top 10 (1986-2015)	IPC Top 10 (2012 & 2013)
1	Preparation methods	Preparation methods
2	Pharmaceutical compositions	Pharmaceutical compositions
3	Pharmaceutically acceptable salts	Pharmaceutically acceptable salts
4	Kinase inhibitors	General formula
5	General formula	Kinase inhibitors
6	Lung cancer	Breast cancer

Table 27. Distribution of the IPC Top 10 (Chinese Inventors in Foreign Countries).

Number	IPC / Group	Application / Piece
1	A61K 31/00 Pharmaceutical preparations containing effective organic components	645
2	A61K 38/00 Pharmaceutical preparations containing peptides	205
3	C07D 487/00 Heterocyclic compounds containing nitrogen atoms in a fused ring system as a heteroatom only, not included in the C07D 451/00, C07D 477/00 groups	159
4	C07D 401/00 Heterocyclic compounds, containing two or more heterocyclic rings, with nitrogen atoms as the only heterocyclic atom. There is at least one hexatomic ring containing only a nitrogen atom.	142
5	C12N 15/00 Mutation or genetic engineering; DNA or RNA involved in genetic engineering, vectors, such as plasmids, or their separation, preparation, or purification; the host	137
6	C07D 471/00 Nitrogen atoms are used as the only heterocyclic atoms in a fused ring system. At least one ring is a six membered heterocyclic compound containing a nitrogen atom and not included in the C07D 451/00, C07D 463/00 groups	128
7	A61K 9/00 Pharmaceutical preparation with special physical shapes	121
8	A61K 36/00 Pharmaceutical preparations containing algae, moss, fungi, or plants such as a traditional herbal medicine	98
9	A61K 39/00 Pharmaceutical preparations containing antigen or antibody (immune test material into G01N 33/53)	94
10	C07D 239/00 Heterocyclic compounds containing 1,3- thiotriazinone or hydro 1,3- thiotriazinone	85

2. Text clustering analysis in the field of anti-cancer drugs

The cluster analysis of the top 10 patents in the IPC sorting is shown in Fig. (**39**). Patent applications of Chinese inventors in foreign countries mostly focused on pharmaceutical compositions, preparation methods, pharmaceutically acceptable salts, tumor cells, kinase inhibitors, tyrosine kinase and side-effects.

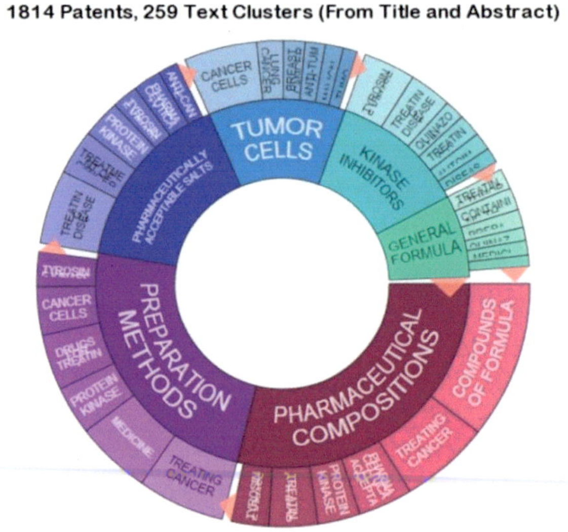

Fig. (39). Distribution of patent technology for the IPC top 10.

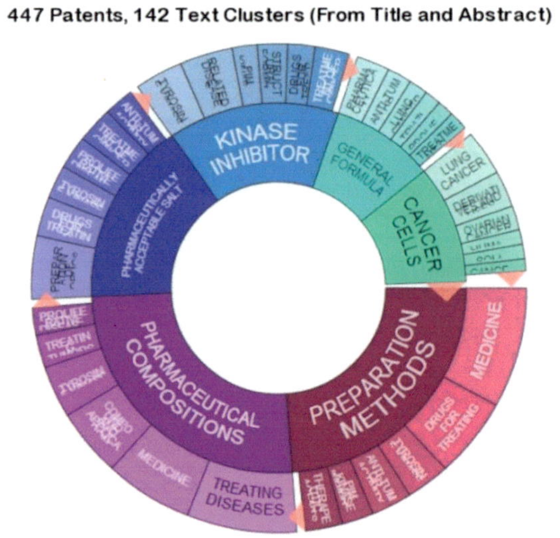

Fig. (40). Distribution of patent technology for the IPC top 10 (2012 & 2013).

Figure **40** shows the cluster analysis of the top 10 patent applications in 2012 and 2013 (IP classification). The main research fields of Chinese inventors pursuing patent applications in foreign countries include preparation methods, pharmaceutical compositions, pharmaceutically acceptable salts, kinase inhibitor, tyrosine kinase and lung cancer.

3.4. Analysis of the Main Applicants

The topic is mainly based on the Innography® bubble chart used to analyze the main applicants. There are 4,036 pieces of patents totally. Roche Holding Ltd. is the most powerful company, whose technical strength and the number of patents put it in a leading position. The patent applications of Medipharma SA are many but the strength is relatively weak. There is a large gap between these two companies and the rest, both in strength and the number of patents.

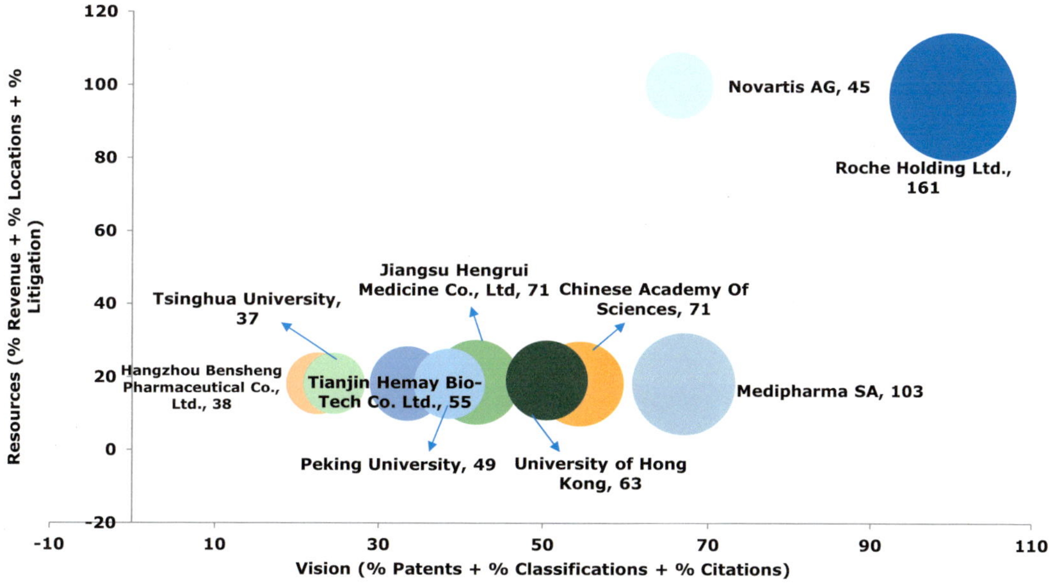

Fig. (41). Bubble analysis of patentees (Chinese inventors in foreign countries).

In addition, Chinese patent applicants in foreign countries include enterprises, universities and research institutions. Roche Holding Ltd., Medipharma SA and Jiangsu Hengrui Medicine Co. Ltd. are the most prominent in Chinese Enterprises for anti-cancer drug research; Chinese universities or scientific institutions such as the Chinese Academy of Sciences, University of Hong Kong and Peking University also have patent applications and have accumulated a certain R & D strength (Fig. (**41**)).

The distribution of Patent Strength for the main applicants (top 10) is shown in Table **28**. The proportion of the important patents for each company is low except for Medipharma SA whose proportion of important patents is up to 25.2%.

Table 28. Distribution of Patent Strength for the Main Applicants (Top 10).

Applicants	General Patent *(Piece /%)	Important Patent *(Piece /%)	Core Patent *(Piece /%)
Roche Holding Ltd.	141/87.6%	20/12.4%	0/0
Medipharma SA	77/74.8%	26/25.2	0/0
Chinese Academy Of Sciences	59/83.1%	12/16.9	0/0
Jiangsu Hengrui Medicine Co., Ltd.	64/90.1%	7/9.9%	0/0
University of Hong Kong	53/84.1%	10/15.9%	0/0
Tianjin Hemay Bio-Tech Co., Ltd.	51/92.7%	4/7.3%	0/0
Peking University	46/93.9%	3/6.1%	0/0
Novartis AG	35/77.8%	10/22.2%	0/0
Hangzhou Bensheng Pharmaceutical Co., Ltd.	36/94.7%	2/5.3%	0/0
Tsinghua University	28/75.7%	9/24.3%	0/0

*Percentage = (general patent or important patent or core patent) / total application amount *100

The distribution of active grants and active applications for the main applicants (top 10) are shown in Table **29**. The proportion of Hangzhou Bensheng Pharmaceutical Co., Ltd. is up to 73.7%.

Table 29. Distribution of Active Grants and Active Applications for the Main Applicants (Top 10).

Applicants	Active Grants and Active Application*(piece/%)
Roche Holding Ltd.	42/26.1%
Medipharma SA	31/30.1%
Chinese Academy Of Sciences	29/40.8%
Jiangsu Hengrui Medicine Co., Ltd.	37/52.1%
University of Hong Kong	27/42.9%

(Table 29) contd.....

Applicants	Active Grants and Active Application*(piece/%)
Tianjin Hemay Bio-Tech Co. Ltd.	8/14.5%
Peking University	19/38.8%
Novartis AG	24/53.3%
Hangzhou Bensheng Pharmaceutical Co., Ltd.	28/73.7%
Tsinghua University	10/27.0%

*Percentage = (grants active + application active) / total applicationamount *100%

The patent applications of the major applicants (top 10) is few. Table **30** shows distribution of patent technology for the main applicants through statistics on the clustering keywords.

Table 30. Distribution of Patent Technology for the Main Applicants (Top 10) (1985-2015).

Applicants	Key Technical Field
Hangzhou Bensheng Pharmaceutical Co., Ltd.	P2X 3 R1 R2 Triazole-substituted arylamides Hdac inhibitors of formula
Tianjin Hemay Bio-Tech Co., Ltd.	Treating an angiogenesis-related disorder Triazolopyridines and triazolopyrazines EGFR Pyrimidinyl indole compounds the present
Chinese Academy of Sciences	EGFR Gleevec R
Peking University	6-Amino quinazoline or 3-cyano quinoline derivatives Pyrrole six-membered heteroaryl ring 1-methyl pyrrolidin-2-yl
Tsinghua University	Nucleic acid Liver cancer Aggregation-induced emission Compounds for inhibiting the MCM complex Cdk5
XuanzhuPharmaco., Ltd.	C1-4 Alkyl F Cl Br C1-4 alkylOHOC1-4 alkylNO2NHC R7 and R8
Taisho Pharmaceutical Co., Ltd.	H and C1-C3 Alkyl Malignant tumor DNA sequences H and C1-C3 Alkyl

(Table 30) contd.....

Applicants	Key Technical Field
Impact Therapeutic Services	Smo Diagnosis and treatment of pathologies
Golden Biotechnology Corporation	Berbamine Acylation derivatives Bisbenzylisoquinoline alkaloids
Inst. of Medication, Chinese Academy of Medicine	DNA or RNA Metastasis

4. CASE STUDY (LIVER CANCER)

4.1. Data Sources

The patent data is from the Innography® platform The retrieval date is updated to September 28, 2015 and the retrieval strategy includes (abstract, claims, title) (Drug or compound or agent or medicine or inhibitor or resistance) and ("liver cancer" or "hepatic carcinoma" or hepatoma or "hepatic cancer"). The retrieval results are 29,510 pieces of patents.

In retrieving Chinese domestic patents about anti-liver cancer drugs, we chose "China Application" to be the source field, which represents Chinese domestic patent applications concerning liver cancer drugs. The total number is 5,582. After screening, we totaled 5,578 pieces of invention patents about anti-liver cancer drugs.

For retrieving the patents of Chinese applicants in foreign countries we chose "Countries other than China" to be the source field. Inventor's location was set to "China". Keywords were "kind_code_a" or "kind_code_a1" or "kind_code_a2" or "kind_code_y" or "kind_code_u". The amount of the patent applications of Chinese inventors in other countries is 738 pieces, which are totally invention patents.

4.2. Analysis of Chinese Domestic Anti-cancer Drug Patents

4.2.1. General Situation of Patents

«CA CANCER J CLIN» published «Global Cancer Statistics, 2012» in 2015.

According to GLOBOCAN statistics, there were 782,000 new cases of liver cancer worldwide in 2012. The new incidence rate for China is about 50% [5]. Based on analysis of the local anti-cancer drug technology in China, it is known that in recent years, the attention of Chinese inventors towards liver cancer has increased.

The development trend of patents for the treatment of liver cancer is shown in Fig. (**42**). The patent applications in this field continue to increase. Since 2004, the growth rate of patent applications has been higher than before, which shows a close relationship with the high incidence of liver cancer in the Chinese.

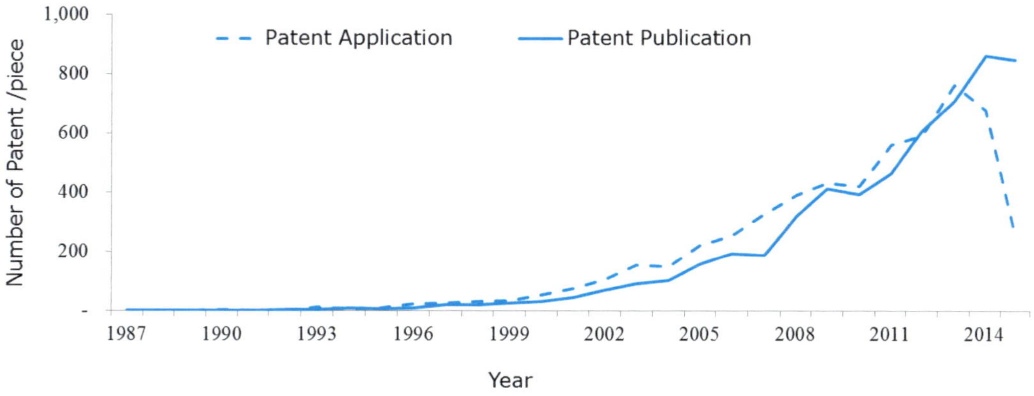

Fig. (42). Development trend of patent technology (liver cancer).

4.2.2. Analysis of Major Competitive Countries and Regions

1. Important patents and core patents account for only 12%

Table 31. Distribution of the Patent Strength.

Patent Strength %	Types	Number of Patents / Pieces	Proportion %
80-100	Core patent	4	0.1%
30-80	Important patent	665	11.9%
0-30	General patent	4,909	88.0%

Generally speaking, the higher the intensity of the patent, the higher the importance and value of the patents are. The correspondence between the intensity of the patent and the patent type is shown in Table **31**. Chinese general domestic patents account for 88%. The core patents and important patents are small, accounting for only 12%.

2. Chinese patent applications account for 74.6% of total applications

Figure **43** shows the distribution of the patent applications for the major countries (top 10). Figure **44** shows the distribution of the patent applications for the top 10 countries (Patent Strength >30%). From the 669 pieces of core and important patents, the patent applications of the top 10 countries are 601 pieces, accounting for about 89.8%. The proportion for the United States is 64.4%.

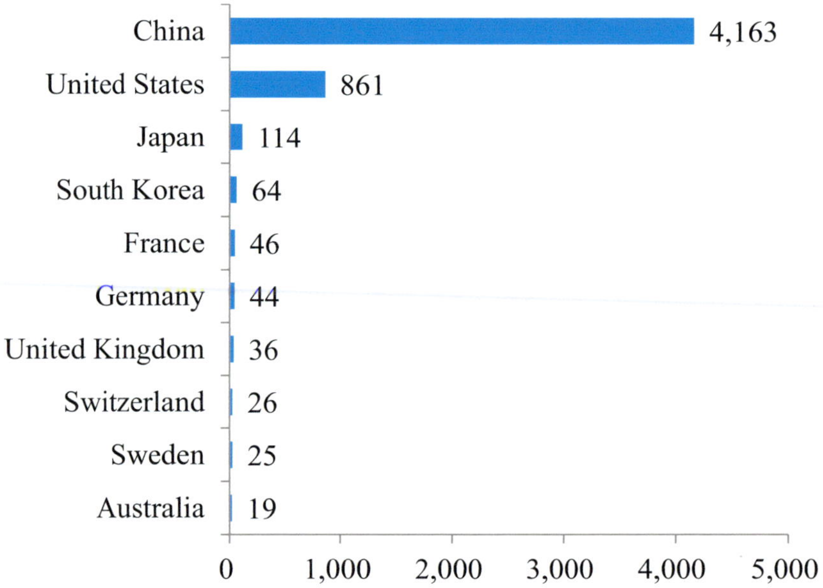

Fig. (43). Distribution of patent applications for major countries (top 10) (Unit: piece).

The Patent Strength of the United States is the highest. Its core patents and important patents account for 50% of its total applications. In the 4,163 pieces of Chinese patents, the core patents and important patents account for only 2%. Chinese patents are at a disadvantage in the Innography® patent strength evaluation due to lack of reference information. However, Chinese inventor's patent applications are first in the inventor's state ranking, but high-level applications are last, which shows that, in China, there are some defects in the technology development for liver cancer.

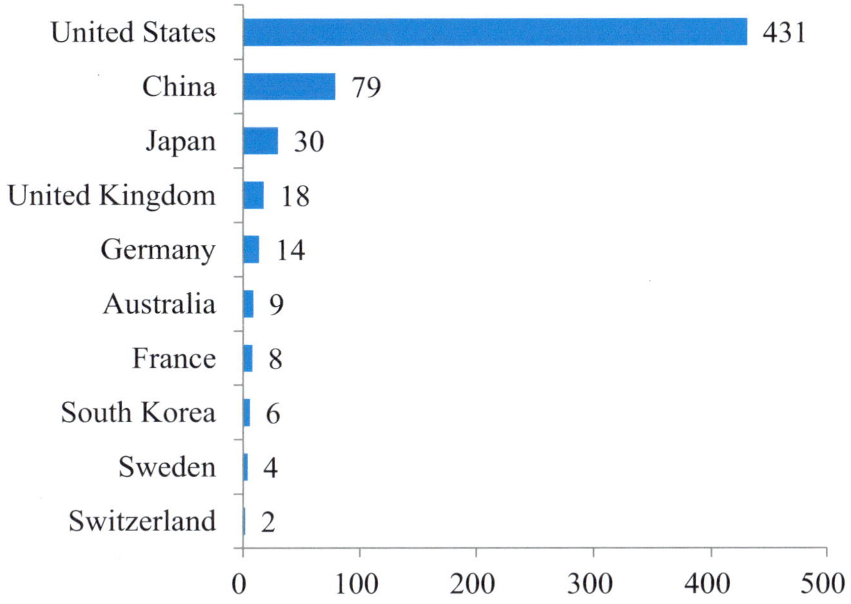

Fig. (44). Distribution of patent applications for the top 10 countries (patent strength >30%).

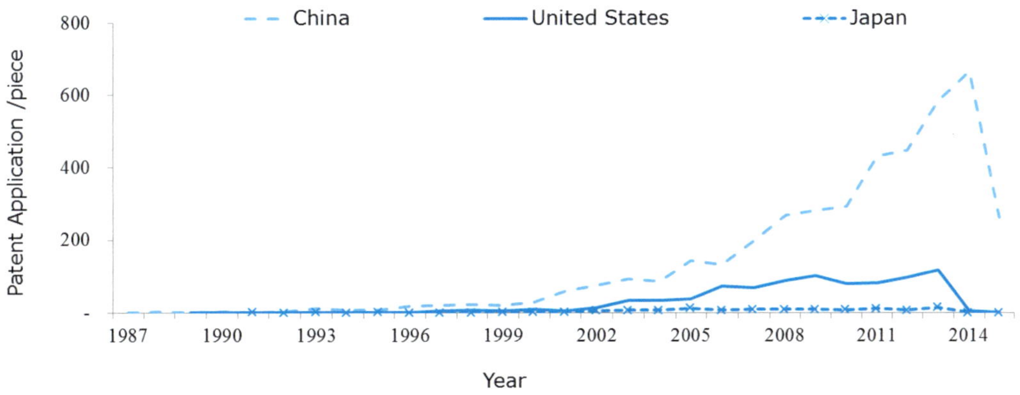

Fig. (45). Trend chart of patent applications for the top 3 countries (liver cancer).

The patent applications of China, the United States and Japan are up to 5,138 pieces, accounting for 92% of the total applications. The trend chart of patent applications for major countries (top 3) is shown in Fig. (**45**). From 2006 to 2009, the United States sped up development in the Chinese market. Then its applications remained stable. Japanese development in the field almost had no change. Affected by the innovation strategy of Chinese science and the improvement of the level of Chinese medical treatment, the Chinese domestic inventors in the field of anti-liver cancer drugs remain on a upward trend.

4.2.3. Analysis of the Characteristics of Technological Development

Table **32** shows the text clustering of patent titles and abstracts in descending order of frequency. We can know that the main research focus of liver cancer drugs has changed little, including mainly cancer cells, traditional Chinese medicine and pharmaceutical compositions. Treating liver cancer became a hot new research topic instead of gene expression.

Table 32. Distribution of the Patent Technology (Liver Cancer).

Number	IPC Top 10 (Since 1985)	IPC Top 10 (2012 & 2013)
1	Preparation methods	Cancer cells
2	Cancer cells	Treating liver cancer
3	Lung cancer	Tumor cells
4	Traditional Chinese Medicine	Lung cancer
5	Pharmaceutical compositions	Traditional Chinese Medicine
6	Gene expression	Pharmaceutical compositions

1. Distribution of the IPC in the field of anti-liver cancer drug

The 5,578 pieces of patent applications were distributed in 283 of the IPC groups. Table **33** is the distribution of the IPC top 10. There are 2,430 pieces of patents, accounting for 43% of the total patent applications.

Table 33. Distribution of the IPC Top 10 (Liver Cancer).

Number	IPC / Group	Applications / Piece
1	A61K 36/00 Pharmaceutical preparations containing algae, moss, fungi, or plants such as a traditional herbal medicine	541
2	A61K 31/00 Pharmaceutical preparations containing effective organic components	528

(Table 33) contd.....

Number	IPC / Group	Applications / Piece
3	C12N 15/00 Mutation or genetic engineering; DNA or RNA involved in genetic engineering, vectors, such as plasmids, or their separation, preparation, or purification; the host	276
4	C12Q 1/00 Methods for the determination or examination of enzymes or microorganisms; compositions thereof; methods for preparing such compositions	210
5	A61K 9/00 Pharmaceutical preparations with special physical shape	181
6	G01N 33/00 Materials are studied or analyzed using special methods not included in the G01N 1/00, G01N 31/00 groups	172
7	C07K 16/00 Immunoglobulin, for example, monoclonal or polyclonal antibodies	158
8	A61K 38/00 Pharmaceutical preparations containing peptides	123
9	C07D 401/00 Heterocyclic compounds, containing two or more heterocyclic rings, with nitrogen atoms as the only heterocyclic atom. There is at least one hexatomic ring containing only a nitrogen atom	122
10	C07D 471/00 Nitrogen atoms are used as the only heterocyclic atoms in a fused ring system. At least one ring is a six membered heterocyclic compound containing a nitrogen atom and not included in the C07D 451/00, C07D 463/00 groups	119

2. Text clustering analysis in the field of liver cancer drugs

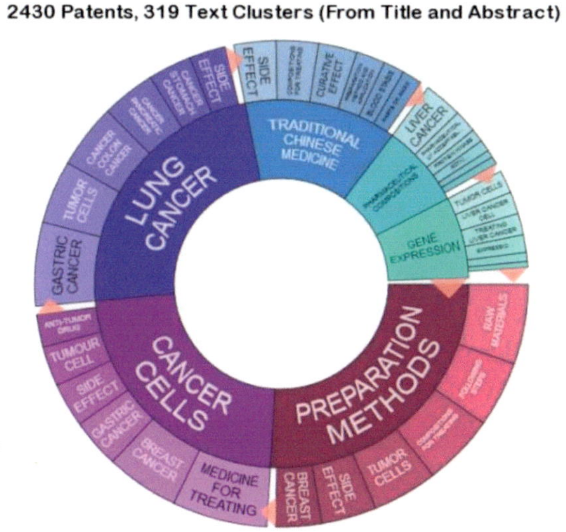

Fig. (46). Distribution of patent technology for the IPC top 10 (1985-2015).

The cluster analysis of the top 10 patents of the IPC sorting is shown in Fig. (**46**) from which we can know the field focuses mostly on preparation methods, cancer cells, lung cancer, traditional Chinese medicine, pharmaceutical compositions and gene expression. Among these, the sub-category keywords of preparation methods include: cancer cells, traditional Chinese medicine, lung cancer, raw materials and pharmaceutical compositions. The sub-category keywords of gene expression include: tumor cells, expression vectors, expression products, nucleic acids, hybrid probes and small interfering RNA.

Figure **47** shows the text clustering for the IPC Top 10 patent applications in 2012 and 2013. These patents include mostly cancer cells (containing tumor cells), treating liver cancer, lung cancer, traditional Chinese medicine and pharmaceutical compositions. Drugs involved in these patents are effective for lung and liver cancer.

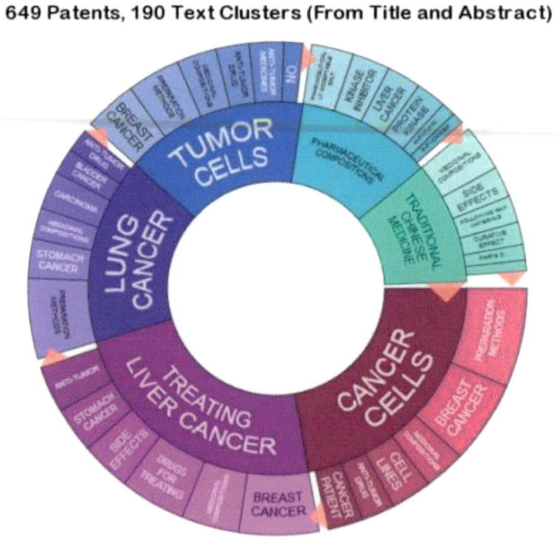

Fig. (47). Distribution of patent technology for the IPC top 10 (2012 & 2013).

Figures **48** and **49** show text clustering for the 115 patents related to tumor cells and the 117 patents related to cancer cells. Moreover, the keywords related to the two technologies are similar.

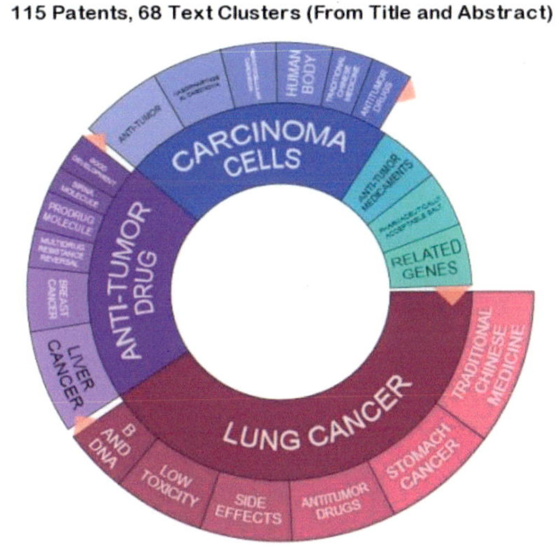

Fig. (48). Distribution of patent technology about tumor cells (2012 & 2013).

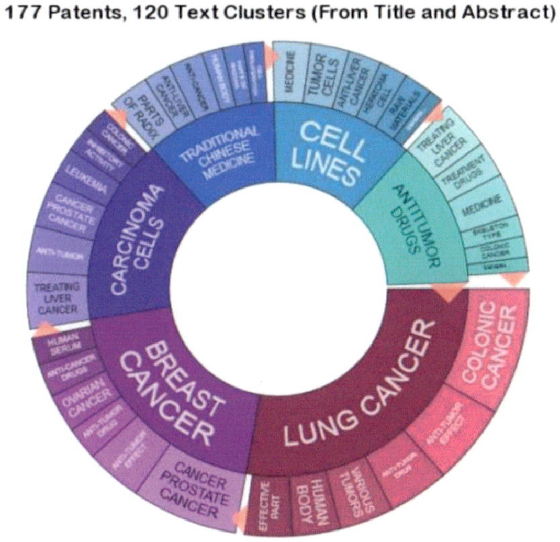

Fig. (49). Distribution of patent technology about cancer cells (2012 & 2013).

4.2.4. Analysis of the Main Applicants

The topic is based mainly on the Innography® bubble chart used to analyze the main applicants. There are 5,578 pieces of patents total. Fudan University and the Chinese Academy of Sciences applied for most. Both have 80 pieces. The patent technology of the Chinese Academy of Sciences is the strongest, while the

GlaxoSmithKline plc. is relatively weak.

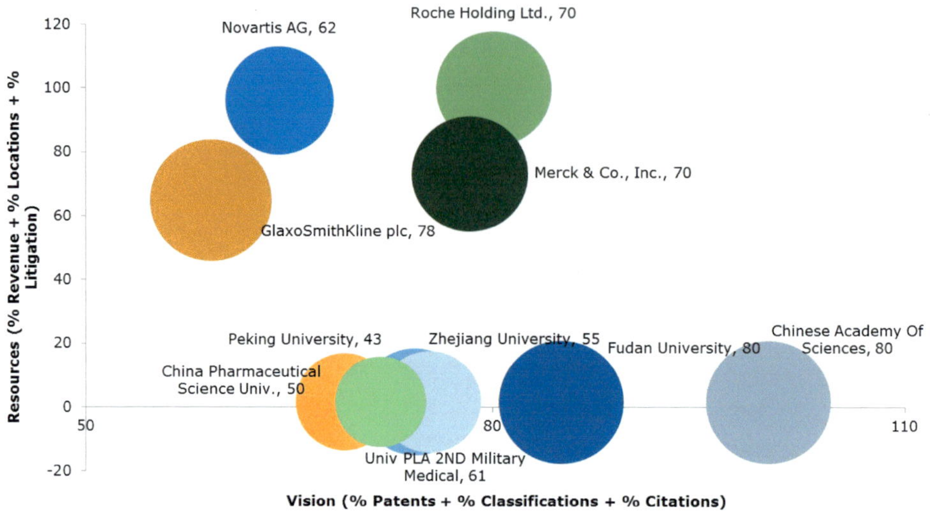

Fig. (50). Bubble analysis of patentees (patent applications top 10).

The sum of active grants and active applications is 2,204, accounting for 39.5% of the total patent applications (Fig. (**50**)).

A detailed analysis of patentees whose patent applications are ranked in the top 5 was based on three aspects: the change of the application trend, the key areas of research and active grants and active applications.

1. Fudan University

The number of patents of Fudan University for the years of 2011-2013 was 2,412 and 28 respectively, accounting for 67.5% of the total applications in this field (Fig. (**51**)).

Figure **52** shows the text clustering for the 80 patents of Fudan University in the field of liver cancer. Technical focus can be classified as anti-tumor drugs (synonyms include anti-tumor medications and antineoplastic drugs), side effects, anti-tumor activities and tumor multi-drug resistance.

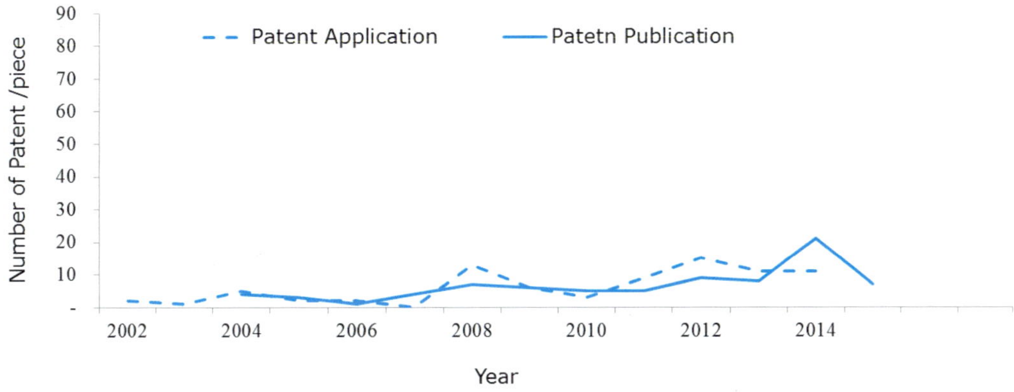

Fig. (51). Development trend of patent technology.

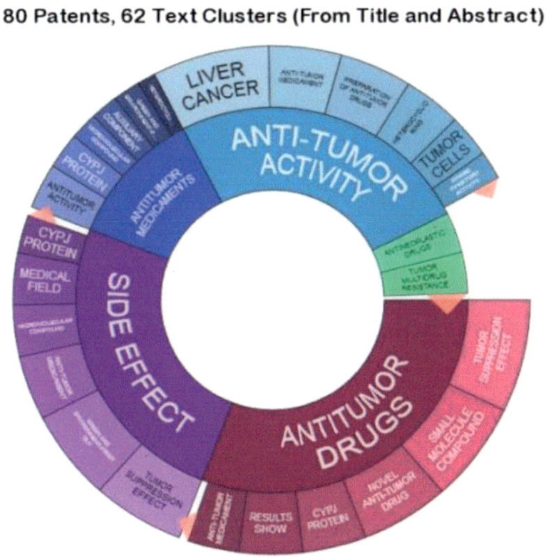

Fig. (52). Distribution of patent technology (1985-2015).

Further analysis on anti-tumor drugs (synonyms include anti-tumor medicaments and antineoplastic drugs) say the patents related to anti-tumor drugs involve anti-tumor medicaments and antineoplastic drugs. The sub categories of anti-tumor drugs include CYPJ protein, small molecule compounds, and tumor suppression effects.

Figure **53** shows the text clustering for patents in 2012 and 2013. The research hotspots of Fudan University include anti-tumor, GSK-3BETA, anti-tumor activity, tumor multi-drug resistance, autophagy inhibitor and hepatitis B.

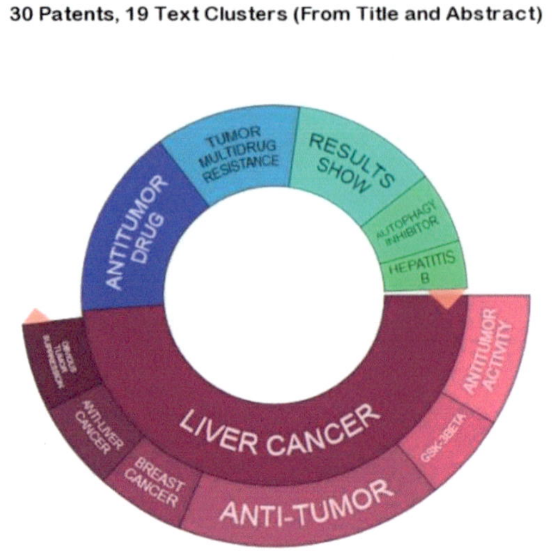

Fig. (53). Distribution of patent technology (2012 & 2013).

At present, the sum of active grants and active applications is 30 pieces, accounting for 37.5% of the total applications, slightly lower than the overall level of anti-liver cancer drug. Figure **54** shows the cluster analysis of the 30 patents. The current effective fields include side-effects, autophagy inhibitor and hepatitis B.

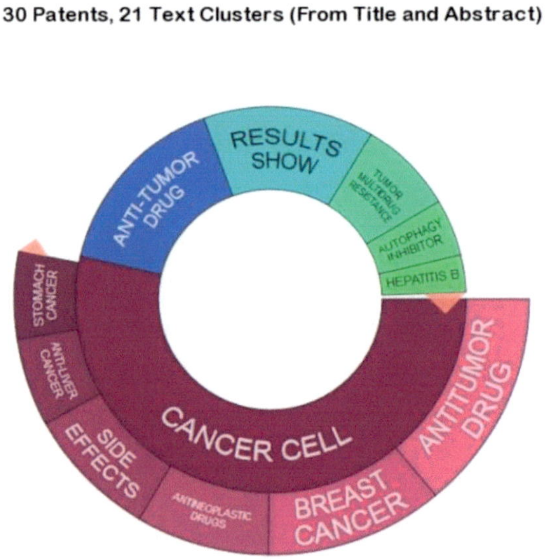

Fig. (54). Distribution of patent technology (active application & active grants).

2. Chinese Academy of Sciences

Figure **55** shows the development trend of patent technologies for the Chinese Academy of Sciences in the field of liver cancer. The patent applications in 2012-2014 remained at more than 10 pieces.

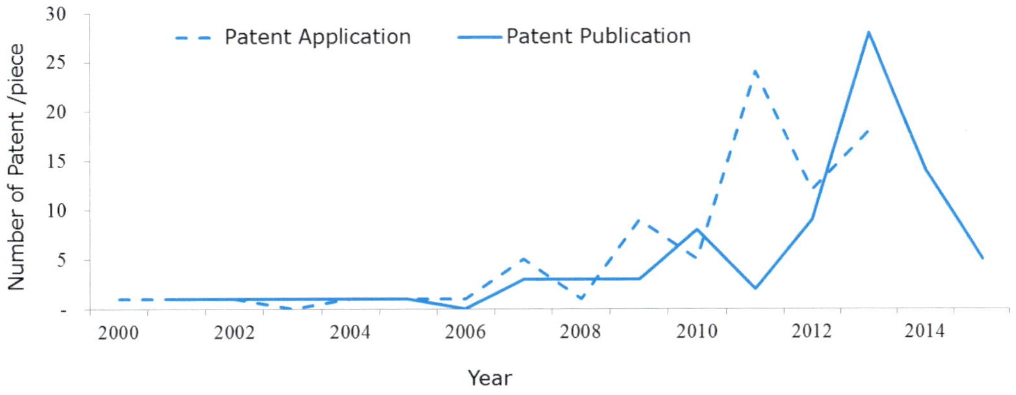

Fig. (55). Development trend of patent technology (liver cancer).

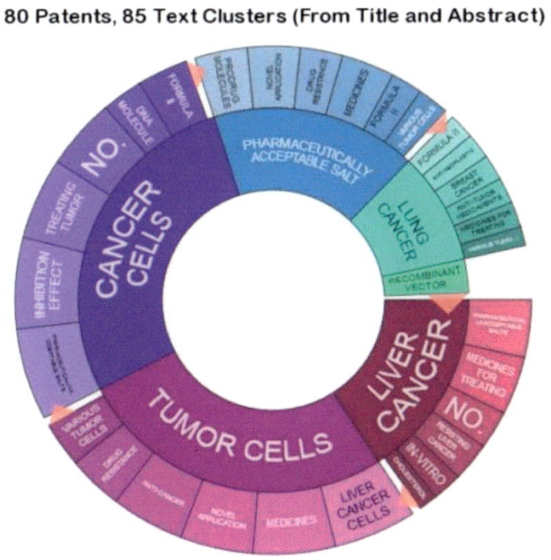

Fig. (56). Distribution of patent technology (1985-2015).

Figure **56** shows the text clustering for the 80 patents of the Chinese Academy of Sciences. The research focus of the patentees includes liver cancer cells, inhibition effects, drug resistance, DAN molecular, pharmaceutically acceptable salts, and *in vitro*.

Figure **57** shows the text clustering for patents in 2012 and 2013. In recent years, the Chinese Academy of Sciences focused on pro-drug molecules, drug resistance, preparation of anti-tumor drugs and pharmaceutical acceptable salts.

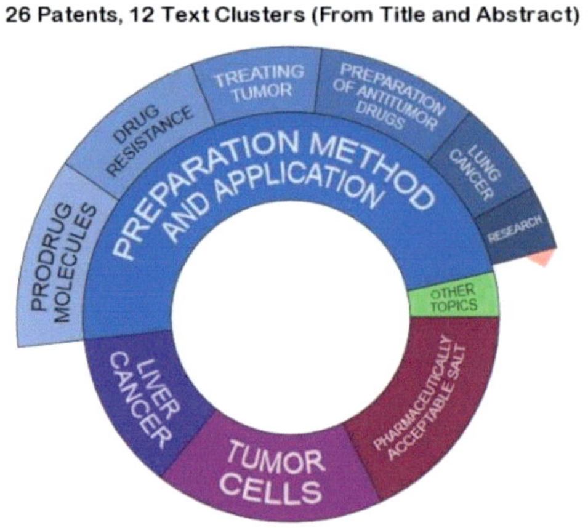

Fig. (57). Distribution of patent technology (2012 & 2013).

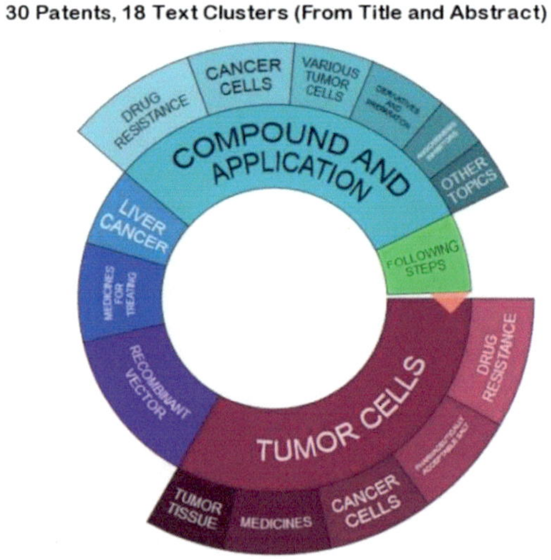

Fig. (58). Distribution of patent technology (active application & active grants).

At present, the sum of active grants and active applications is 30 pieces, accounting for 37.5% of the total applications, slightly lower than the overall level of liver cancer drugs. Figure **58** shows the cluster analysis of the 30 patents. The current effective fields include drug resistance, derivatives and preparations, angiogenesis inhibitors, pharmaceutically acceptable salts and recombinant vectors.

3. GlaxoSmithKline plc.

Figure **59** shows the development trend of patent technologies for GlaxoSmithKline plc. in the field of anti-liver cancer. The total number of applications is 78. The amount of applications in 2008 was 28 pieces, reaching the peak in this year. The number of patents has dropped in recent years.

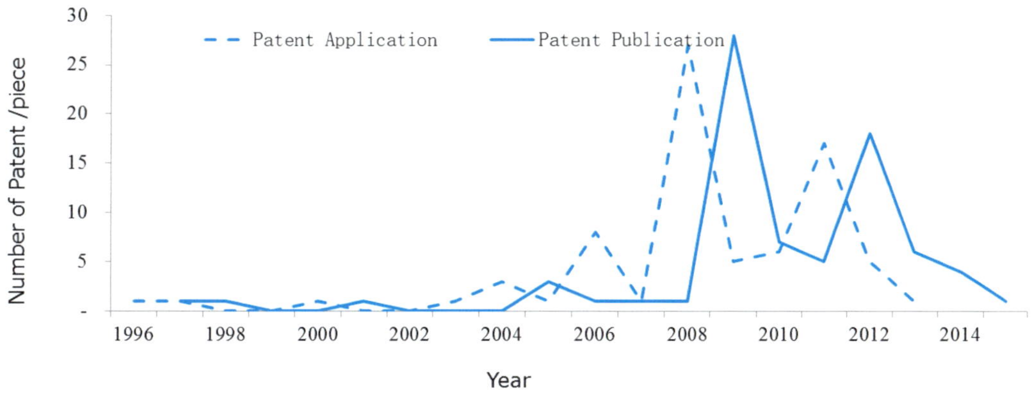

Fig. (59). Development trend of patent technology.

Figure **60** shows the text clustering for the 78 patents of patentees in the field of liver cancer. The focus areas of the patents include liver cancer diagnosis, coding protein, target points, expression products, inhibiting genes, target genes for preparing medicaments treating liver cancer, novel symmetrical triphenyl compounds and pharmaceutically acceptable salts.

In 2012 and 2013, patent applicants only applied for 6 patents in the field of liver cancer. Among these, patents concerning gene expression accounted for half.

At present, the sum of active grants and active applications is 11 pieces, accounting for 14.1% of the total application amount. This is below the overall level of liver cancer drugs.

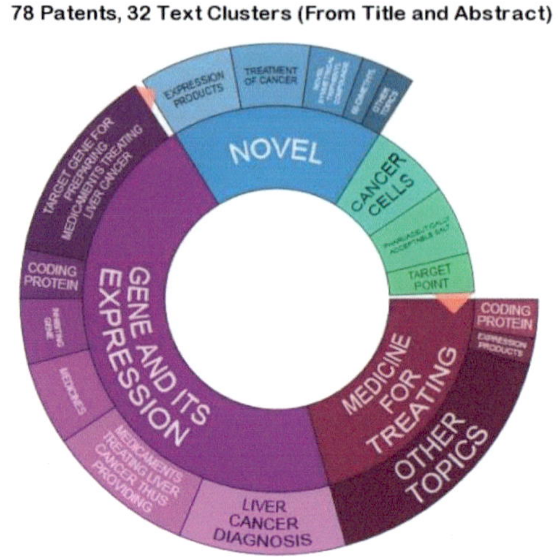

Fig. (60). Distribution of patent technology (1985-2015).

4. Roche Holding Ltd.

The patent applications of Roche Holding Ltd. in China are not stable every year, as shown in Fig. (**61**). But the upward trend is obvious.

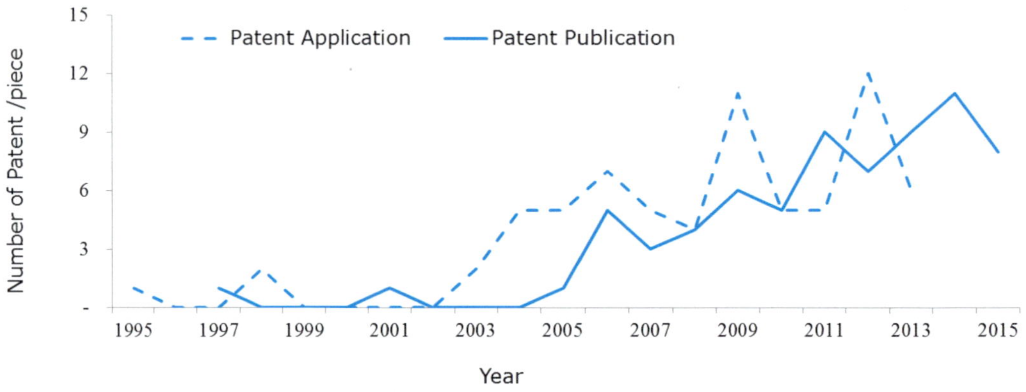

Fig. (61). Development trend of patent technology.

Figure **62** shows the text clustering for the 70 patents of Roche Holding Ltd. The focus is on lipid kinases, IA and IB, RAF kinase, PI3 kinase and BTK.

70 Patents, 34 Text Clusters (From Title and Abstract)

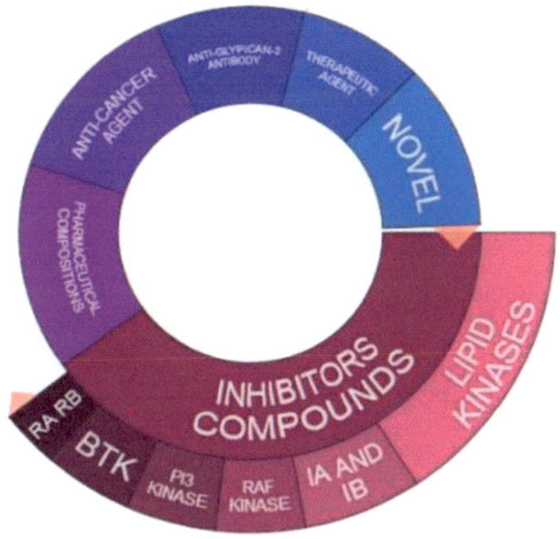

Fig. (62). Distribution of patent technology (1985-2015).

At present, the sum of active grants and active applications are 30 pieces, accounting for 37.5% of the total application amount. As shown in Fig. (**63**), the technical points include BTK, RA & RB, R1 & R2 and anti-glypican 3 anti-body.

30 Patents, 12 Text Clusters (From Title and Abstract)

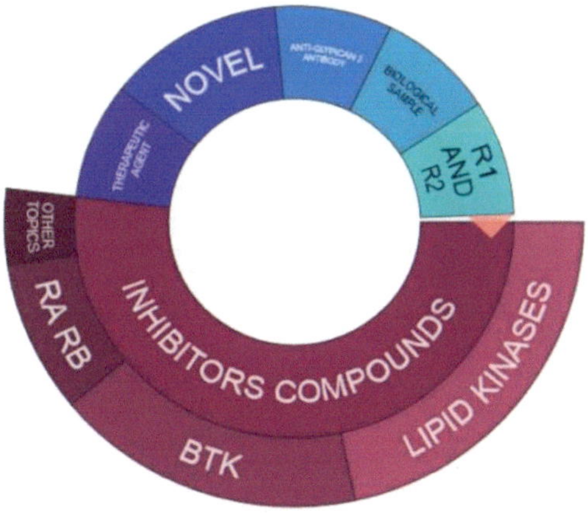

Fig. (63). Distribution of patent technology (active application & active grants).

5. Merck & Co., Inc.

Figure **64** show the development trend of patent technologies for Merck & Co., Inc. The time from 2006 to 2008 is the peak for patent applications. There were 47 pieces of patents total, accounting for 67% of total applications. However, there were no applications concerning liver cancer in China in the recent 2 years.

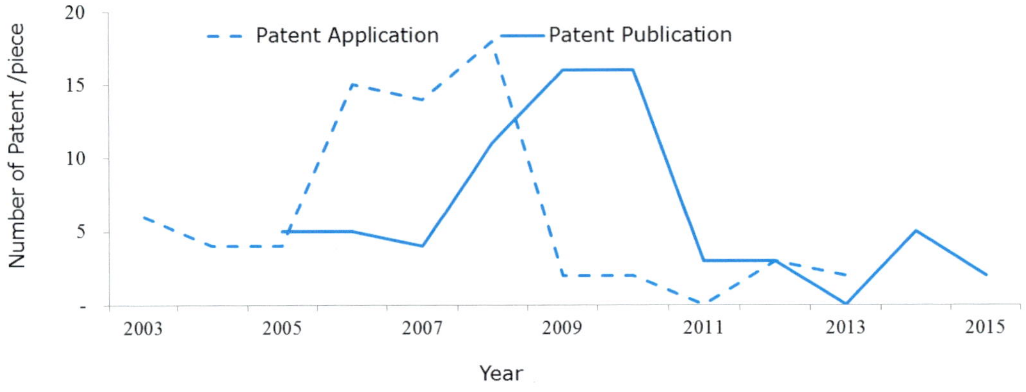

Fig. (64). Development trend of patent technology.

Figure **65** shows the text clustering for the 70 patents for Merck & Co., Inc. The focus is on kinase inhibitors, pharmaceutically acceptable salts, ERK inhibitors, cyclin dependent kinases, HS90 inhibitors and derivatives and methods.

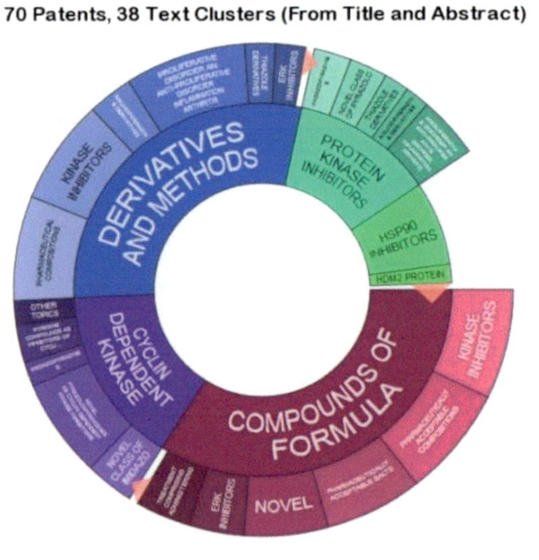

Fig. (65). Distribution of patent technology (1985-2015).

At present, the sum of active grants and active applications is 9 pieces, accounting for 12.8% of the total applications. As shown in Fig. (**65**), the technical points include BTK, RA & RB, R1 & R2 and anti-glypican 3 antibody, far below the overall level of liver cancer drugs.

4.3. Analysis of Patent Applications in Foreign Countries by Chinese Inventors

4.3.1. General Situation of the Development of Anti-cancer Drugs

The development trend for Chinese inventors in foreign markets is shown in Fig. (**66**). From 1985 to 2015, Chinese inventors provided 738 patents for liver cancer drugs in foreign countries. It maintained a sustained trend increase. Since 2011, the annual applications were more than 100 pieces.

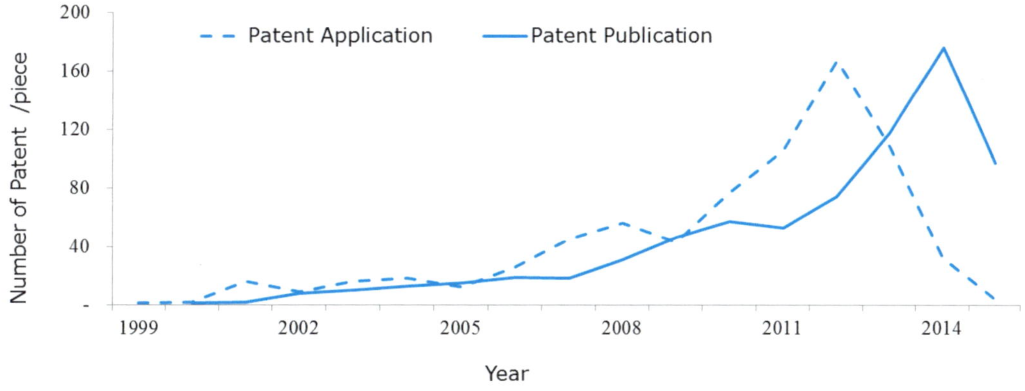

Fig. (66). Development trend of patent technology (Liver cancer).

4.3.2. Analysis of Major Competitive Countries and Regions

The distribution of the Patent Strength for Chinese inventors is shown in Table **34**. The proportion of core patents and important patents is 20.3%. However, the proportion of Chinese inventors in the Chinese domestic markets is only 2%. The only piece of core patent was by Bioscience Jenken, Inc. and is invalid because the priority does not meet the requirements.

Figure **67** shows the distribution of patent applications for the major technology applying countries. The United States, Japan, South Korea, Canada and Australia are the main markets for Chinese inventors. The five countries account for 67.8% of total applications.

Table 34. Distribution of the Patent Strength.

Patent Strength %	Types	Number of Patents / Pieces	Proportion%
80-100	Core patent	1	0.01%
30-80	Important patent	149	20.2%
0-30	General patent	588	79.7%

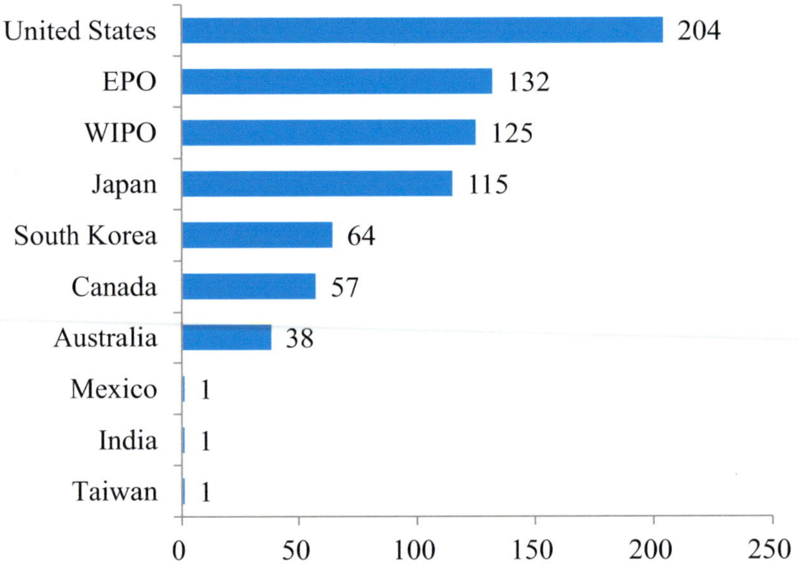

Fig. (67). Distribution of patent applications for major countries (top 10) (unit: piece).

Since 2005, patent applications of Chinese inventors through EPO and the WIPO continued to rise, as shown in Fig. **(68)**.

4.3.3. Analysis of the Characteristics of Technological Development

In 738 patent applications, the distribution of the top 10 IPCs is shown in Table **35**. There are 371 pieces of patents, accounting for 50.3% of total patent applications.

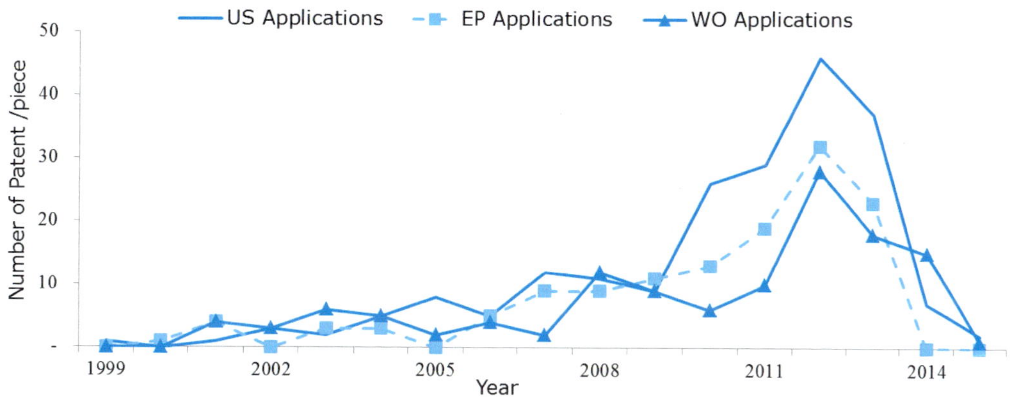

Fig. (68). Distribution of patent technologies for major countries (Top 3) (Liver cancer).

Table 35. Distribution of the IPC Top 10 (Liver Cancer).

Number	IPC / Group	Applications / Piece
1	A61K 31/00 Pharmaceutical preparations containing effective organic components	127
2	A61K 38/00 Pharmaceutical preparations containing peptides	46
3	C07D 487/00 Heterocyclic compounds containing nitrogen atoms in fused ring system as heteroatom only, not included in the C07D 451/00, C07D 477/00 groups	37
4	C07D 491/00 Heterocyclic compounds which contain 1 or more oxygen atoms as the only heterocyclic atom in a fused ring system, and contains 1 or more nitrogen atoms as the only heterocyclic atom in a fused ring system, not included in the C07D 451/00, C07D 459/00, C07D 463/00, C07D 477/00 and C07D 489/00 groups	30
5	A61K 9/00 Pharmaceutical preparation with special physical shapes	22
6	C07D 495/00 Heterocyclic compounds: there is at least 1 heterocyclic compound with sulfur atoms which are used as the only heterocyclic atoms in the fused ring system	19
7	C07D 471/00 Nitrogen atoms are used as the only heterocyclic atoms in a fused ring system. At least one ring is a six membered heterocyclic compound containing a nitrogen atom and not included in the C07D 451/00, C07D 463/00 groups	19
8	C07K 14/00 Immunoglobulin, for example, monoclonal or polyclonal antibodies	19
9	C07D 401/00 Heterocyclic compounds, containing two or more heterocyclic rings, with nitrogen atoms as the only heterocyclic atom. There is at least one hexatomic ring containing only a nitrogen atom	18

(Table 35) contd.....

Number	IPC / Group	Applications / Piece
10	C07K 16/00 Immunoglobulin, for example, monoclonal or polyclonal antibodies	17
11	A61P 35/00 Anti-cancer drugs	17

Figure **69** shows the cluster analysis for the top 10 patents in the IPC classification. The main fields include pharmaceutical methods, pharmaceutically acceptable salts, liver cancer and cancer cells (including tumor cells).

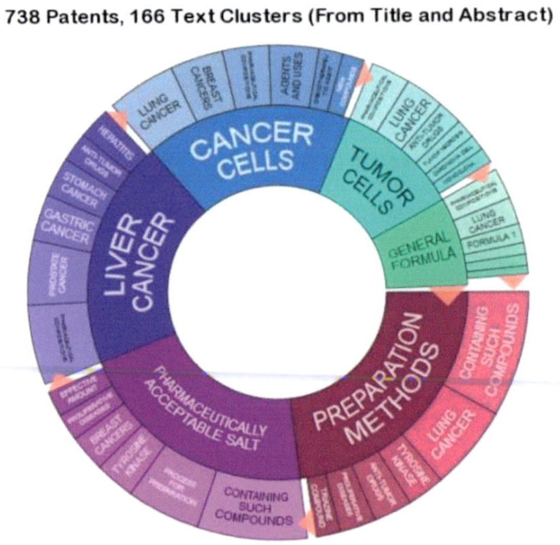

Fig. (69). Distribution of patent technology for the IPC top 10 (1985-2015).

After the statistics for each keyword, we eliminated some noise words such as "Containing Such Compounds". Table **36** shows the Top 5 keywords ranking in the frequency statistics.

Table 36. Word Frequency Statistics for Patent Technology Top 5 (1985-2015).

Pharmaceutical Methods	Pharmaceutically Acceptable Salt	Liver Cancer	Cancer Cells
Lung cancer	Tyrosine kinase	Prostate/gastric/stomach cancer	Chemotherapeutic agent
Tyrosine kinase	Breast cancers	Raw materials	Monoclonal antibody
Proliferative diseases	Proliferative diseases	Nucleic acid	Therapeutic effect

(Table 36) contd.....

Pharmaceutical Methods	Pharmaceutically Acceptable Salt	Liver Cancer	Cancer Cells
Triazine compound	c-Met kinase	Sterol derivatives	Tyrosine kinase
Nucleic acid	Oleanolic acid	Monoclonal antibody	C1-4 Alkyl

Figure **70** shows the cluster analysis for the top 10 patents (2012 & 2013) from the IP classifications. The main fields include preparation methods, general formulas, PARP inhibitors, tyrosine kinase, monoclonal antibodies and cancer screenings.

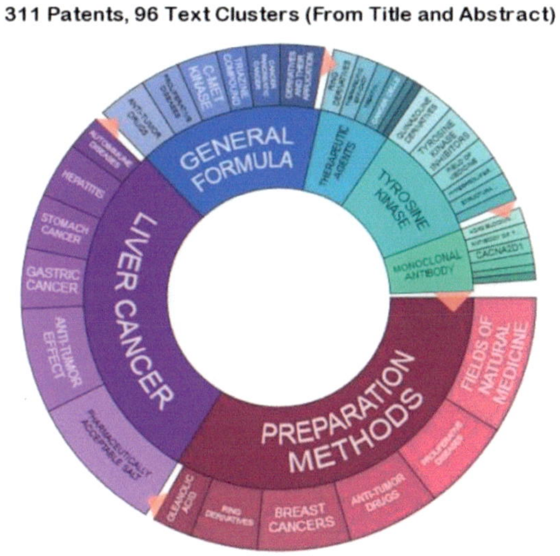

Fig. (70). Distribution of patent technology for the IPC top 10 (2012 & 2013).

After screening the word frequency in each aspect and eliminating the interference, the top 5 keywords are shown in Table **37**.

Table 37. Word Frequency Statistics for Patent Technology Top 5 (2012 & 2013).

Preparation Methods	General Formula	PARP Inhibitors	Tyrosine Kinase	Monoclonal Antibody	Screening Cancers
Fields of natural medicine	Derivatives and their application	Ar R1-R6	Tyrosine kinase inhibitors	CACNA2D1	Pyrimidine compound
Ring derivatives	Proliferative diseases	Pharmaceutical compositions	Quinazoline derivatives	Antibody of the present	Cell lines

(Table 37) contd.....

Preparation Methods	General Formula	PARP Inhibitors	Tyrosine Kinase	Monoclonal Antibody	Screening Cancers
Breast cancers	c-Met kinase	4-diones and analogs	Stereoisomer	AGR2 blocking antibody	Danshen
Oleanolic acid	Triazine compound	Hedgehog	Structural formula	Antibodies protein	Chemotherapeutic agent
Triazine compound	Inhibitory activity		Proliferative diseases	Growth factor	6-dione derivatives

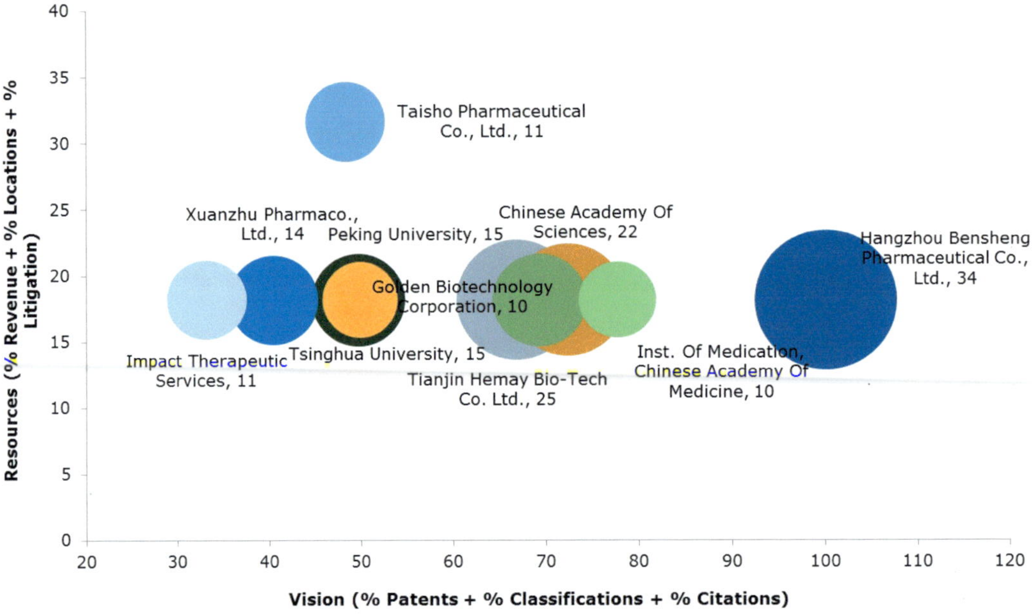

Fig. (71). Bubble analysis of patentees (patent applications top 10).

4.3.4. Analysis of the Main Applicants

The topic is mainly based on the Innography® bubble chart used to analyze the main applicants. Figure **71** shows the statistical analysis of 378 patents. The bubble of Hangzhou Bensheng Pharmaceutical Co., Ltd. is the largest, which indicates that its application is up to 34. It is located at the far right side of the horizontal axis, which indicates the patentee has the strongest technical strength. In addition to Taisho Pharmaceutical Co., Ltd., we did not get revenue information of the other patentees. The system sets it to 0 automatically. Therefore, the vertical coordinate values are the same, all of which are arranged on the same horizontal line.

The distribution of the Patent Strength for the main applicants (top 10) is shown in Table **38**. There are 18 important patents, accounting for only 12.1% of total important patents.

Table 38. Distribution of Patent Strength for the Main Applicants (Top 10).

Applicants	General Patent *(Piece/%)	Important Patent *(Piece/%)	Core Patent *(Piece/%)
Hangzhou Bensheng Pharmaceutical Co., Ltd.	32/94.1%	2/5.9%	0/0
Tianjin HemayBio-Tech Co., Ltd.	23/92.0%	2/8.0%	0/0
Chinese Academy Of Sciences	21/95.5%	1/4.5%	0/0
Peking University	14/93.3%	1/6.7%	0/0
Tsinghua University	14/93.3%	1/6.7%	0/0
XuanzhuPharmaco., Ltd.	12/85.7%	2/14.3%	0/0
Taisho Pharmaceutical Co., Ltd.	9/81.8%	2/18.2	0/0
Impact Therapeutic Services	9/81.8%	2/18.2	0/0
Golden Biotechnology Corporation	9/90.0%	1/10.0%	0/0
Inst. of Medication, Chinese Academy of Medicine	8/80.0%	2/10.0%	0/0

* Percentage = (general or important or core patent) / total application *100

The distribution of active grants and active applications for the main applicants is shown in Table **39**. Among the 14 patent applications of the Xuanzhu Pharmaco., Ltd., there are 13 pieces in a valid state. After analysis of its patents, it can be found that the applicant has begun to apply for liver cancer drug patents in the United States, Japan, or through the EPO since 2011. However, there was no applications for a patent since 2013.

Table 39. Distribution of Active Grants and Active Application for the Main Applicants.

Applicants	Active Grants and Active Application*(Piece/%)
Hangzhou Bensheng Pharmaceutical Co., Ltd.	28/82.4%
Tianjin Hemay Bio-Tech Co., Ltd.	5/20.0%
Chinese Academy of Sciences	11/34.4%

(Table 39) contd.....

Applicants	Active Grants and Active Application*(Piece/%)
Peking University	5/33.3%
Tsinghua University	8/53.3%
XuanzhuPharmaco., Ltd.	13/92.9%
Taisho Pharmaceutical Co., Ltd.	5/45.5%
Impact Therapeutic Services	8/72.7%
Golden Biotechnology Corporation	1/10.0%
Inst. of Medication, Chinese Academy of Medicine	3/30.0%

*Percentage = (Active Grants + Active Application) / total application *100%

As the patent applications of the main applicants (top 10) are less, we counted the clustering keywords. Finally, the distribution of the patent technology (1985-2015) for each applicant is obtained, as shown in Table **40**.

Table 40. Distribution of Active Grants and Active Application for the Main Applicants (Top 10) (1985-2015).

Applicants	Key Technical Fields
Hangzhou Bensheng Pharmaceutical Co., Ltd.	Berbamine Tanshinone Tetrandrine Acylation derivatives Homoharringtonine Oleanolic acid amidate derivatives
Tianjin Hemay Bio-Tech Co., Ltd.	C1-4 Alkyl Tetracyclic anthraquinones PyridylCyanoguanidines R2 R3 R4 R5 R6 R7 and R8 Doxorubicin Thiophene derivatives
Chinese Academy of Sciences	Triazine compound Gleevec
Peking University	Pharmaceutically acceptable salt PDCD5 polypeptides Tripeptide boronic acid
Tsinghua University	Pharmaceutically acceptable salt PDCD5 polypeptides Tripeptide boronic acid
XuanzhuPharmaco., Ltd.	Quinazoline derivatives
Taisho Pharmaceutical Co., Ltd.	Submicron emulsion

(Table 40) contd.....

Applicants	Key Technical Fields
Impact Therapeutic Services	AR R1-R6 4-Diones and analogs
Golden Biotechnology Corporation	AntrodiaCamphorata
Inst. of Medication, Chinese Academy of Medicine	NA.

5. CURRENT & FUTURE DEVELOPMENTS

In the Chinese domestic market, there are the same characteristics for anti-cancer and anti-liver cancer drugs. The growth of patent applications is fast. The number of patent applications in China is greater. However, core patents and important patents are few relative to foreign applications. Chinese applications are mainly from universities or research institutes, but for foreign applications enterprises apply more often. That indicates the lower industrialization of Chinese patents.

For the whole anti-cancer drug field, American patents stay ahead in quality. From the competition aspect, Bode Gene Dev. Co. Ltd. Shanghai has 1,960 patent applications, holding first place. Pfizer Inc. has the most patents in the field of anti-cancer drugs. Roche Holding Ltd. has the most abundant resources. All the players have their areas of focus. The main research hotspots and focus for anti-cancer drugs has changed little, mainly including cancer cells, traditional Chinese medicine, pharmaceutical compositions, liver cancer and raw materials.

Especially for anti-liver cancer drugs in the Chinese market, since 2004 the growth rate of patent applications has been higher than before, which has a close relationship with the high incidence of liver cancer in the Chinese. Chinese patent applications account for 74.6% of total applications, but important patents and core patents account for only 12%. The sum of active grants and active applications is 2,204, accounting for 39.5% of the total patent applications. The main research focus for liver cancer drugs mainly includes cancer cells, traditional Chinese medicine, and pharmaceutical compositions.

With the increasing strength of research and development, Chinese applicants prefer to improve their global layout through patents. In this thesis, Chinese patent applications have begun to grow rapidly since 2001 and reached a peak for anti-cancer drugs in 2012, with more than 100 pieces per year for anti-liver cancer drugs since 2011. Chinese applicants focus on the WIPO and EPO to carry out the layout of their patents, and the United States is the largest applying country. Enterprises contribute more compared to universities or research institutes, which is the opposite of the domestic market.

In recent years, lower health brought on by the rapid aging of the Chinese population and urbanization caused the morbidity and mortality of Chinese cancers patients to increase gradually. The demand for anti-cancer drugs will keep growing fast. At the same time, the amount of patent applications in the field of anti-cancer drugs will maintain its rising trend with gradual improvements in the Chinese legal system. That means intellectual property protection systems will become mature. Patent analysis will be more important if there is a business layout in China.

CONFLICT OF INTEREST

The authors confirm that they have no conflict of interest to declare for this publication.

ACKNOWLEDGEMENTS

Declared none.

REFERENCE

[1] China 13th Five Year Plan. Available at: http://www.gov.cn/xinwen/2016-03/17/content_5054992.htm, 2016 [Accessed on: March, 2016];

[2] The number of patent application in China is the first all over the world. Available at: http://news.xinhuanet.com/2012-12/12/c_113999683.htm, 2016 [Accessed on: March, 2016];

[3] The number of patent application in China is over 1,000 thousand. Available at: http://news.xinhuanet.com/2016-01/14/c_1117779338.htm, 2016 [Accessed on: March, 2016];

[4] The patent application number by PCT reaches new height in 2015. Available at: http://www.sipo.gov.cn/mtjj/2016/201603/t20160323_1254407.html, 2016 [Accessed on: March, 2016];

[5] World Health Organization. World Cancer Report 2014 [R]. 2014.

[6] Patent and IP Analytics Solutions. Available at: https://www.innography.com/solutions, 2016 [Accessed on: October 09, 2016];

[7] PatentStrength. Patent Value. Available at: https://www.innography.com/why-innography/patentstrength, 2016 [Accessed on: October 09, 2016];

[8] Allison JR, Lemley MA, Moore KA. Derek Trunkey Valuable Patents Law and Economics Working Paper Series, George Mason University School of Law & University of California at Berkeley School of Law. 2003.

[9] CFDA website. Medicine Administration Law of the People's Republic of China. Available at: http://www.sda.gov.cn/WS01/CL0784/124980.html, 2015 [Accessed on: October, 2016];

[10] CFDA website. Regulations for the Implementation of Drug Administration Law of the People's Republic of China. Available at: http://www.sda.gov.cn/WS01/CL0784/23395.html, 2015 [Accessed on: October, 2015];

[11] CFDA website. Rules for the Implementation of the Regulations on the Administration of Pharmaceuticals. Available at: http://www.sda.gov.cn/WS01/CL0053/24463.html, 2015 [Accessed on: October, 2015];

[12] CFDA website. Rules for the Implementation of the Regulations on the Administration of Pharmaceuticals. Available at: http://www.sda.gov.cn/WS01/CL0053/24463.html, 2015 [Accessed on: October, 2015];

[13] CFDA website. Provisions on the Supervision and Administrative Punishment Procedures of Drugs. Available at: http://www.sda.gov.cn/WS01/CL0053/24471.html, 2015 [Accessed on: October, 2015];

[14] CFDA website. The quality control standard for drug clinical trials. Available at: http://www.sda.gov.cn/WS01/CL0053/24473.html, 2015 [Accessed on: October, 2015];

[15] CFDA website. Good Laboratory Practice. Available at: http://www.sda.gov.cn/WS01/CL0053/24472.html, 2015 [Accessed on: October, 2015];

[16] CFDA website. Measures for the Administration of Drug Import. Available at: http://www.sda.gov.cn/WS01/CL0053/31658.html, 2015 [Accessed on: October, 2015];

[17] CFDA website. Measures for the Administration of Drug Business License. Available at: http://www.sda.gov.cn/WS01/CL0053/24476.html, 2015 [Accessed on: October, 2015];

[18] CFDA website. Measures for the Supervision and Administration of Drug Production. Available at: http://www.sda.gov.cn/WS01/CL0053/24501.htm, 2015 [Accessed on: October, 2015];

[19] CFDA website. Administrative Measures for Supervision and Administration of Medical Institutions" (Trial Implementation). Available at: http://www.sda.gov.cn/WS01/CL0053/24515.html, 2015 [Accessed on: October, 2015];

[20] CFDA website. Administrative Measures for the Registration of Medical Institutions. Available at: http://www.sda.gov.cn/WS01/CL0053/24518.html, 2015 [Accessed on: October, 2015];

[21] CFDA website. State Food and Drug Administration Drug Special Approval Procedures. Available at: http://www.sda.gov.cn/WS01/CL0053/24520.html, 2015 [Accessed on: October, 2015];

[22] CFDA website. Measures for the Administration of Imported Medicinal Materials" (Trial Implementation). Available at: http://www.sda.gov.cn/WS01/CL0053/24519.html, 2015 [Accessed on: October, 2015];

[23] CFDA website. Measures for the Examination of Drug Advertisements. Available at: http://www.sda.gov.cn/WS01/CL0053/24527.html, 2015 [Accessed on: October, 2015];

[24] CFDA website. Drug Advertisement Examination and Issue Standard. Available at: http://www.sda.gov.cn/WS01/CL0053/24526.html, 2015 [Accessed on: October, 2015];

[25] CFDA website. Measures for the Supervision and Administration of Drug Circulation. Available at: http://www.sda.gov.cn/WS01/CL0053/24525.html, 2015 [Accessed on: October, 2015];

[26] CFDA website. Provisions for Drug Registration. Available at: http://www.sda.gov.cn/WS01/CL0053/24529.html, 2015 [Accessed on: October, 2015];

[27] CFDA website. Provisions for Drug Recall. Available at: http://www.sda.gov.cn/WS01/CL0053/26913.html, 2015 [Accessed on: October, 2015];

[28] CFDA website. Good Practices in the Manufacture and Quality Control of Drugs. Available at: http://www.sda.gov.cn/WS01/CL0053/58500.html, 2015 [Accessed on: October, 2015];

[29] SIPO website. Patent Law. Available at: http://english.sipo.gov.cn/laws/lawsregulations/201101/t20110119_ 566244.html, 2016 [Accessed on: October 09, 2016];

[30] SIPO website. Implementing Regulations of the Patent Law of the People's Republic of China. Available at: http://english.sipo.gov.cn/laws/lawsregulations/200804/t20080416_380326.html, 2016 [Accessed on: October 09, 2016];

[31] SIPO website. Regulations on the Protection of Layout-Designs of Integrated Circuits. Available at: http://english.sipo.gov.cn/laws/lawsregulations/200804/t20080416_380325.html, 2016 [Accessed on: October 09, 2016];

[32] SIPO website. Regulations on Patent Commissioning. Available at: http://english.sipo.gov.cn/laws/lawsregulations/200804/t20080416_380324.html, 2016 [Accessed on: October 09, 2016];

CHAPTER 5

Recent Developments in Anticancer Agents Targeting Heat Shock Proteins

Aykut Özgür[1], **Banu Bayram**[2], **Lütfi Tutar**[3] and **Yusuf Tutar**[2,4,*]

[1] *Gaziosmanpaşa University, Faculty of Natural Sciences and Engineering, Department of Bioengineering, Tokat, Turkey*

[2] *University of Health Sciences, Faculty of Health Sciences, Department of Nutrition and Dietetics, Istanbul, Turkey*

[3] *Ahi Evran University, Faculty of Arts and Sciences, Department of Molecular Biology and Genetics, Kırşehir, Turkey*

[4] *Cumhuriyet University, Faculty of Pharmacy, Department of Basic Pharmaceutical Sciences, Division of Biochemistry, Sivas, Turkey*

Abstract: Proteins are metabolic factors to perform biochemical functions. For proper protein function, these macromolecules must be in their properly folded-native states. Under stress, cells employ Heat Shock Proteins (Hsps) to overcome this folding problem. For this reason, Hsp proteins play essential roles in the metabolic processes. In cancer cells the situation is different than healthy cells. Since the metabolic rates of cancer cells are faster than that of healthy cells, cancer cells overexpress Hsps to rescue unfolded proteins to perform biochemical functions. Thus, several research groups have been focused on Hsps. This protein family consists of several members and interacts with several cell signaling proteins, kinases, and transcriptional factors. All these interactions provide key controlling points to inhibit cancer cells and drive them to apoptosis for therapeutic purposes. Different approaches on Hsp mechanism were employed for cancer cell inhibition either by interrupting Hsp90-apoptosis inhibitor protein interactions or by blocking Hsp90-proteasome function. In a similar way, topoisomerase-Hsp90 interaction was perturbed. Small molecules as well as peptides

* **Corresponding author Yusuf Tutar:** Cumhuriyet University, Faculty of Pharmacy, Department of Basic Pharmaceutical Sciences, Division of Biochemistry, Sivas, Turkey; Tel: +90 346 219 10 10 ext 3907; Fax: +90 346 219 16 34; E-mails: ytutar@cumhuriyet.edu.tr, ytutar@yahoo.com

Atta-ur-Rahman and Khurshid Zaman (Eds.)

were employed to inhibit functions of Hsp70 and Hsp27. Several designs were performed and patented using Hsp cascade and this study summarizes the innovative patents in the area.

Keywords: Antigenic peptide complex, apoptosis, berberine, cancer, chimeric peptide, delivering an anticancer agent, heat shock protein targeted therapy, hepatitis, hepatoma, Hsp27, Hsp70 inhibitors, Hsp90 NTD inhibitors, Hsp90 CTD inhibitors, oncogenic client proteins, peptides, proteasome, protein folding, protein-protein interaction inhibitor, secreting modified heat shock protein, topoisomerase I.

INTRODUCTION

Heat shock proteins (Hsps) are highly conserved chaperone protein family and Hsps are essential biomolecules for the maintenance of cell viability. Hsps are involved in protein hemostasis pathways (folding and stabilization of proteins, prevention of protein aggregation, degradation of aggregated proteins, and protein translocation) in all living organisms. The molecular weights of Hsps are between 10 and 110 kDa, and Hsps can be divided into six groups according to their molecular weights (small Hsps, Hsp40, Hsp60, Hsp70, Hsp90, and Hsp110). Hsps are localized at different compartments of the cell and their expression level is highly increased in response to cellular and external stress factors (metal ions, tumorogenesis, UV light, pH alterations, oxidative stress, fever, and temperature variation). Hsps and their different isoforms are expressed either inductively or constitutively in the cell [1 - 4].

Pathogenesis of diseases is related with expression level of the Hsps and therefore, Hsps are considered as target biomolecules for drug design studies. To protect and repair cellular proteins against stress factors, Hsp inducers have been developed for the treatment of neurodegenerative diseases, cardiovascular diseases, febrile diseases, and gastrointestinal diseases [5]. Expression of Hsps in cancer cells has been extensively investigated in relation to the pathogenesis of tumorogenesis. Especially, Hsp27, Hsp70, and Hsp90 are key chaperone proteins in all phases of tumorogenesis (apoptosis, angiogenesis, metastases, invasion, and cell differentiation), and their expression level is increased significantly in cancer cells. Hsp27, Hsp70, and Hsp90 provide stabilization and proper folding of the oncogenic proteins in cancer cells. Several methods of inhibition were designed. Small molecule inhibition as well as peptide dependent inhibition gave promising results and an innovative approach interrupted protein-protein interaction through blocking key steps in biochemical pathways by designed compounds. Protein-protein interactions are important in Hsp coordinating-cooperating mechanism. Therefore, inhibition of chaperone activity of Hsp27, Hsp70, and Hsp90 has been a remarkable therapeutic strategy for target specific cancer treatment [5 - 7].

Heat Shock Protein 90

Commonly investigated macromolecule in chaperone inhibition is Hsp90. Hsp90 is a 90 kDa chaperone protein which plays vital roles in stabilization and proper folding of oncogenic client proteins (transcriptional factors, transmembrane tyrosine kinases, metastable/chimeric/mutated signaling proteins, and cell cycle regulators) for the growth and survival of cancer cells.

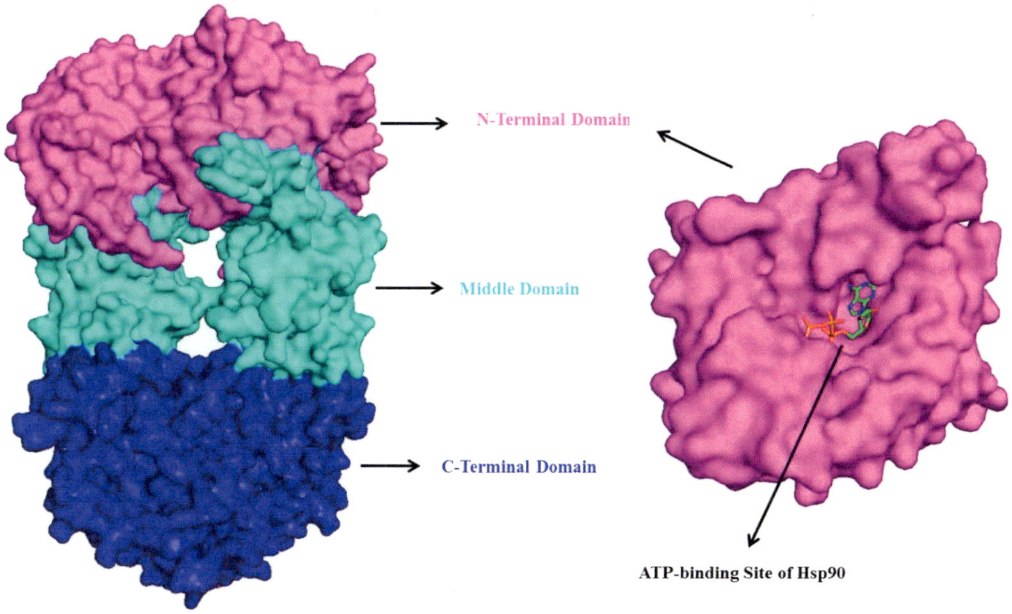

Fig. (1). Structure of Hsp90 (PDB ID 2CG9).

Hsp90 has four isoforms: Hsp90AA1, Hsp90AB1, TRAP1, and Grp94. Hsp90AA1 and Hsp90AB1 are localized in cytoplasm and they are expressed inductively and constitutively, respectively. TRAP1 is found in mitochondrial matrix and Grp94 is localized in endoplasmic reticulum. Hsp90 consists of three highly conserved domains: N-terminal domain (NTD), middle domain (MD), and C-terminal domain (CTD) [5, 8, 9]. ATPase activity of Hsp90 is essential process to perform chaperone activity. NTD contains a high-affinity ATP-binding cavity that binds both ATP and ADP nucleotides (Fig. (**1**)). ATP hydrolysis energy leads to conformational changes for interaction between oncogenic client proteins and Hsp90 CTD. CTD has conserved EEVD motif which regulates Hsp90 ATPase process and interacts with co-chaperones. MD contains binding site for client proteins. Hsp90 is the most expressed protein in unstressed eukaryotic and prokaryotic cells (1-2% of cellular proteins). In tumorogenesis, its expression level increases to 4-6% of cellular proteins [5, 8 - 11]. Due to this expression increase, drug designers employ Hsps as innovative drug targets to drive cancer cells to apoptosis.

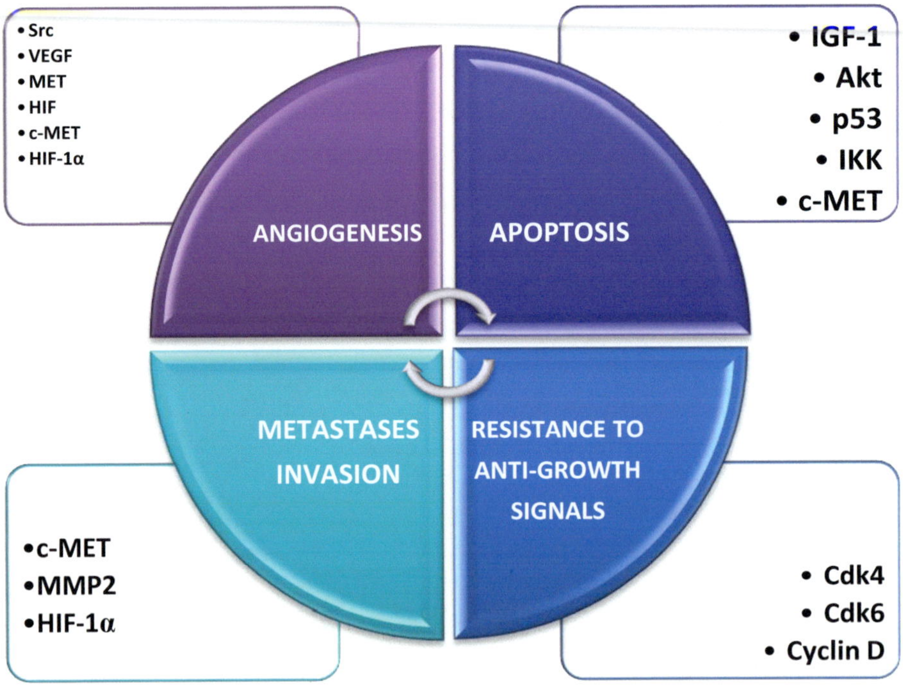

Fig. (2). Important oncogenic client proteins and their roles in tumorogenesis.

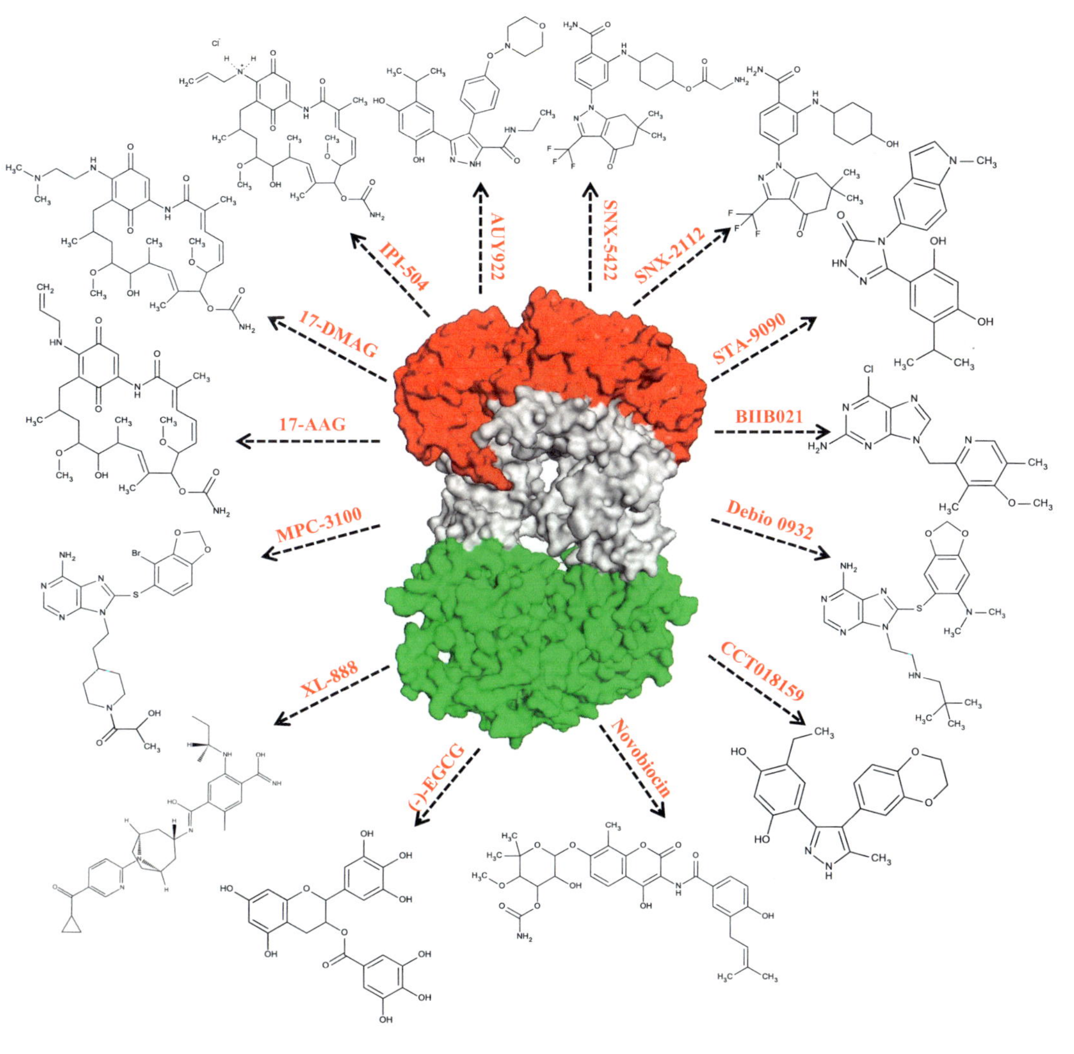

Fig. (3). Important Hsp90 inhibitors in clinical phase studies.

Cancer cells are exposed to unfavorable conditions (oxidative stress, low pH, poor nutritional status). These stress factors induce destabilization and misfolding of the oncogenic client proteins (Cdk4, Bcr-Abl, EGFR, ErbB2, Akt, p53,c-MET) in cancer cells (Fig. (**2**)). Client proteins at different biochemical pathways were summarized in Fig. (**2**). There are several proteins involved and therefore, cancer cells need more chaperone activity of the Hsps than normal healthy cells [5]. Therefore, inhibition of Hsp90 has been a remarkable therapeutic approach for the treatment of cancer. There are two strategies for the inhibition of Hsp90 chaperone activity: perturbation of the Hsp90 ATPase activity and inhibition of dimerization process of the Hsp90 CTD. Numerous compounds have been evaluated as Hsp90 inhibitors and some of these compounds displayed antiproliferative activity for cancer cells and they are in clinical phase studies. Geldanamycin is the first Hsp90 inhibitor which binds NTD ATP binding region and blocks Hsp90 ATPase activity. However, hepatotoxic features and poor water solubility of geldanamycin limit its clinical evaluation. For this reason, synthetic geldanamycin analogs, 17-AAG, 17-DMAG, and IPI-504, were designed and synthesized as Hsp90 inhibitors, and now their anticancer potentials are evaluated in clinical phase studies. According to the clinical studies, orally available and water soluble new generation Hsp90 NTD inhibitors (Fig. (**3**)) will be used for the treatment of cancer in the near future [2, 5, 7, 12, 13].

Hsp90 CTD inhibitors have also been developed by researchers including our laboratory and a CTD inhibitor patent was discussed at the end of this chapter.

Heat Shock Protein 70

Hsp90 cooperates and coordinates with Hsp70. And Hsp70 is a central protein in heat shock response. Hsp70 is a member of the chaperone protein family and it has an important place in the protection of cellular hemostasis. Hsp70 functions in various biological processes: degradation and translocation of proteins, proper protein folding, and protein-protein interactions. Hsp70 has a highly conserved ATPase domain (ATD) and a substrate binding domain (SBD). During stress conditions, Hsp70 is over-expressed in cell and binds to the substrate protein for stabilization of its native structure and disruption of protein aggregation [1]. Hsp70 has 16 isoforms and these different isoforms are localized in different parts of the cell. Hsp70 needs ATP hydrolyzes energy in order to participate in protein folding processes. ATP is hydrolyzed to ADP in the ATD of Hsp70 and this hydrolysis energy provides conformational changes in Hsp70 SBD. SBD consists of a β-barrel cavity to provide substrate proteins a hydrophobic environment and α-helix lid to cover the cavity (Fig. (**4**)). The lid connects to the cavity by a hinge region and ATPase activity regulates opening-closing of the lid during substrate protein processing. Closing of the lid over the cavity provides substrate proteins a hydrophobic environment for proper folding to reach their native conformation. Hsp70 ATD interacts with J-domain of Hsp40 and this interaction stimulates Hsp70 ATPase activity [1, 14 - 16].

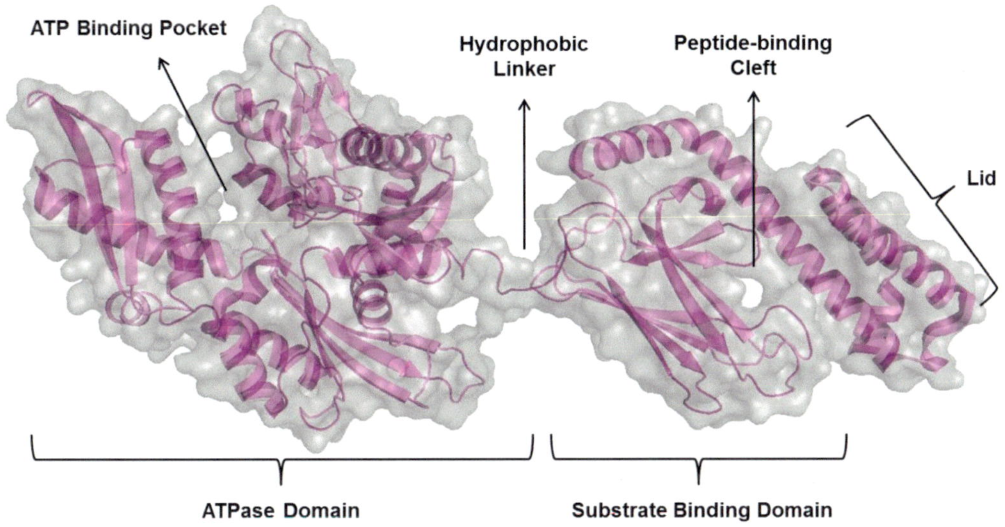

Fig. (4). Structure of Hsp70. ATP hydrolyses in ATPase domain is transmitted to substrate binding domain to help client proteins to fold their native state (PDB ID 2KHO).

Normal expression level of Hsp70 has prominent cytoprotective roles however, cancer cells increase Hsp70 expression level since higher metabolic rates of cancer cells accumulate more client proteins and increase in Hsp70 helps these proteins folding to their native-functional forms. An innovative method in cancer cell inhibition is to block Hsp70 expression and perturb client protein folding - function to induce apoptosis. Several research groups design Hsp70 inhibitors to drive cancer cells to apoptosis. Thus, increased expression of Hsp70 means either poor prognosis or resistance to cancer chemotherapy in cancer cells. Hsp70 stimulates cell proliferation and suppresses apoptotic and senescence pathways. Apoptosis is activated and regulated by caspase-independent processes. Hsp70 interacts with apoptosis protease activating factor-1 (Apaf-1) and prevents activation of the apoptosome, the Apaf-1/cytochrome c/caspase-9 activation complex 1,2 [14]. As reported in the literature, inhibition of Hsp90 alone is not enough because inhibition of Hsp90 chaperone activity stimulates Hsp70 expression and complements inhibited Hsp90 function [17]. Therefore, inhibition of Hsp70 has been extensively studied for blocking tumorigenesis in recent years. By the same token, researchers designed inhibitors to block Hsp70 ATPase activity however, Hsp70 ATD has a deep hydrophobic structure and the ATP binds with polar interactions. Thus, the structure and the polar interactions are not proper for ATPase inhibition. For this reason, Hsp70 ATD is not a suitable target for drug development. Recently, researchers have focused on Hsp70 SBD to design efficient Hsp70 inhibitors [17].

Heat Shock Protein 27

Another key molecule in heat shock response is Hsp27. Hsp27 (also known as Heat Shock Protein beta-1) is an important member of the small Hsp group and participates in protein folding, cell differentiation, inhibition of apoptosis, regulation of cell proliferation, and signal transduction. Hsp27 is constitutively expressed in normal healthy cells. Like other Hsps, expression of Hsp27 is greatly increased in response to stress factors [18].

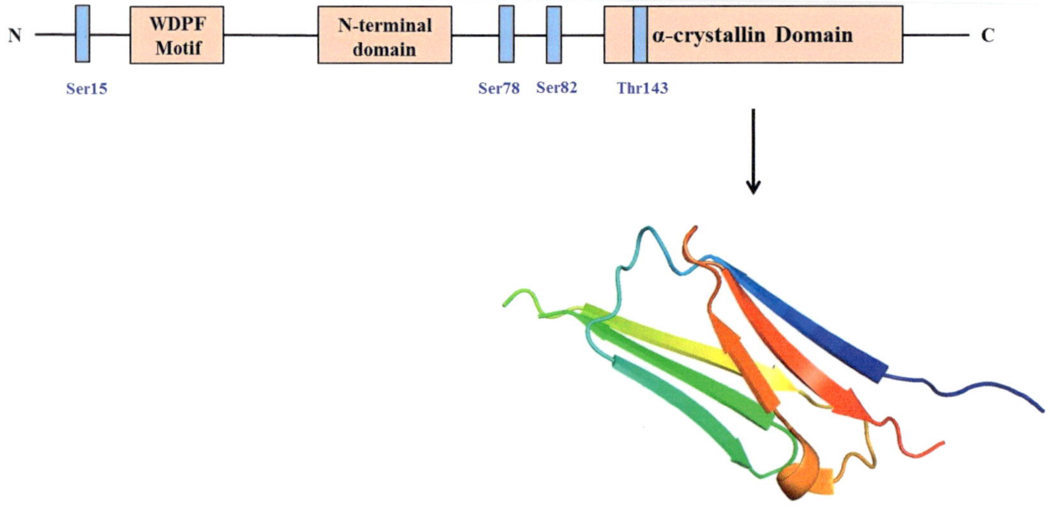

Fig. (5). Structure of Hsp27 (Modified from Ref 18).

Hsp27 contains a highly conserved α-crystalline domain which is involved in constitution of stable dimers (Fig. (**5**)). Unlike other Hsps, Hsp27 performs chaperone function using ATP independent way. Hsp27 inhibits protein aggregation and facilitates irreversible denaturation of substrate proteins. To tangle unfolded substrate proteins in bigger aggregates, Hsp100 chops off a big chunk and sends it for further processing to cooperating chaperones. In either case, Hsp70-Hsp40 chaperone complex executes refolding of these submitted substrate proteins (Fig. (**6**)) [18 - 20].

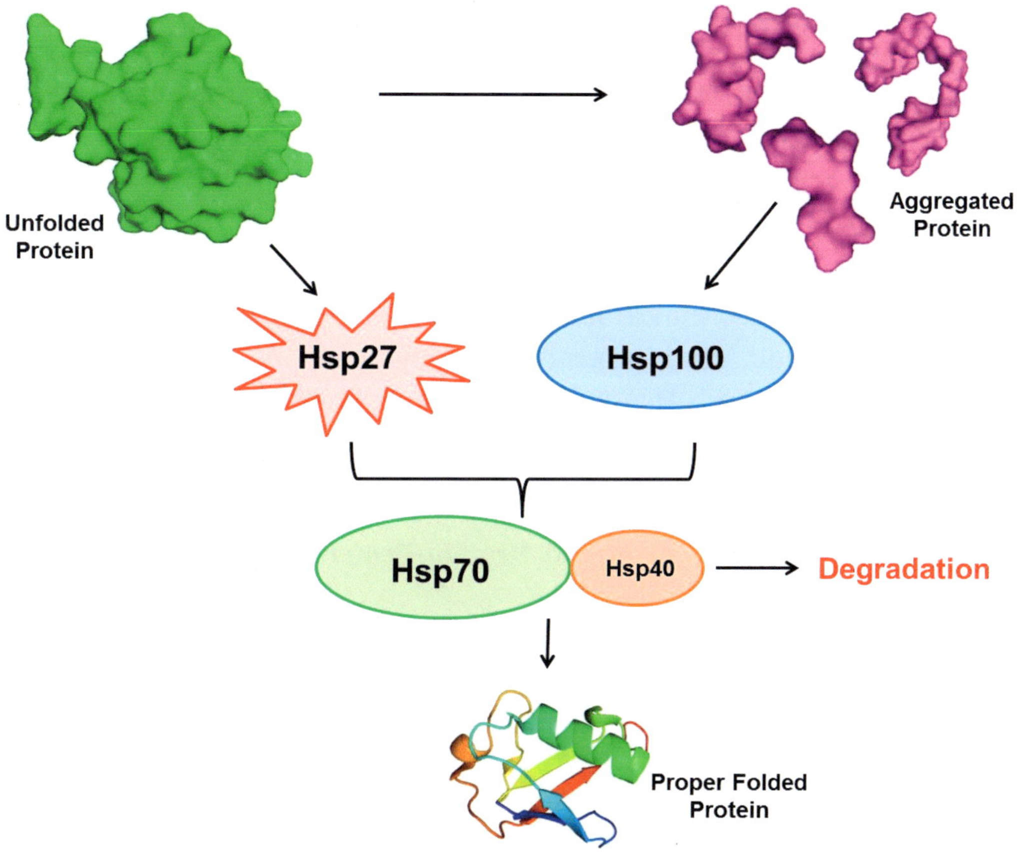

Fig. (6). Proper protein folding mechanism of Hsp complexes (Modified from Ref 18). Hsp27 blocks hydrophobic patches interaction of the client proteins and Hsp100 dissolves protein aggregates to smaller chunks. These smaller parts are folded by Hsp70-Hsp90 complex. If a client protein may not be folded to its native structure then it is transported to proteasome. Hsp27 has more biochemical functions beside its role in client protein folding-please see text for details.

Hsp27 is over-expressed in cancer cells and especially it takes a part at inhibition of apoptosis pathways. Hsp27 controls and regulates several key points in the apoptotic pathway. Overexpression of Hsp27 supports cancer cell survival and interrupts senescence program of the cell. There are two essential points regarding Hsp27 expression during tumorigenesis. Inhibition of Hsp27 phosphorylation suppresses tumor cell migration and invasion. Further, Hsp27 regulates transcription of metalloproteases that are essential for metastases. Therefore, inhibition of Hsp27 takes place in target specific cancer drug design studies as an alternative treatment model for Hsp90 and Hsp70 inhibition [18, 21, 22].

Using these strategies summarized above, several patents were submitted and this review covers these recently submitted key patents for Hsp inhibition.

IMPORTANT PATENTS IN MODULATION OF HEAT SHOCK RESPONSE

Hsps have different biochemical functions. However, Hsp inhibitors only block Hsps and/or Hsp interacting proteins either by small molecules or peptides. Different isoforms of each Hsp make complex interaction network but Hsp90, Hsp27, and Hsp70 function at the key steps of the network. Thus, most patents depend on inhibition of these key proteins.

1. Compounds That Inhibit Hsp90 Protein-Protein Interactions with IAP Proteins

Tumor cells may survive and proliferate in adverse conditions. Further, the cells prevent normal cells from dividing by downregulating cellular pathways in hostile environment. Tumor cells inactivate apoptotic pathways and upregulate pathways for active proliferation. Cellular stress response is one of the pathways involved in proliferation in tumor cells and allows the tumor cells to synthesize and maintain the required proteins for proliferation. Some of the Hsp proteins are upregulated in cellular stress response and Hsp90 is upregulated in several cancer types. Hsp90 maintains several client proteins structure in a proper conformation so that the client proteins can be functional. If this is not possible Hsp90 sends the client proteins to degradation-proteasome. The client proteins are involved in signal transduction and cell proliferation. Faster metabolic rates of cancerous cells overexpress Hsps to maintain client proteins in their properly folded functional form. Patent US20060035837 utilizes Hsp90 interaction with client proteins-

Inhibitor of Apoptosis (IAP). IAP proteins-Survivin, cIAP1, cIAP2, and XIAP-interaction with Hsp90 suppress apoptosis in tumor cells. The invention provides peptides and peptide derivatives of IAP proteins to disrupt Hsp90-IAP interaction. This process stops cell proliferation and help induction of apoptosis in cancer cells. The cancer cells may not avoid cell death through perturbation of protein-protein interaction [23]. Enhancing protein-protein interaction through Hsp provides a mechanism for cancer cell removal.

2. Methods for Inhibiting Proteasome and Heat Shock Protein 90

US20070249540 patent uses Hsp90 monitoring function and blocks Hsp90 forwarding client proteins to proteasome by inhibiting proteasome. Proteasome is a protein complex for destruction of proteins. Regulatory client proteins control key cellular functions such as cell cycle, transcription activation, and apoptosis. If these client proteins may not properly folded by Hsp mechanism, then misfolded, damaged, or improperly assembled client proteins are send to proteasome. Proteasome catalytic core has a hollow cylindrical structure and the active sites are located in the inner side of this structure. The cylinder is flanked by two identical proteins that control the access of client proteins to the core of the cylinder. Destruction process occurs only if the protein is ubiquitin labelled. Labelled proteins are recognized by the receptors and degraded at inner core.

Currently proteasome inhibition is an alternative emerging anticancer treatment strategy in pharmaceutical industry. Rapidly growing cells are more likely to proteasome inhibition than differentiated cells. Tumor cells exhibit susceptible to increased proteolytic activity compared to the healthy cells. Higher metabolic rates and genetic instability of the tumor cells may increase protein degradation levels to remove misfolded-unfolded proteins to prevent toxicity to the cell [24]. Accumulation of unfolded proteins drives the cell to apoptosis and this unique method inhibits cancer cell proliferation.

3. Treatment of Cancer by Inhibition of Hsp27

Hsp27 is a key chaperone protein for survival of cancer cells. There is a close relation between the overexpression of Hsp27 and metastases, invasion, cell differentiation, and anti-apoptotic pathways in tumorogenesis. Therefore, inhibition of Hsp27 has been disclosed as a significant aspect in the treatment of cancer.

US20090281166 patent manifests inhibitory activity of berberine derivatives on Hsp27 chaperone activity. The Hsp27 inhibition activity of the compounds was evaluated in human lung, gastric, colon, prostate, uterus and neuroblastoma cancer cell lines. Berberine derivatives extremely induced Hsp27 expression in these cancer cells [25].

4. Small Molecule Hsp70 Inhibitors

Hsp70 is one of the most important members of the Hsp protein family and it is mainly involved in protein quality control and protection of protein hemostasis. Hsp70 is a critical chaperone protein to survival of all cells and disruption of pathogenesis of diseases. Under stress conditions, cellular proteins show a tendency to aggregate and they lose their native conformation. In this case, expression of Hsp70 is increased to prevent protein aggregation and protein misfolding. Especially, cancer cells are exposed to intensive stress conditions and therefore, cancer cells need more Hsp70 chaperone activity compared with healthy cells. Increased expression of Hsp70 is correlated with poor prognosis of cancer. Inhibition of Hsp90 stimulates up-regulation of Hsp70 in cancer cells. Then, Hsp70 participates in oncogenic signaling pathways and protein quality control network in tumor cell. For this reason, inhibition of Hsp70 has an important place in development of target specific cancer agents. Hsp70 and Hsp90 need ATP hydrolyze energy to perform chaperone activity. ATPase domains of Hsp70 and Hsp90 are target regions of the proteins for inhibition. However, inhibition of ATPase activity of Hsp70 has been less amenable to this strategy. Therefore, inhibition of Hsp70 SBD is suitable for blocking of Hsp70 activity. US2015017736 patent comprises inhibition of Hsp70 SBD with small molecular weight compounds for cancer treatment. The Hsp70 inhibition activity of the small compounds was evaluated in human cancer cell lines. Obtained results indicate that inhibition of Hsp70 SBD interrupts tumorogenesis [26].

5. Combination of an Agent That Attenuates Topoisomerase 1 Activity and an Agent That Inhibits Heat Shock Protein 90 for Use in Chemotherapy

Hsp90 is an ATP-dependent chaperone protein which is the most highly expressed protein in almost all species. Hsp90 expression increases in response to internal and external stress factors (tumorogenesis, infection, oxidative stress, metal ions, etc.). Hsp90 plays vital roles in stabilization and proper folding of cellular proteins. Oncogenic client proteins are assigned in oncogenic signaling pathways (apoptosis, angiogenesis, invasion, metastases, and cell differentiation) for tumor formation and survival of cancer cells. Oncogenic client proteins require Hsp90 chaperone activity in order to gain proper three dimensional structures. Topoisomerases catalyze the overwinding or underwinding of DNA and play key roles in DNA replication.Topoisomerases are overexpressed and provide cell proliferation in cancer cells.

The importance of interaction between Hsp90 and topoisomerases was highlighted in US20050239720 patent. Inhibition of topoisomerases is a significant cancer treatment method and many topoisomerase inhibitors have been applied in cancer patients. However, its side effects emerges limitations in cancer treatment. Interruption of Hsp90-topoisomerases interaction triggers DNA damage and decreases cancer cell proliferation. Therefore, combined inhibition of Hsp90 and topoisomerases has been an effective method for cancer treatment [27].

6. Use of Heat Shock Protein Inhibitor in Preparing Pharmaceutical Composition for Treating Hepatitis and Hepatoma

The patent US20150366892 aims to use a heat shock protein inhibitor in pharmaceutical compositions to treat hepatitis B by scavenging hepatitis B virus infected cells. The gene of hepatitis B virus and the proteins expressed by hepatitis B virus are regarded as important carcinogenic factors. Thus, hepatoma may be caused by hepatitis virus B and any invention treating hepatitis B may enable the treatment of hepatoma. Hepatitis B is hard to be cured effectively as the drugs on the markets are unable to scavenge the virus. They can only inhibit the reproduction of hepatitis B virus in the liver. Hence, there is a need of a drug which has a mechanism of action through scavenging hepatitis B virus infected cells.

The invention stated in patent US20150366892, can scavenge the virus of hepatitis B, leading to treatment or control of hepatitis B as well as hepatoma. The mechanism under that invention is to use of a Hsp inhibitor to be used in pharmaceutical compositions, that is selected from a group including VER155008, Pifithrin-μ, and pharmaceutical acceptable salts thereof (pharmaceutical solvates, pharmaceutical esters, and prodrugs thereof). Both inhibitors are able to modulate specific heat shock proteins and cytotoxically kill the Hepatitis B Virus infected liver cells specifically. The chemical name of VER155008 is 5′O [(4-cyanophenyl) methyl]8[[(3,4dichlorophenyl) methyl]amino]adenosine, which is an effective Hsp70 family inhibitor. The chemical name of Pifithrin-μ is 2-phenylethynesulfonamide, which is a p53 specific inhibitor, decreasing the affinity of p53 to BclxL and Bcl2 and inhibits the function of Hsp72 and autophagy. It has been found that VER155008 and Pifithrin-μ can specifically kill the virus infected liver cells and reduce the viral load in mice. Furthermore, intravenous injection of VER15500 and Pifithrin-μ in mice successfully reduced hepatitis B surface antigen in the blood serum of mice at concentration of 20 mg/mL.

Development of a drug containing these Hsp inhibitors which can scavenge the cells infected by hepatitis B virus will enable them to be used in cancer treatment leading to prevention/treatment of hepatoma. As Pifithrin-μ can selectively inhibit carcinoma through plasmolysis, protein aggregation, peel off from the substrate, and autophagy, the Hsp inhibitor of this invention can be applied in cancer treatment. It has been stated that it is the first time of using Pifithrin-μ in treating hepatitis B and hepatoma [28].

7. Novel Hsp90 Targeted Anticancer Chimeric Peptide

Immonotoxicologic way of cancer treatment caused by bacterial toxins is a potent way of treatment. However the hepatotoxicity caused by the bacterial toxin and the immunogenicity induced by the toxin protein makes it restricted. Additionally, immunotoxins affect the penetration of the medicine into the tumor mass due to their large molecular size. In order to overcome these problems, a new generation of immunotoxin is required. Apart from that it has been focused on the inhibition of Hsp90 protein in cancer treatments. However, inhibition of Hsp90 protein function by the compound causes side effects and functional disorders in normal cells, as this protein is present widely in every cell and takes part in regulation of cell functions. There is a need for the design of a highly efficient new anticancer agent or new structure that is effective even at low doses, and working selectively in cancer cells.

The patent US20120003299 works on the invention of a Hsp90 targeted delivery anticancer agent containing a chimeric peptide. It has been found that Hsp90 only shows its chaperone function when a partner protein, Hop, is bound. This invention focuses on the amino acids in the TPR (tetratricopeptide repeat) domain, which is important for binding of Hop to Hsp90. Furthermore, it provides a delivery agent for delivering an objective substance containing an Hsp90 TPR domain binding peptide to cancer cells and a relevant drug delivery system as TPR peptide alone does not have the cell killing effect. Through this invention, it will be possible to regulate cancer cells containing an Hsp90 TPR domain binding peptide present on a vehicle as a delivery system, namely liposome, and an objective substance.

A new peptide with higher in efficiency and efficacy having a cell killing ability specifically for cancer cells was invented by combining the amino acids with a conventionally reported cell penetrating peptide Antp and introducing the chimeric peptide containing an Hsp90 TPR domain binding peptide into cells. This chimeric complex binds to Hsp90 specifically and exerts no influence on normal cells, whereas it induces death selectively in cancer cells particularly via an apoptotic mechanism. The chimeric peptide AntpTPR according to the present invention has a cell killing effect similar to Hsp90 inhibitors. The peptide penetrated into the cell without destruction of the cell membrane and also the membrane was not destructed even after penetration of the peptide [29].

8. Methods for Delivering an Anticancer Agent to a Tumor

In the treatment of tumors, the application of local heat generated by high energy laser excitation of their surface plasmons has some restrictions due to the limited tissue penetration depths of light. In addition, the lethality of photothermal therapy that uses passive diffusion of their nanoconstructs for delivery to the tumor, decreases at low laser energies caused by low intratumoral concentrations and large plasma membrane separation distances of nanoconstructs. In order to overcome these problems new photothermal strategies are required with maximized efficacy using minimal light energy.

A new photothermal therapy is described in the patent US20160129111 that use gold particles for delivering anticancer agents to treat cancer and reduce tumor proliferation. It aims to deliver an anticancer agent to a tumor through administering gold particles and at least one anticancer agent directly or indirectly bonded to the macromolecule and/or unbound to the macromolecule. This enables the formulation of different pharmaceutical compositions depending on the mode of administration to enhance selectivity and uptake of the particles by cancer cells. Topical, ophthalmical, vaginal, rectal, intranasal, intravenous, and intraperitoneal administrations of particles are possible that enhances the ability of anticancer agents to penetrate cancer cells. After contacting the cancer cells, the tumor or cancer cells are exposed to light for a sufficient time and wavelength for the gold particles to achieve surface plasmon resonance and heating. A minimally invasive laser light source whose wavelength overlaps with the localized surface plasmon resonance peak can cause hyperthermia and at higher temperatures extensive vascular damage. In one aspect, plasmonic photothermal therapy can induce tumor hyperthermia, increase tumor penetration of macromolecular therapeutics at controlled temperatures, and also act as an effective antivascular therapy. Hyperthermia enabled drug delivery has several limitations due to the difficulty in the maintenation of tumor temperature and nonspecific heating of surrounding healthy tissue. It has been demonstrated that presence of gold particles significantly amplified the degree of heat generation immediately after laser treatment. In the present invention, it has been shown that hyperthermia caused by plasmonic photothermal therapy, enhances delivery of polyn(2-hydr--xypropyl)methacrylamide (HPMA) copolymer conjugates in solid tumors. The heat shock targeted and -untargeted copolymers were injected and allowed to accumulate. After 24h, the untargeted copolymers diffused back out of the tumor to the same level as the tumors left untreated, whereas the heat shock targeted copolymers were retained [30].

9. Recombinant Cancer Cell Secreting Modified Heat Shock Protein-Antigenic Peptide Complex

The use of immunogenic stress protein-peptide complexes which consist of Hsps and antigenic peptides for the treatment and prevention of cancer and infectious diseases has been reported. An example of this method is the use of Hsps in combination with a defined antigen. These Hsp-peptide complexes are formed from cancer cells or pathogen infected cells, inducing a specific immune response, and therefore, are applicable for the prevention and treatment of the cancer or infectious diseases. There are also attempts to prepare a vaccine from Hsp-peptide complexes against cancer. But, these complexes are not secreted in bulk quantities and a constant supply is required for their commercial production. In summary, it is not feasible to extract desirable amount of Hsp-peptide complexes from either cancer cells or infected cells.

The patent US8685384 presents an invention to obtain Hsps involved in antigen presentation by employing recombinant technologies. This includes preparation of immunogenic material for vaccine to prevent and treat the diseases. The material comprised of noncovalent complexes of modified Hsps, including, Hsp70, Hsp90, and antigenic (or immunogenic) peptides. Accordingly, the invention introduces methods for producing immunogenic Hsp-peptide complexes to be secreted continuously by antigenic cells into the culture medium then they are conveniently harvested from the culture medium. Moreover, the invention gives the possibility of enhancing the immunogenic properties of the aforementioned cells to administer as a vaccine. The invention eases culturing recombinant cells and provides bulk amounts of modified Hsp or modified Hsp-peptide complexes. This facilitates to obtain vaccine preparation [31].

10. C-Terminal Hsp90 Inhibitors to Treat Pituitary Adenomas

Recently, development of Hsp90 CTD inhibitors has become crucial in cancer treatment as an alternative to Hsp90 NTD inhibitors. CTD inhibitors perturb Hsp90 dimerization process and disrupt proper folding of oncogenic client proteins. Therefore, CTD inhibition strategy provides significant opportunities for next generation target specific cancer therapy.

The patent US20150335613 presents inhibitory activity of silibinin and novobiocin analogs on Hsp90 CTD. Hsp90 CTD inhibition activity and pharmaceutical activities of the compounds were studied in human pituitary adenomas. Experimental results demonstrated that, these compounds block Hsp90 CTD and block pituitary cancer cell proliferation [32].

CURRENT & FUTURE DEVELOPMENTS

Cancer therapy has several modes of action. Different approaches for anticancer treatments provide novel inhibitors. Higher metabolic rates of cancer cells make Hsp proteins valuable targets for cancer treatment. Hsp proteins coordinate and cooperate with each other and other essential cellular proteins. These wide biochemical pathways provide key points to disrupt cancer cell survival as summarized in this review and novel methods for next generation drug design have yet to be discovered.

CONFLICT OF INTEREST

The authors confirm that they have no conflict of interest to declare for this publication.

ACKNOWLEDGEMENTS

Declared none.

REFERENCES

[1] Tutar L, Tutar Y. Heat shock proteins; An overview. Curr Pharm Biotechnol 2010; 11(2): 216-22. [http://dx.doi.org/10.2174/138920110790909632] [PMID: 20170474]

[2] Ozgur A, Tutar Y. Heat shock protein 90 inhibitors in oncology. Curr Proteomics 2014; 11(1): 2-16. [http://dx.doi.org/10.2174/1570164611666140415224635]

[3] Richter K, Haslbeck M, Buchner J. The heat shock response: Life on the verge of death. Mol Cell 2010; 40(2): 253-66. [http://dx.doi.org/10.1016/j.molcel.2010.10.006] [PMID: 20965420]

[4] Kakkar V, Meister-Broekema M, Minoia M, Carra S, Kampinga HH. Barcoding heat shock proteins to human diseases: Looking beyond the heat shock response. Dis Model Mech 2014; 7(4): 421-34.

[http://dx.doi.org/10.1242/dmm.014563] [PMID: 24719117]

[5] Özgür A, Tutar Y. Heat shock protein 90 inhibition in cancer drug discovery: From chemistry to futural clinical applications. Anticancer Agents Med Chem 2016; 16(3): 280-90. [http://dx.doi.org/10.2174/1871520615666150821093747] [PMID: 26295332]

[6] Koca İ, Özgür A, Er M, Gümüş M, Açikalin Coşkun K, Tutar Y. Design and synthesis of pyrimidinyl acyl thioureas as novel Hsp90 inhibitors in invasive ductal breast cancer and its bone metastasis. Eur J Med Chem 2016; 122: 280-90. [http://dx.doi.org/10.1016/j.ejmech.2016.06.032] [PMID: 27376491]

[7] Jego G, Hazoumé A, Seigneuric R, Garrido C. Targeting heat shock proteins in cancer. Cancer Lett 2013; 332(2): 275-85. [http://dx.doi.org/10.1016/j.canlet.2010.10.014] [PMID: 21078542]

[8] Trepel J, Mollapour M, Giaccone G, Neckers L. Targeting the dynamic HSP90 complex in cancer. Nat Rev Cancer 2010; 10(8): 537-49. [http://dx.doi.org/10.1038/nrc2887] [PMID: 20651736]

[9] Li J, Buchner J. Structure, function and regulation of the hsp90 machinery. Biomed J 2013; 36(3): 106-17. [http://dx.doi.org/10.4103/2319-4170.113230] [PMID: 23806880]

[10] Neckers L. Hsp90 inhibitors as novel cancer chemotherapeutic agents. Trends Mol Med 2002; 8(4) (Suppl.): S55-61. [http://dx.doi.org/10.1016/S1471-4914(02)02316-X] [PMID: 11927289]

[11] Maloney A, Workman P. HSP90 as a new therapeutic target for cancer therapy: The story unfolds. Expert Opin Biol Ther 2002; 2(1): 3-24. [http://dx.doi.org/10.1517/14712598.2.1.3] [PMID: 11772336]

[12] Fukuyo Y, Hunt CR, Horikoshi N. Geldanamycin and its anti-cancer activities. Cancer Lett 2010; 290(1): 24-35. [http://dx.doi.org/10.1016/j.canlet.2009.07.010] [PMID: 19850405]

[13] Gorska M, Popowska U, Sielicka-Dudzin A, *et al.* Geldanamycin and its derivatives as Hsp90 inhibitors. Front Biosci (Landmark Ed) 2012; 17: 2269-77. [http://dx.doi.org/10.2741/4050] [PMID: 22652777]

[14] Tutar Y. Hsp70 in oncology. Recent Pat DNA Gene Seq 2011; 5(3): 214-8. [http://dx.doi.org/10.2174/187221511797636293] [PMID: 21892920]

[15] Ozgur A, Tutar L, Coskun KA, Tutar E, Tutar Y. Toxoplasma gondii and heat shock proteins. In: Méndez-Vilas A, Ed. Microbial pathogens and strategies for combating them: Science, technology and education. 4th ed. Berlin: Formatex 2008; pp. 1969-79.

[16] Goloudina AR, Demidov ON, Garrido C. Inhibition of HSP70: A challenging anti-cancer strategy. Cancer Lett 2012; 325(2): 117-24. [http://dx.doi.org/10.1016/j.canlet.2012.06.003] [PMID: 22750096]

[17] Tutar Y. Inhibition of heat shock protein 70 and 90 (Hsp70 and Hsp90) in target specific cancer treatment. Adv Tech Biol Med 2015; 3.

[18] Tutar Y, Özgür A, Tutar E, Coskun KA, Tutar L. Anti-apoptotic and oncogenic function of HSP27. In: Dunn BM, Ed. Frontiers in Protein and Peptide Sciences. Bentham Publication 2014; pp. 75-90.

[19] Laskowska E, Matuszewska E, Kuczyńska-Wiśnik D. Small heat shock proteins and protein-misfolding diseases. Curr Pharm Biotechnol 2010; 11(2): 146-57. [http://dx.doi.org/10.2174/138920110790909669] [PMID: 20166966]

[20] Kim KK, Kim R, Kim SH. Crystal structure of a small heat-shock protein. Nature 1998; 394(6693): 595-9. [http://dx.doi.org/10.1038/29106] [PMID: 9707123]

[21] Sherman M, Multhoff G. Heat shock proteins in cancer. Ann NY Acad Sci 2007; 1113: 192-201. [http://dx.doi.org/10.1196/annals.1391.030] [PMID: 17978282]

[22] Vargas-Roig LM, Gago FE, Tello O, Aznar JC, Ciocca DR. Heat shock protein expression and drug resistance in breast cancer patients treated with induction chemotherapy. Int J Cancer 1998; 79(5): 468-75. [http://dx.doi.org/10.1002/(SICI)1097-0215(19981023)79:5<468::AID-IJC4>3.0.CO;2-Z] [PMID: 9761114]

[23] Altieri DC, Plescia J, Salz W. Compounds that inhibit Hsp90 protein-protein interactions with IAP proteins. US20060035837, 2006.

[24] Papathanassiu A. Methods for inhibiting proteasome and heat shock protein 90. US20070249540, 2007.

[25] Gleave M, Ong C, Hayashi N. Treatment of cancer by inhibition of Hs. US20090281166, 2009.

[26] George DL, Murphy ME, Leu J. Small molecule Hsp70 inhibitors. US2015017736, 2015.

[27] Jenkins J. Combination of an agent that attenuates topoisomerase 1 activity and an agent that inhibits heat shock protein 90 for use in chemotherapy. US20050239720, 2005.

[28] Wang HC, Yen TC, Huang LR. 6-Use of Heat shock protein inhibitor in preparing pharmaceutical composition for treating hepatitis and hepatoma. US20150366892, 2015.

[29] Kawakami K, Masayuki K, Horibe T. Novel Hsp90 targeted anticancer chimeric peptide. US20120003299, 2012.

[30] Ghandehari H, Gormley A, Ray A, Larson N. Methods for delivering an anticancer agent to a tumor. US20160129111, 2016.

[31] Podack ER, Spielman J, Yamazaki K. Recombinant cancer cell secreting modified heat shock protein-antigenic peptide complex. US8685384, 2014.

[32] Paez-Pereda M, Stalla G. C-terminal hsp90 inhibitors to treat pituitary adenomas. US20150335613, 2014.

AUTHOR INDEX

SUBJECT INDEX

Atta-ur-Rahman and Khurshid Zaman (Eds.)

Made in the USA
Las Vegas, NV
03 November 2026

57425092R00143